Keratoconus

This is an updated and comprehensive treatise on optical, medical, and surgical management of keratoconus with an exclusive panoramic view of all existing modalities for confronting this serious disabling morbidity affecting people in their youth. Early diagnosis and proper treatment can salvage vision and help patients to get back to their routines and enhance their quality of life. The contents include optical and glass prescription and contact lens fitting; CXL alone; and combined surgeries, phakic IOLs, and corneal transplantation. The illustrated and organized 360-degrees approach makes this a must-have manual for ophthalmology trainees, fellows, and professionals.

Key Features:

1. Focuses on optical management for keratoconus, with the latest updates on surgical management

2. Covers a very interesting and relevant topic for ophthalmologists and cornea specialists, using a practical case-based format

3. Uses evidence-based algorithms from updated published data and insights from experienced authors

Keratoconus

Optical and Surgical Management

Edited by
Mehrdad Mohammadpour and Masoud Khorrami-Nejad

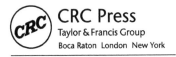

CRC Press
Taylor & Francis Group
Boca Raton London New York

CRC Press is an imprint of the
Taylor & Francis Group, an **informa** business

Designed cover image: www.shutterstock.com/image-vector/staphyloma-keratoconus-pellucid-vintage-engraved-illustration-155930051

First edition published 2025
by CRC Press
2385 NW Executive Center Drive, Suite 320, Boca Raton FL 33431

and by CRC Press
4 Park Square, Milton Park, Abingdon, Oxon, OX14 4RN

CRC Press is an imprint of Taylor & Francis Group, LLC

© 2025 selection and editorial matter, Mehrdad Mohammadpour and Masoud Khorrami-Nejad; individual chapters, the contributors

Library of Congress Cataloging-in-Publication Data
Names: Mohammadpour, Mehrdad, editor. | Khorrami-Nejad, Masoud, editor.
Title: Keratoconus: optical and surgical management / edited by Mehrdad
Mohammadpour and Masoud Khorrami-Nejad.
Other titles: Keratoconus (Mohammadpour)
Description: First edition. | Boca Raton: CRC Press, 2024. |
Identifiers: LCCN 2024022050 (print) | LCCN 2024022051 (ebook) |
ISBN 9781032443256 (hbk) | ISBN 9781032443232 (pbk) |
ISBN 9781003371601 (ebk)
Subjects: MESH: Keratoconus–therapy | Corneal Cross-Linking–methods |
Refractive Surgical Procedures–methods | Keratoconus–diagnosis
Classification: LCC RE339 (print) | LCC RE339 (ebook) | NLM WW 225 |
DDC 617.7/19–dc23/eng/20240703
LC record available at https://lccn.loc.gov/2024022050
LC ebook record available at https://lccn.loc.gov/2024022051

ISBN: 9781032443256 (hbk)
ISBN: 9781032443232 (pbk)
ISBN: 9781003371601 (ebk)

DOI: 10.1201/9781003371601

Typeset in Palatino
by Deanta Global Publishing Services, Chennai, India

Contents

Preface

It's a great honor for me to have a pivotal role as both co-editor and contributorin this all-in-one textbook on medical and surgical management for keratoconus, now recognized as a common disease in the era of advanced corneal imaging and diagnostic modalities for early diagnosis and treatment.

This book includes all one needs from zero to hundred in all aspects to gain a new horizon in the field of diagnostic tools and medical and surgical options, from prescribing glasses to fitting contact lenses, corneal cross-linking in different situations and various methods and techniques alone or combined with other surgeries, intracorneal ring segments, and complete 360-degree rings with and without cross-linking, various types of corneal transplantations, including deep anterior lamellar keratoplasty and penetrating keratoplasty by both conventional and femtosecond laser-assisted keratoplasty.

The common complications of corneal transplantation, from corneal astigmatism to suture-related problems, ocular surface morbidities, graft rejection, and post-keratoplasty infections, are well discussed in detail in specific chapters.

Additionally, the new horizons for the management of keratoconus, consisting of gene therapy, synthetic allografts, bioengineering, novel modalities, and translational sciences, are also discussed in two separate chapters.

I cordially thank all the well-known professors of ophthalmology for dedicating their time and experience to contribute a must-have book for all who care for patients with keratoconus, by bringing hope and joy to the life of a great community of young people who deserve better vision and a higher quality of life.

Sincerely,
Mehrdad Mohammadpour, MD
Professor of Ophthalmology,
Cornea Department,
Farabi Excellency Eye Hospital,
Tehran University of Medical Sciences, Iran

Welcome to our comprehensive guide on keratoconus, a condition that can significantly impact upon quality of life if left untreated. As authors, we found it essential to create this book to provide a deeper understanding of keratoconus, its diagnosis, treatment options, latest advancements, and future perspectives.

The book is divided into three main parts, each focusing on a different aspect of keratoconus. In the first part, we delve into the introduction, definition, diagnosis, and classification of keratoconus. Second part focuses on optical management options for keratoconus. It explores considerations for managing vision and the role of contact lenses and spectacles. A variety of contact lens types and fitting approaches, as well as optical treatment strategies by spectacles, are evaluated. The last part is dedicated to surgical management for keratoconus, which begins with the indications and contraindications of corneal cross-linking (CXL), a fundamental treatment option. This is followed by several chapters discussing various CXL techniques, CXL combined with other procedures, and other surgical options such as intracorneal rings and corneal transplantation. The final chapters of the book provide a look into other treatment options and a glimpse into the future of keratoconus management, offering hope and anticipation for the advancements to come.

I have written many chapters in this book. I have collaborated closely on producing this comprehensive textbook under Professor Mohammadpour's supervision. In addition, we are honored to include contributions from other distinguished experts in keratoconus from around the world. Their insights and expertise help provide a truly global perspective on recent advances and best practices in managing this important ocular condition. Collectively, we hope this textbook serves as an invaluable resource to equip eyecare professionals worldwide with the knowledge needed to deliver the highest quality, evidence-based care to patients affected by keratoconus.

We hope our work will be a valuable resource for ophthalmologists, optometrists, medical professionals, and researchers seeking to better understand and treat keratoconus. We believe that knowledge and understanding are the first steps towards effective management and ultimately improving the quality of life for patients with keratoconus.

Thank you for embarking on this journey with us.

Masoud Khorrami-Nejad, PhD
Head of Optometry Department,
Tehran University of Medical Sciences, Iran

About the Editors

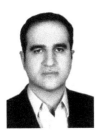

Professor Mehrdad Mohammadpour, MD

He graduated from Alborz College in 1989 as the first-ranked student and, in the same year, was accepted as a medical student at the Tehran University of Medical Sciences, School of Medicine. In 1996, he graduated from the TUMS as an excellent student and, in 1998, he started the Cornea Fellowship and, after that, he succeeded in completing the corneal subspecialty course. Since 2003, he has performed more than ten thousand eye surgeries in the field of kerato-conus, cataract, and refractive surgery and corneal cross-linking, and inventor of many techniques in combined corneal cross-linking and refractive surgeries and intrastromal corneal ring implantation with long follow-up and success He has published more than 100 scientific articles in the field of ophthalmology in the most prestigious ophthalmological journals.

He has also trained more than 200 ophthalmologists and subspecialists as a faculty member in Tehran University of Medical Sciences. He is also a reviewer for most ophthalmology journals around the world and has given several lectures at high-level ophthalmology international congresses

He is the inventor of several new ophthalmic surgical techniques and the inventor of the first nano-ophthalmology eye drop. Currently, he is an official scientific member of the Department of Ophthalmology, Faculty of Medicine, Tehran University of Medical Sciences, Farabi Hospital. He teaches fellows and residents of ophthalmology. He also has one of the highest H-index values in ophthalmology articles in the world. He is also the main author of the *Diagnostics in Ocular Imaging Cornea, Retina, Glaucoma and Orbit* published by Springer and the *Updates of Diagnosis and Managements for Dry Eye* book published by TUMS Publishing Group.

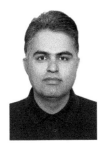

Assistant Professor Masoud Khorrami-Nejad, PhD

He was born and raised in Tehran, Iran in 1985. After completing his BSc degree, he went on to pursue graduate studies in the field of optometry and vision science. He obtained his MSc degree and later secured the top rank in his PhD program, demonstrating his exceptional academic abilities.

Over the past years, he has established himself as a prolific researcher and author in ophthalmology and optometry, with over 80 papers published in reputable international journals. He has played a lead role in many of these publications, being either the first author or corresponding author in more than 70% of his papers. He has also written or edited four academic books, sharing his expertise with students and fellow researchers.

In addition to his robust research portfolio, he is also an experienced educator. Since 2013, he has taught at various Iranian universities training over 300 optometry students. He currently holds a head of optometry department at the international campus of Tehran University of Medical Sciences. To date, he has delivered over 20 presentations at major global conferences and has served as the scientific secretary for seven congress and seminars. He has successfully supervised upwards of 40 Masters and PhD candidates, guiding the next generation of academics studying visual sciences.

List of Contributors

Parisa Abdi
Farabi Eye Hospital
Tehran University of Medical Sciences
Tehran, Iran

Rua Abulhosein
Tehran University of Medical Sciences
Tehran, Iran

Mehdi Aminizadeh
Farabi Eye Hospital
Tehran University of Medical Sciences
Tehran, Iran

Renato Ambrósio Jr.
Federal University of the State of Rio de Janeiro
  (UNIRIO)
Rio de Janeiro, RJ, Brazil

Timothy J. Archer
Biomedical Science Research Institute
Ulster University
Coleraine, UK

Asieh Aslani
Isfahan Eye Research Center
Department of Ophthalmology
Isfahan University of Medical Sciences
Isfahan, Iran

Mehrnaz Atighehchian
Eye Research Center
Farabi Eye Hospital
Tehran University of Medical Sciences
Tehran, Iran

Elham Azizi
Department of Optometry and
  Vision Sciences
University of Melbourne
Melbourne, Australia

Zahra Bibak Bejandi
Translational Ophthalmic Research Center
Farabi Eye Hospital
Tehran University of Medical Sciences
Tehran, Iran

Alireza Eslampoor
Eye Research Center
Mashhad University of Medical Sciences
Mashhad, Iran

Sadegh Ghafarian
Eye Research Center
Farabi Eye Hospital
Tehran University of Medical Sciences
Tehran, Iran

Leila Ghiasian
Eye Research Center, Eye Department
The Five Senses Health Institute
School of Medicine
Iran University of Medical Sciences
Tehran, Iran

Mohammad Ghoreishi
Isfahan University of Medical Sciences
Co-founder, Parsian Vision Research
  Institute
Isfahan, Iran

Yasaman Hadi
Eye Research Center
Five Senses Institute, Rassoul Akram
  Hospital
Iran University of Medical Sciences
Tehran, Iran

Farhad Hafezi
ELZA Institute
Dietikon/Zurich, Switzerland
and
Laboratory of Ocular Cell Biology
Center for Applied Biotechnology and
  Molecular Medicine
University of Zurich, Zurich,
  Switzerland
Faculty of Medicine
University of Geneva
Geneva, Switzerland
and
USC Roski Eye Institute
University of Southern California
Los Angeles, CA, USA
and
Department of Ophthalmology
Medical University of Wenzhou
Wenzhou, China

Hassan Hashemi
Noor Ophthalmology Research Centre
Noor Eye Hospital
Tehran, Iran

Seyed Javad Hashemian
Eye Research Center
Five Senses Institute
Rassoul Akram Hospital
Iran University of Medical Sciences
Tehran, Iran

Mohammad Naser Hashemian
Eye Research Center
Farabi Eye Hospital
Tehran University of Medical Sciences
Tehran, Iran

Kiana Hassanpour
Ophthalmic Research Center
Research Institute for Ophthalmology and Vision
*   Sciences*
Shahid Beheshti University of Medical
*   Sciences*
Tehran, Iran

Zahra Heidari
Psychiatry and Behavioral Sciences Research Center
Mazandaran University of Medical Sciences
Sari, Iran
and
Functional Neurosurgery Research Center
Shohada Tajrish Comprehensive Neurosurgical
*   Center of Excellence*
Shahid Beheshti University of Medical Sciences
Tehran, Iran

Mark Hillen
ELZA Institute
Dietikon/Zurich, Switzerland

Khosrow Jadidi
Vision Health Research Center
Semnan University of Medical Sciences
Semnan, Iran
and
Vision Health Research Center
Bina Eye Hospital
Tehran, Iran

Mohammad-ali Javadi
Ophthalmic Research Center
Research Institute for Ophthalmology and Vision
*   Sciences*
Shahid Beheshti University of Medical Sciences
Tehran, Iran

Aydano P Machado
Federal University of Alagoas (UFAL)
Maceió, Alagoas, Brazil

Ahmad Masoumi
Eye Research Center
Farabi Eye Hospital
Tehran University of Medical Sciences
Tehran, Iran

Seyed Farzad Mohammadi
Translational Ophthalmology Research Center
Farabi Hospital
Tehran University of Medical Sciences
Tehran, Iran

Hossein Mohammad-Rabei
Ophthalmic Research Center
Research Institute for Ophthalmology and Vision
*   Sciences*
Shahid Beheshti University of Medical Sciences
Tehran, Iran

Seyed Aliasghar Mosavi
Vision Health Research Center
Semnan University of Medical Sciences
Semnan, Iran
and
Vision Health Research Center
Bina Eye Hospital
Tehran, Iran

M. Hossein Nowroozzadeh
Department of Ophthalmology
Shiraz University of Medical Sciences
Shiraz, Iran

Alireza Peyman
Isfahan Eye Research Center
Department of Ophthalmology
Isfahan University of Medical Sciences
Isfahan, Iran

Mohsen Pourazizi
Isfahan Eye Research Center
Department of Ophthalmology
Isfahan University of Medical Sciences
Isfahan, Iran

Kiana Raeesdana
School of Optometry
University of Montreal
Montréal, Canada

Saeed Raeisi
Translational Ophthalmic Research Center
Farabi Eye Hospital
Tehran University of Medical Sciences
Tehran, Iran

Dan Z. Reinstein
Reinstein Vision
and
London Vision Clinic
London, UK
and
Columbia University Medical Center
New York, USA
and
Sorbonne Université
Paris, France
and
Biomedical Science Research Institute
Ulster University
Coleraine, UK

Javad Sadeghi
Eye Research Center
Mashhad University of Medical Sciences
Mashhad, Iran

Ramin Salouti
Department of Ophthalmology
Shiraz University of Medical Sciences
and
Salouti Cornea Research Center
Salouti Eye Clinic
Shiraz, Iran

Mohammad-Reza Sedaghat
Eye Research Center
Mashhad University of Medical Sciences
Mashhad, Iran

Saeid Shahhosseini
Noor Ophthalmology Research Centre
Noor Eye Hospital
Tehran, Iran

Yasir Adil Shakor
Azadi Teaching Hospital
Kirkuk, Iraq

Mehrdad Motamed Shariati
Eye Research Center
Mashhad University of Medical Sciences
Mashhad, Iran

Mohammad Soleimani
Eye Research Center
Farabi Eye Hospital
Tehran University of Medical Sciences
Tehran, Iran

Sara Taghizadeh
Translational Ophthalmology Research Center
Farabi Hospital
Tehran University of Medical Sciences
Tehran, Iran

Emilio A Torres-Netto
ELZA Institute
Dietikon/Zurich
Zurich, Switzerland
and
Laboratory of Ocular Cell Biology
Center for Applied Biotechnology and Molecular
  Medicine
University of Zurich
Zurich, Switzerland
and
Faculty of Medicine
University of Geneva
Geneva, Switzerland

Siamak Zarei-Ghanavati
Eye Research Center
Mashhad University of Medical Sciences
Mashhad, Iran

1 Keratoconus Definition, Epidemiology, and Risk Factors

Leila Ghiasian

INTRODUCTION

Keratoconus derives from the words 'Keras', meaning cornea, and 'cōnus', defined as cone, collectively conveying a sense of a 'cone-shaped' cornea.[1] Keratoconus is a progressive, bilateral and asymmetric ectatic disorder characterized by changes in corneal structure, which results in focal thinning and cone-like steepening of the cornea, leading to astigmatism, especially the irregular type.[2–4] Most commonly, the progressive stromal thinning occurs at the paracentral part of the cornea, especially the inferotemporal part.[5] Asymmetricity on the surface of the cornea can cause various amounts of visual loss, image distortion, and increased sensitivity to light and glare.

The manifestation as well as the progression of this ectatic disorder could be highly variable between the two eyes.[6–7] Most experts admit that a real unilateral keratoconus does not exist.

Multiple hypotheses have been proposed including genetics, environment, age, sex, inflammation and immune factors, hormones, nutrition, pollution, and even specific behavioral traits, which may affect unknown pathophysiology of the keratoconus.[8] Despite many studies, the enigmatic pathophysiology of keratoconus is due to complex relations between genetic and epigenetic components that are triggered by environment factors.[9–11]

Several recent studies have shown the important role of inflammation and changes in some inflammatory mediators and probable effects of oxidative stress in the cause and also its progression.[12–14] Specifically, it affects different ethnicities and both genders.[15] It usually appears as an isolated ocular disorder, yet it may sometimes occur as a part of an ocular or systemic problem.[16]

EPIDEMIOLOGY

Determining the prevalence and occurrence of keratoconus in any region is an important part of keratoconus evaluation.[17] It affects the decisions, goals, and actions that determine how care is administered and who accesses the healthcare policies.[18]

Over the years, studies have shown that both the prevalence and occurrence of keratoconus have been highly variable in different regions.[19–20] In addition to, the important role of genetics, the environment, ethnicity and geographic location, there could be other reasons for this obvious variability including dissimilarity of epidemiologic studies and their study design, lack of similar specified criteria for keratoconus definition and classification, and lack of newer diagnostic imaging information and artificial intelligence for diagnosis in older studies.[13,21–22]

Keratoconus prevalence varies among different ethnicities. Studies on the Caucasian population report the prevalence rate of keratoconus, at approximately 1,000 per 100,000 persons. Studies related to Asian and the Middle Eastern populations report an incidence of one per1,500 to 5,000, which seems much higher. The keratoconus incidence also shows a higher rate in Asian and the Middle Eastern population compared with Caucasians (2-4 per 100,000 in comparison with 20 per 100,000 persons/year, respectively).[23–24] In different studies, based on diagnostic criteria for the keratoconus confirmation, the prevalence was reported differently. The diagnostic criteria have varied from Scissor reflex in retinoscopy to diagnosis based on Scheimflug tomography images.[25] The population-based studies seem more accurate than hospital-based ones in determining the prevalence and incidence of keratoconus. Population-based studies tend to show a lower prevalence rate due to selection bias, including only symptomatic patients who have visited the hospitals.[23,26] The global prevalence rate ranges from 0.2/100,000 in Russia to 3300/100,000 in Iran.[18,27] In studies conducted on children, a higher prevalence of the disease has been reported with the highest report being from Saudi Arabia with a prevalence of 4,790/100,000.[28] A recent meta-analysis study, having analyzed more than 50 million individuals from 15 different countries, reports the keratoconus prevalence as 138/100,000.[29]

COMORBIDITIES

Although several studies have linked keratoconus to other systemic and ocular disorders, the possibilities of association could not be ruled out. Table 1.1 summarizes some of these comorbidities.

Several studies reported that several types of atopic diseases, especially atopic dermatitis, are associated with keratoconus.[30]

DOI: 10.1201/9781003371601-1

Table 1.1   Keratoconus-Linked Systemic and Ocular Disorders

Ocular disorders	Leber congenital amaurosis
	Retinitis pigmentosa
	Pigmentary keratopathy
	Vernal keratoconjunctivitis
	Cataract
	Avellino dystrophy
	Granular dystrophy
	Fuchs endothelial dystrophy
Connective tissue disorders	Mitral valve prolapse
	Floppy eyelid syndrome
	Ehlers–Danlos syndrome
	Osteogenesis imperfecta
	Pseudoxanthoma elasticum
	Congenital hip dysplasia
Genetic syndromes	Atopic diseases
	Down syndrome
	Marfan syndrome
	Tourette syndrome
	Noonan syndrome
	Apert syndrome
	Crouzon syndrome
	Turner syndrome
	Bardet–Biedl syndrome
	Ichthyosis
	Neurofibromatosis
	Xeroderma pigmentosum
	Neurocutaneous angiomatosis
Other	Obesity and obstructive sleep apnea

Vernal keratoconjunctivitis is strongly associated with keratoconus. Nearly 70% of keratoconus cases show abnormal topographic patterns, but roughly 11–23% are diagnosed as a keratoconus case.[31–32]

Obesity affects keratoconus patients more frequently and there is an association between BMI (body mass index) and keratoconus.[33–34] Studies reported that obstructive sleep apnea occurs twenty times more frequently than in the general population.[34]

There is a strong correlation between mitral valve prolapse and keratoconus.[35] Studies found mitral valve prolapse in 38–58% of keratoconus patients and an estimated 22% of mitral valve prolapse cases suffer from keratoconus.[26]

Down syndrome has a potent association with keratoconus. The prevalence of keratoconus in this genetic syndrome is about 21–70%. Studies also reported steeper and thinner cornea in Down syndrome patients compared with the general population.[36–37]

In Tourette syndrome, as a psychiatric disorder, eye-rubbing in an obsessive-compulsive manner may justify its association with keratoconus.[38]

Diabetes may be considered a protection for keratoconus possibly due to acceleration in normal cross-linking processes.[39]

CHARACTERISTICS AND RISK FACTORS

Genetics

Keratoconus is genetically complex and heterogeneous with a varied inheritance pattern.[40] It follows an autosomal dominance or recessive inheritance but, in some families, sporadic keratoconus shows no Mendelian pattern.[29] Genetic studies hypothesized that mutations in the presence of a predisposed genetic background are required to draw out the keratoconus trait.[29] It seems that, in patients with a positive family history, early onset, and a more severe form of the disease, genetics may play a much greater role.[29]

Studies have found the incidence of keratoconus in the first-degree relatives is about 11% compared with a value of 0.05% in the general population. It has been estimated that relatives have a 15–67 times greater risk of developing keratoconus.[41]

Genetic testing is the future trend for keratoconus as well as in medicine as a whole. These tests help us to spot the individuals who are at risk and diagnose the condition earlier to guide a follow-up or treatment plan that fits their specific genetic markers and provides better care.[41]

There are scenarios where genetic testing has become an invaluable practice:

1. Refractive surgery should be conducted in suspected cases, choosing the specific type of surgery or deciding to avoid any kind of corneal refractive surgery.

2. Siblings and children of patients should undergo risk assessment and decisions made on how they should be followed-up.

Since keratoconus needs polygene testing, as we test more patients and upgrade the genetic database, artificial intelligence (AI) also can be applied to help us adopt more efficient and practical decisions and treatments.[42]

Two different types of studies for keratoconus gene identification are available:[26,29]

1. Linkage studies: family-based studies that identify the linkage regions throughout the genome which are probably linked to keratoconus.[29] The studies reported more than 19 loci linked to keratoconus, the most famous of which are micro RNA184, located on chromosome 15, DOCK9 (dedicator of cytokinesis 9) on chromosome 13, LOX (collagen crosslinking lysyl oxidase), the enzyme responsible for collagen crosslinking in the cornea and CAST (calpastatin-encoding gene), which introduces calpastatin as a calpain inhibitor playing the role of intercellular proteases.[26,29]

2. Candidate studies: case–control and cohort studies that screen the candidate genes for their presence in cases and absence in controls or identify any significant difference of allele frequencies between them.[26] Candidate genes related to keratoconus include VSX1 (visual system homeobox1), mutations in which are reported in some corneal dystrophies and keratoconus, SOD1 (superoxide dismutase1), which is located on chromosome 21 and affected in Down syndrome, and ZNF469 (zinc finger protein469), variants of which may increase the risk of keratoconus in the general population.[26,29]

3. Other genes: IL1 (interleukin1), with an important role in the ocular surface inflammatory response, may cast doubt on its role in keratoconus;[26] TGF1B (transforming growth factor 1-beta), with various mutations reported in corneal dystrophies and the expression of this gene is also decreased in keratoconus.[26]

4. Mitochondrial DNA is an interesting target due to its role in inflammation. A large number of mutations were present in keratoconus patients.[26]

A new FDA-approved genetic test, introduced by Avellino Lab USA, Inc., considered approximately 2,000 variants in the 75 genes related to keratoconus, which can calculate the degree of keratoconus risk for any suspected cases.[43]

Environment

Age

The manifest clinical onset may occur early in life, e.g., at puberty, and usually progress until the fourth decade.[26,44,45] The highest incidence rate of keratoconus is at the ages of 20 and 30 years.[46] Some reports indicate the occurrence of the disease at a later age or even infancy or as a part of change in an endocrinological status like pregnancy.[47–48] Individual cases can appear at any age and progress at any time. The incidence of the aggressive form of keratoconus is higher at younger ages, especially in children;[47] the younger the age, the more severe the disease and its progression and the higher the likelihood of requiring surgery.[47] Some studies reported shorter life in keratoconus patients due to comorbidities namely mitral valve prolapse, obesity, and sleep apnea.[49]

Gender

Some studies show a higher prevalence in women, whereas others show a greater occurrence in men, yet taking all together into consideration, it seems that keratoconus affects both genders at relatively similar rates.[50] Nevertheless, there may be a tendency for women to develop the disease earlier.[45] This variation in gender predominancy may depend on geographic zone and specific environmental factors.[47]

Eye-Rubbing

Many studies report eye-rubbing as an important independent risk factor for keratoconus and its progression. Eye-rubbing is reported in about half of keratoconic patients.[44,51] Studies also showed that keratoconis patients rub their eyes repeatedly and more forcefully, not to mention for much longer, than non-keratoconic patients. Rubbing has been shown to induce ocular surface inflammation, thinning of the epithelium, keratocyte loss, and stromal weakening, and also it could affect the keratometry.[52–54] Some studies confirmed that rubbing may decrease the tear break-up time.[26,44] Another theory for the role of repeated eye-rubbing, especially for the progression is related to increased intraocular pressure intermittently. This may affect corneal rigidity and viscosity and secondary curvature changes.[53] Studies also debated the theory of any progression in pellucid marginal degeneration and post-refractive surgery ectasia with eye-rubbing.[55–56] Although some studies do not attribute the main role to eye-rubbing, most of them strongly recommend avoiding this habit.

Contact Lens Wear

Contact lenses have played an important role in raising visual acuity in keratoconus patients recently. There are certain theories proposing that contact lens usage (soft contact lens or rigid contact lens) may play a role in the development or progression of the keratoconus.[26,44] Microtrauma due to constant movement on corneal surface could release the inflammatory mediators in tear film. Contact lens-induced dry eye also elevates these inflammatory markers.[57] Furthermore, contact lenses may promote eye-rubbing with all its aforementioned effects.[57] Finally, long-term use of contact lenses may induce keratocyte apoptosis and stromal structural changes, which may play a role in keratoconus induction or progression at least in susceptible subjects.[58] There is little consensus whether these changes are contact lens-induced or that all of them are secondary to the keratoconus disease process as a progressive disease.

Atopia

Atopia traits, such as any type of allergy, asthma, and eczema, are more common in keratoconus patients.[8] Studies showed that keratoconus appears at younger ages in patients with atopic traits. Thus, it may suggest the accelerating role of atopy in the course of the disease as a factor for induction and progression of keratoconus.[44] As the atopia is the main culprit for eye-rubbing, studies suggest that it may have an indirect role due to its association with eye-rubbing.[26]

Sun (Ultraviolet) Exposure

Some studies proposed UV exposure as a risk factor for keratoconus development or progression. They showed that it could be a contributing factor in keratocyte apoptosis as an oxidative stress process and secondary stromal thinning.[26] On the other hand, UV is a main component of the cross-linking procedure as a successful method for halting a progressive keratoconus.[59] Although studies pointed out the higher prevalence of keratoconus in hot and sunny climates, this relationship is unclear and needs further data to be evaluated.[60]

Floppy Eyelid Syndrome

Floppy eyelid syndrome is a confirmed risk factor for keratoconus. Secondary ocular surface inflammation, and dry eye may play a role in the development or progression of keratoconus.[26,61]

Hormones (Thyroid and Sex Hormones)

Studies reported a possible association between keratoconus and thyroid diseases. They reported that changes in thyroid hormones could be a risk factor as a structural stromal changer, which may affect keratoconus progression.[62] In keratoconus patients, there was a rise in thyroxin hormone (T4) level in tears and aqueous humor.[63] It should also be mentioned that, in some studies, increased expression of thyroxine receptors in keratocytes was reported.[44] Other conditions, like pregnancy, thyroidectomy, or iodine therapy, could also be a reason for thyroid dysfunction and may have a role in changing the keratoconus course, yet a causal relationship needs further studies.[64]

Studies supported a potential relationship between sex hormones and keratoconus. They reported an increased expression of estrogen and androgen receptors instead of a decrease in expression of progesterone receptors in the corneal epithelium of keratoconus patients.[44] These relationships must be confirmed by future studies.

Pregnancy

It has been proposed that changes in hormonal status in pregnant women can affect corneal biomechanics, which may induce progression in a stable keratoconus.[65] A prospective cohort study has shown significant progression during pregnancy compared with the control group.[44] Other studies proposed that keratoconus progression during pregnancy is a temporary effect and disappears a few months after delivery.[66] As a practical point, studies suggested that pregnant women with keratoconus should be followed-up closely during pregnancy. Due to cross-linking procedure challenges during pregnancy, it is not recommended.[67] Therefore, some clinicians consider cross-linking for keratoconus patients as a prophylactic procedure before deciding for pregnancy.[26,68]

Cigarette Smoking

Some studies reported smoking as an either negatively correlated or non-correlated factor with keratoconus.[69] They demonstrated that smoking cigarettes may promote natural corneal cross-linking, which leads to beneficial effects on the keratoconus.[69]

Personality

The correlation between personality disorders and keratoconus has been proposed for a long time by ophthalmologists.[26] There are reports of concurrent keratoconus and schizophrenia, but these lack supporting evidence.[26] Some studies described a relationship between keratoconus and compulsive behavior or psychiatric disorders because of the relationship with chronic eye-rubbing.[26]

Nutritional Imbalance

Vitamins

1. Vitamin D: Studies reported that low levels of vitamin D (<10 ng/mL) may play an important role in increasing the risk of keratoconus, an association which requires further investigation.[70]

2. Vitamin C: Impaired collagen synthesis in the course of keratoconus may lead to an increased level of vitamin C in keratoconic corneas. This kind of compensatory process may happen after cross-linking.[70]

3. Vitamin A: studies reported that a retinoic acid supplement, as an active metabolite of vitamin A, could promote the cross-linking process in the cornea.[70]

4. Others: Some studies suggested the role of B_9 and B_{12} in the keratoconus pathogenesis due to their effect on collagen synthesis enzymes.[70]

Minerals

Metal ions, such as iron, copper, selenium, and zinc, play crucial roles in collagen synthesis and cross-linking.[70] Thus, any imbalance of these minerals in a malnourished subject could be a risk factor for keratoconus development.

Keratoconus is a multifactorial and complex disease with an important role for genetics and many environmental factors. Genes and the gene × environment interaction are not fully understood in the keratoconus setting. Understanding all the risk factors in depth could help in the prevention, diagnosis, prognosis, and treatment of this disease.

REFERENCES

1. Grzybowski A, Mcghee CNJ. The early history of keratoconus prior to Nottingham's landmark 1854 treatise on conical cornea: A review. *Clin Exp Optom* 2013;96:140–5.

2. Li X, Rabinowitz YS, Rasheed K, Yang H. Longitudinal study of the normal eyes in unilateral keratoconus patients. *Ophthalmology* 2004;111:440–6.

3. Zadnik K, Barr JT, Gordon MO, Edrington TB. Biomicroscopic signs and disease severity in keratoconus. *Cornea* 1996;15:139–46.

4. Kennedy RH, Bourne WM, Dyer JA. A 48-year clinical and epidemiologic study of keratoconus. *Am J Ophthalmol* 1986;101:267–73.

5. Romero-Jiménez M, Santodomingo-Rubido J, Gonzá lez-Meijome JM. The thinnest, steepest, and maximum elevation corneal locations in noncontact and contact lens wearers in keratoconus. *Cornea* 2013;32:332–7.

6. Nichols JJ, Steger-May K, Edrington TB, Zadnik K. The relation between disease asymmetry and severity in keratoconus. *Br J Ophthalmol* 2004;88:788–91.

7. Zadnik K, Steger-May K, Fink BA, Joslin CE, Nichols JJ, Rosenstiel CE, et al. Between-eye asymmetry in keratoconus. *Cornea* 2002;21:671–9.

8. Lucas SE, Burdon KP. Genetic and environmental risk factors for keratoconus. *Annu Rev Vis Sci* 2020;6:25-46.

9. Davidson AE, Hayes S, Hardcastle AJ, Tuft SJ. The pathogenesis of keratoconus. *Eye* 2014;28(2):189–95.

10. Li X, Yang H, Rabinowitz YS. Longitudinal study of keratoconus progression. *Exp Eye Res* 2007;85(4):502–7.

11. Millodot M, Shneor E, Albou S, Atlani E, Gordon-Shaag A. Prevalence and associated factors of keratoconus in jerusalem: A cross-sectional study. *Ophthalmic Epidemiol* 2011;18(2):91–7.

12. Wisse RPL, Kuiper JJW, Gans R, Imhof S, Radstake TRDJ, Van Der Lelij A. Cytokine expression in keratoconus and its corneal microenvironment: A systematic review. *Ocul Surf* 2015;13:272–83.

13. Galvis V, Sherwin T, Tello A, Merayo J, Barrera R, Acera A. Keratoconus: An inflammatory disorder? *Eye* 2015;29:843–59. https://doi.org/10.1038/eye.2015.63.

14. McMonnies CW. Inflammation and keratoconus. *Optom Vis Sci* 2015;92:e35–41.

15. Li X, Rabinowitz YS, Rasheed K, Yang H. Longitudinal study of the normal eyes in unilateral keratoconus patients. *Ophthalmology* 2004;111(3):440–6.

16. Rabinowitz YS. Keratoconus. *Surv Ophthalmol* 1998;42:297–319.

17. Epidemiology is a science of high importance. *Nat Commun* 2018;9, 1703 (2018). https://doi.org/10.1038/s41467-018-04243-3

18. Spronk I, Korevaar JC, Poos R, Davids R, Hilderink H, Schellevis FG, et al. Calculating incidence rates and prevalence proportions: Not as simple as it seems. *BMC Public Health* 2019;19. https://doi.org/10.1186/s12889-019-6820-3.

19. Salomão MQ, Esposito A, Dupps WJ Jr. Advances in anterior segment imaging and analysis. *Curr Opin Ophthalmol* 2009;20:324–32.

20. Stapleton F, Alves M, Bunya VY, Jalbert I, Lekhanont K, Malet F, et al. TFOS DEWS II epidemiology report. *Ocul Surf* 2017;15:334–65.

21. Gordon-Shaag A, Millodot M, Kaiserman I, Sela T, Barnett Itzhaki G, Zerbib Y, et al. Risk factors for keratoconus in Israel: A case-control study. *Ophthalmic Physiol Opt* 2015;35:673–81.

22. Godefrooij DA, de Wit GA, Uiterwaal CS, Imhof SM, Wisse RP. Age-specific incidence and prevalence of keratoconus: A nationwide registration study. *Am J Ophthalmol* 2017;175:169–72.

23. Pearson AR, Soneji B, Sarvananthan N, Sanford-Smith JH. Does ethnic origin influence the incidence or severity of keratoconus? *Eye* 2000;14:625–8.

24. Georgiou T, Funnell CL, Cassels-Brown A, O'Conor R. Influence of ethnic origin on the incidence of keratoconus and associated atopic disease in Asians and white patients. *Eye* 2004;18:379–83.

25. Santodomingo-Rubido J, Carracedo G, Suzaki A, Villa-Collar C, Vincent SJ, Wolffsohn JS. Keratoconus: An updated review. *Cont Lens Anterior Eye* 2022;45(3):101559.

26. Ferrari G, Rama P. The keratoconus enigma: A review with emphasis on pathogenesis. *Ocul Surf* 2020;18(3):363–73.

27. Ziaei H, Jafarinasab MR, Javadi MA, Karimian F, Poorsalman H, Mahdavi M, et al. Epidemiology of keratoconus in an Iranian population. *Cornea* 2012;31:1044–7.

28. Torres Netto EA, Al-Otaibi WM, Hafezi NL, Kling S, Al-Farhan HM, Randleman JB, et al. Prevalence of keratoconus in paediatric patients in Riyadh, Saudi Arabia. *Br J Ophthalmol* 2018;102:1436–41.

29. Lucas SE, Burdon KP. Genetic and environmental risk factors for keratoconus. *Annu Rev Vis Sci* 2020;6:25–46.

30. Pietruszyńska M, Zawadzka-Krajewska A, Duda P, Rogowska M, Grabska-Liberek I, Kulus M. Ophthalmic manifestations of atopic dermatitis. *Postepy Dermatol Alergol* 2020;37(2):174–9.

31. Gautam V, Chaudhary M, Sharma AK, Shrestha GS, Rai PG. Topographic corneal changes in children with vernal keratoconjunctivitis: A report from Kathmandu, Nepal. *Contact Lens Anterior Eye* 2015;38:461–5.

32. Correa Dantas PE, Alves MR, Nishiwaki-Dantas MC. Topographic corneal changes in patients with vernal keratoconjunctivitis. *Arq Bras Oftalmol* 2005;68:593–8.

33. Pihlblad MS, Schaefer DP. Eyelid laxity, obesity, and obstructive sleep apnea in keratoconus. *Cornea* 2013;32:1232–6.

34. Slater JA, Misra SL, Braatvedt G, McGhee CNJ. Keratoconus and obesity: Can high body mass alter the shape of the cornea? *Clin Exp Ophthalmol* 2018;46:1091–3.

35. Siordia JA, Franco JC. The association between keratoconus and mitral valve prolapse: A meta-analysis. *Curr Cardiol Rev* 2020;16:147–52.

36. Marsack JD, Benoit JS, Kollbaum PS, Anderson HA. Application of topographical keratoconus detection metrics to eyes of individuals with Down syndrome. *Optom Vis Sci* 2019;96:664–9.

37. Alio JL, Vega-Estrada A, Sanz P, Osman AA, Kamal AM, Mamoon A, et al. Corneal morphologic characteristics in patients with Down syndrome. *JAMA Ophthalmol* 2018;136:971–8.

38. Mashor RS, Kumar NL, Ritenour RJ, Rootman DS. Keratoconus caused by eye rubbing in patients with Tourette syndrome. *Can J Ophthalmol* 2011;46:83–6.

39. Naderan M, Naderan M, Rezagholizadeh F, Zolfaghari M, Pahlevani R, Rajabi MT. Association between diabetes and keratoconus: A case-control study. *Cornea* 2014;33:1271–3.

40. Hao XD, Gao H, Xu WH, Shan C, Liu Y, Zhou ZX, Wang K, Li PF. Systematically displaying the pathogenesis of Keratoconus *via* multi-level related gene enrichment-based review. *Front Med (Lausanne)* 2022;8:770138. https://doi.org/10.3389/fmed.2021.770138.

41. Chen S, Li XY, Jin JJ, Shen RJ, Mao JY, Cheng FF, et al. Genetic screening revealed latent keratoconus in asymptomatic individuals. *Front Cell Dev Biol* 2021;9:650344.

42. Vandevenne MMS, Favuzza E, Veta M, Lucenteforte E, Berendschot T, Mencucci R, et al. Artificial intelligence for detecting keratoconus. *Cochrane Database Syst Rev* 2021;2021(12):CD014911.

43. Linda Charters, Genetic testing: Key to identifying keratoconus suspects, Ophthalmology times Europe, Mar 10, 2022, 18(3).

44. Crawford AZ, Zhang J, Gokul A, McGhee CNJ, Ormonde SE. The enigma of environmental factors in keratoconus. *Asia Pac J Ophthalmol (Phila)* 2020;9(6):549–6.

45. Ertan A, Muftuoglu O. Keratoconus clinical findings according to different age and gender groups. *Cornea* 2008;27(10):1109–13.

46. Gomes JAP, Rodrigues PF, Lamazales LL. Keratoconus epidemiology: A review. *Saudi J Ophthalmol* 2022;36(1):3–6.

47. Gordon-Shaag A, Millodot M, Shneor E, Liu Y. The genetic and environmental factors for keratoconus. *Biomed Res Int* 2015;2015:795738.

48. Bilgihan K, Hondur A, Sul S, Ozturk S. Pregnancy-induced progression of keratoconus. *Cornea* 2011;30(9):991–4.

49. McMonnies CW. Quo vadis older keratoconus patients? Do they die at younger ages? *Cornea* 2013;32:496–502.

50. Hashemi H, Heydarian S, Hooshmand E, Saatchi M, Yekta A, Aghamirsalim M, et al. The prevalence and risk factors for keratoconus: A systematic review and meta-analysis. *Cornea* 2020;39:263–70.

51. Najmi H, Mobarki Y, Mania K, Altowairqi B, Basehi M, Mahfouz MS, Elmahdy M. The correlation between keratoconus and eye rubbing: A review. *Int J Ophthalmol* 2019;12(11):1775–81.

52. Balasubramanian SA, Pye DC, Willcox MD. Effects of eye rubbing on the levels of protease, protease activity and cytokines in tears: Relevance in keratoconus. *Clin Exp Optom* 2013;96:214–8.

53. McMonnies CW. Mechanisms of rubbing-related corneal trauma in keratoconus. *Cornea* 2009;28:607–15.

54. McMonnies CW, Alharbi A, Boneham GC. Epithelial responses to rubbing-related mechanical forces. *Cornea* 2010;29:1223–31.

55. Martínez-Abad A, Piñero DP. Pellucid marginal degeneration: Detection, discrimination from other corneal ectatic disorders and progression. *Cont Lens Anterior Eye* 2019;42(4):341–9.

56. Giri P, Azar DT. Risk profiles of ectasia after keratorefractive surgery. *Curr Opin Ophthalmol* 2017;28(4):337–42.

57. Lopez-de la Rosa A, Gonzalez-Garcia MJ, Calonge M, Enríquez-de-Salamanca A. Tear inflammatory molecules in contact lens wearers: A literature review. *Curr Med Chem* 2020;27:523–48.

58. Ferdi AC, Nguyen V, Gore DM, Allan BD, Rozema JJ, Watson SL. Keratoconus natural progression: A systematic review and meta-analysis of 11 529 eyes. *Ophthalmology* 2019;126:935–45.

59. Chan E, Snibson GR. Current status of corneal collagen cross-linking for keratoconus: A review. *Clin Exp Optom* 2013;96:155–64.

60. Hashemi H, Khabazkhoob M, Fotouhi A. Topographic keratoconus is not rare in an Iranian population: The Tehran eye study. *Ophthalmic Epidemiol* 2013;20:385–91.

61. Mastrota KM. Impact of floppy eyelid syndrome in ocular surface and dry eye disease. *Optom Vis Sci* 2008;85:814–6.

62. Stival LRS, Giacomin NT, Santhiago MR. The role of thyroid gland dysfunction in the development of keratoconus. In: Almodin E, Nassaralla BA, Sandes J (eds) *Keratoconus*. Springer, Cham, 2022.

63. Stachon T, Stachon A, Hartmann U, Seitz B, Langenbucher A, Szentmáry N. Urea, uric acid, prolactin and fT4 concentrations in aqueous humor of keratoconus patients. *Curr Eye Res* 2017;42:842–6.

64. Lee R, Hafezi F, Randleman JB. Bilateral keratoconus induced by secondary hypothyroidism after radioactive iodine therapy. *J Refract Surg* 2018;34(5):351–3.

65. Naderan M, Jahanrad A. Topographic, tomographic and biomechanical corneal changes during pregnancy in patients with keratoconus: a cohort study. *Acta Ophthalmol* 2017;95:e291–6.

66. Sarac O, Yesilirmak N, Caglayan M, Yaman D, Ozdas D, Toklu Y, Cagil N. Dynamics of keratoconus progression after a previous successful accelerated crosslinking treatment during and after pregnancy. *J Cataract Refract Surg* 2022;48(5):599–603.

67. Photrexa and Photrexa Viscous [package insert]. Waltham, MA: Avedro; 2016.

68. Taneja M, Vadavalli PK, Veerwal V, Gour R, Reddy J, Rathi VM. Pregnancy-induced keractesia: A case series with a review of the literature. *Indian J Ophthalmol* 2020;68(12):3077–81.

69. Spoerl E, Raiskup-Wolf F, Kuhlisch E, et al. Cigarette smoking is negatively associated with keratoconus. *J Refract Surg* 2008;24:S737–40.

70. Lasagni Vitar RM, Bonelli F, Rama P, Ferrari G. Nutritional and metabolic imbalance in keratoconus. *Nutrients* 2022;14(4):913.

2 Keratoconus Classification

Mohammad Ghoreishi and Alireza Eslampoor

INTRODUCTION

Keratoconus classification has evolved over the past decades due to significant advances in the diagnosis and management approaches. In the past, the path to keratoconus management was mainly limited to the advanced forms of the disease with typical clinical findings (Vogt's striae, Munson's sign, hydrops, etc.) and significant visual loss. The need to recognize more subtle or subclinical forms of the disease was neither appreciated nor needed because of the lack of effective modalities for halting progression or achieving treatment at the early stage, except for optical correction.[1] However, emerging cases of keratectasia following keratorefractive surgery highlight the need for more detailed pre-operative diagnostic systems to better classify and exclude subclinical and suspect cases (Figure 2.1).[2,3] The evolution of the corneal collagen crosslinking (CXL) procedure to stabilize the disease was another indication of the need to develop updated classification systems.[4]

This chapter reviews different classification systems currently available for assessing keratoconus severity based on both historical and newer perspectives and proposes a new approach to classifying mild forms of the disease.

CLASSIFICATION SYSTEMS

Historically, older classification systems were based on imaging modalities existing at the time. The main available data had been central corneal curvature and central pachymetry. However, the development of tomography-based systems has provided detailed tomographic data, as well as precise thickness profiles of the entire cornea and corneal aberrometric information. Availability of these parameters promoted the development of more comprehensive systems. In 2015, four major multinational cornea societies (Asia Cornea, The Cornea Society, EuCornea, and PanCornea) published an influential paper, entitled the Global Consensus on Keratoconus and Ectatic Corneal Diseases, which showed that abnormal posterior elevation, abnormal corneal thickness distribution, and clinical non-inflammatory corneal thinning are mandatory criteria for keratoconus diagnosis.[5] This novel consensus exposed the inadequacies of the older classification systems, which suffer from the lack of tomographic data and, as such, do not recognize the early or subclinical disease.

Amsler–Krumeich Classification (AK)[6]

This 70-year-old classification system, of all the systems available, is the one most used in clinical practice to classify keratoconus, employs apex anterior corneal curvature, apex corneal thickness, manifest refraction, and the presence or absence of corneal scarring (Table 2.1). The main disadvantages (or constraints) of this system are the limited and focused data obtained from the corneal apex and its dependence on the subjective refraction that could affect the staging and progression monitoring by fitting the diseased corneas into more than one stage.

Morphological (Buxton) Classification[7]

This system utilizes the morphology of the cone for its classification (Table 2.2).

Keratometric Classification[8]

This system classifies keratoconus based on the central corneal power into four grades: (1) mild (<45 diopters [D]); (2) moderate (between 46 D and 52 D); (3) advanced (between 53 D and 59 D); and (4) severe (>59 D).

Hom's Classification[9]

This system classifies keratoconus into four grades based on clinical signs: (A) preclinical cases indicate that no keratoconus signs are detected; (B) mild keratoconus displays mild corneal thinning and scissors reflex; (C) moderate keratoconus indicates poor visual quality and corneal thinning without corneal scarring; and (D) severe keratoconus includes the presence of scars, unreliable refraction, and severe corneal thinning.

DOI: 10.1201/9781003371601-2

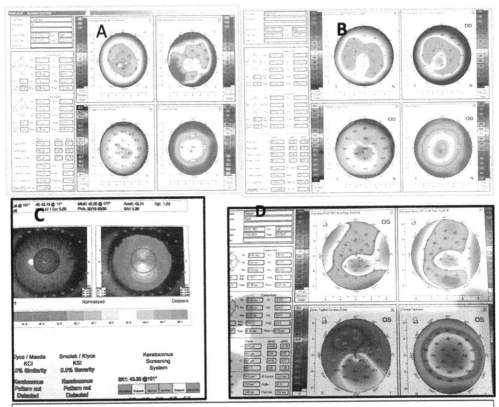

Preop (A) and post op (B) maps of a 38 y/0 male with a refraction around – 2.25 SE and thin flap Femto-Lasik who developed ectasia. RSB and PTA were around 330 and 30% respectively. Mildly abnormal axial map and relatively thin cornea may have risk factors. C (perop) and D(postop) belongs to a patient who developed ectasia following thin flap Femto-Lasik. He had no risk factor except keratoconus in his brother which was disclosed later on. RSB = residual stromal bed. PTA = percent tissue altered.

Figure 2.1 Keratectasia in KC suspect cases.

Table 2.1 Grading System and Parameters Used in the Amsler–Krumeich Classification

Grade	Apical Keratometry	Apical Pachymetry	Refraction (Myopia & Astigmatism)	Central Scar
1	<48	>500	<5 D	No
2	48–53	400–500	5–8 D	No
3	53–55	200–400	8–10 D	No
4	>55	<200	Not measurable	Yes

Fernandez–Alfonso Classification[10]

A new classification of keratoconus proposed by Luis Fernandez-Vega and Jose Alfonso (Oviedo, Spain) is mainly aimed at the implantation of intra-stromal corneal rings. Five phenotypes of keratoconus are defined according to the following variables: location of the cone, the relationship between the three main diagnostic axes (flat refractive, flat topographic, and coma), astigmatism topographic orthogonality, astigmatic symmetry, and the topographic pattern of the curvature

Table 2.2   Grading System and Parameters Used in the Buxton Classification

Stage	Size of the Cone	Location of the Cone
Nipple Keratoconus (KC)	<5 mm	Central or paracentral, usually inferonasal
Oval KC	5–6 mm	Central or paracentral, usually inferotemporal
Globe KC	>6 mm or >75% of anterior cornea	Generalized

Table 2.3   Grading System and Parameters Used in the Alio–Shabayek Classification

Severity	Mean Central Keratometry	Thickness	Spherical Equivalent	RMS of Coma-like Aberration	Corneal Scar
1	<48 D	>500 μm	<−5 D	1.5–2.5	No
2	<53 D	401–500 μm	−5 to −8 D	2.5–3.5	No
3	53–55 D	300–400 μm	>−8 D	3.5–4.5	No
4	>55 D	<300 μm	Not measurable	>4.5	Central scar

map. These phenotypes symbolically represent the disease as snowman, croissant, duck, nipple, or bowtie patterns and the authors proposed their ring implantation nomogram based on these patterns and other parameters.

Alio–Shabayek Classification[11]

This system is similar to the Amsler–Krumeich system but also includes the root mean square (RMS) of anterior corneal coma-like aberrations by which to grade keratoconus severity (Table 2.3).

The problem that may arise with this classification is that values for coma and spherical equivalents may not correspond with corneal keratometric and pachymetric parameters and consequently may designate one cornea into different classes, based on discrepant severity stages.

Keratoconus Severity Score (KSS)[12]

This system grades the severity of keratoconus based on slit-lamp findings (including apical scarring), corneal topographic map characteristics, and two easily determined topographic indices, namely average corneal power (ACP) and anterior corneal high-order RMS from 0 (suspect) to 5 (severe).

RETICS Classification[13]

In addition to clinical signs and optical and visual function variables, this classification system considers corneal biomechanical parameters (i.e., hysteresis and resistance factor)

Belin ABCD Grading System[14]

This novel classification system is based on tomographic and topographic parameters derived from Scheimpflug imaging of the cornea. The ABCD classification uses four parameters: "A" represents the anterior radius of curvature taken from a 3.0-mm zone centered on the thinnest point; "B" (for back) is the posterior radius of curvature from a 3.0-mm zone centered on the thinnest point; "C" is the minimal corneal thickness; and "D" is the best corrected distance visual acuity. The first three parameters are machine-generated (objective), whereas the "D" value (vision) is subjective and operator-entered. Each parameter is independently staged from 0 to 4. The four ABCD parameters are displayed in three ways; graphically, as the actual radius of curvature and pachymetry values, or in a five-step staging ranging from 0 to 5. This grading system is included in the OCULUS Pentacam system (OCULUS GmbH, Wetzlar, Germany) (Table 2.4).

ARTIFICIAL INTELLIGENCE–BASED SYSTEMS

Machine learning has enormous potential in image processing and task classification with acceptable sensitivity and specificity. Therefore, several AI-based keratoconus-detection systems have been included in various instruments. These methods are based on different algorithms for keratoconus detection and typically use cut-off values to allow differentiation between normal

Table 2.4   Grading System and Parameters Used with Belin ABCD Classification

Stage	A ARC (3-mm zone)	B PRC (3-mm zone)	C Thinnest Pachymetry	D CDVA
0	>7.25 (<46.5 D)	>5.9	>500	≥20/20 (≥1.00)
1	>7.05 (<48 D)	>5.70	>470	<20/20 (<1)
2	>6.35 (<53 D)	>5.15	>435	<20/40 (<0.5)
3	>6.15 (<55 D)	>4.95	>400	<20/100 (<0.2)
4	<6.15 (>55 D)	<4.95	≤400	<20/400 (<0.05)

ARC = anterior radius of curvature; PRC = posterior radius of curvature; CDVA = corrected distance visual acuity

corneas, keratoconus suspects, and clinical keratoconus. Smolek and Klyce have developed a Keratoconus Severity Index (KSI) using Placido-based topography and artificial intelligence (AI).[15] The Belin/Ambrósio Enhanced Ectasia Display (BAD) available on the OCULUS Pentacam,[16] the Screening Corneal Objective Risk of Ectasia Analyzer in ORBSCAN,[17] keratoconus screening display in Sirius,[18] the Keratoconus Prediction Index in Galilei,[19] and the keratoconus screening display in MS-39[20] are some of these AI systems. In addition, KeratoScreen is a novel deep-learning algorithm based on Zernike polynomials that may be a valuable tool for detecting early keratoconus and other corneal ectasias during pre-operative screening for corneal refractive surgery.[21]

DETERMINING ECTASIA PROGRESSION

Monitoring keratoconus progression and documenting stable or progressive forms is as important as early detection and severity staging. K_{max} (maximum anterior sagittal curvature) used to be an indicator of ectatic progression in the earlier literature. Some evidence defined ectatic progression as an increase in K_{max} of 1 D, or even 0.75 D in more recent studies.[22,23] However, K_{max} changes are not fully representative of the changes in the entire cornea. Moreover, there are reports of progressive cases despite no change in K_{max}.[24,25] The Global Consensus on Keratoconus and Ectatic Corneal Diseases (2015) defined ectasia progression as a consistent change in at least two of the following parameters: steepening of the anterior corneal surface, steepening of the posterior corneal surface, thinning and/or an increase in the rate of corneal thickness change from the periphery to the thinnest point. They also stated that a change in uncorrected and best spectacle-corrected visual acuity is optional when documenting progression.[5]

It seems that the Belin ABCD Progression Display meets the ectasia progression criteria defined by the aforementioned consensus. It allows up to eight examinations to be monitored over time. Each ABCD parameter is presented graphically, with one-sided confidence intervals of change shown for normal and keratoconic populations as green and red lines, respectively (with dashed and solid lines representing 80% and 95% confidence intervals (CIs), respectively)[26] (Figure 2.2).

The most recent progression display map also incorporates CIs for CXL-treated eyes. The post-CXL CIs (shown in blue, with dashed and solid lines representing 80% and 95% CIs, respectively) only appear at post-operative examinations with a minimal 12-month follow-up to allow for the normal variation in measurements seen in the first-year healing period.[27]

Recent evidence represents the clinical benefit of the ABCD Progression Display compared with previous criteria based on K_{max} changes.[28,29] The ABCD Progression Display provides the clinician with a better method of diagnosis, classification, and monitoring of disease progression than earlier systems based on the anterior corneal surface. In addition, this allows earlier interventions that can preserve vision or even improve optical performance, not just stabilize visual loss after it has already occurred.

Definition and Classification of Keratoconus-like Patterns

The aforementioned classifications are mainly used in the cases where keratoconus (KC) diagnosis is not disputed. There are a group of cases that are not eligible for being labeled as evident keratoconus but this pathology cannot be completely ruled out or in due to sharing some criteria and hence some similarity with true KC. Several terminologies have been used to define and classified these cases, such as forme fruste keratoconus (FFKC), subclinical keratoconus, keratoconus suspect (KCS), pre-keratoconus, early keratoconus, false keratoconus, and so on.[30–35]

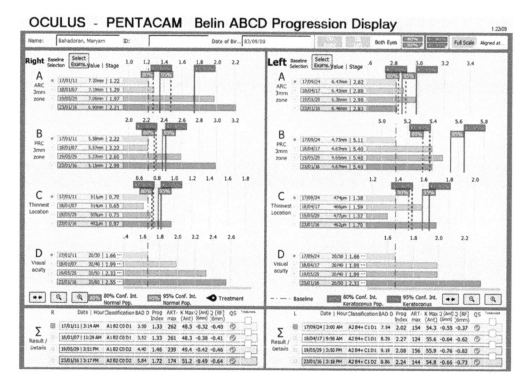

Figure 2.2 An example of Belin ABCD Progression Display.

Using some of these terms not only has no clinical benefits but also causes more confusion and complexity.[30,31] In the following subsections, we will review currently-used terminologies and classifications in this context and propose a term (keratoconus suspect) that we think is more appropriate and beneficial clinically. We will also propose a rational approach (keratoconus risk assessment spectrum and pyramid, KRASP) to risk assessment in this group of patients. Before any judgment is made, it is essential that the quality of the image has been assessed. Examiners should follow the guidelines of the manufacturer of each instrument to acquire a qualified image.[32]

Forme Fruste Keratoconus

This term was first proposed by Amsler in 1961 to define the apparently normal contralateral eye in unilateral KC. The nominated eye was normal clinically and topographically, while the fellow eye had frank keratoconus.[33] However, this term has been frequently and inappropriately used to describe a wide spectrum of findings from mild abnormality to obvious ectasia. Contrary to the initial application, many colleagues use this term for some types of KC that are considered to be aborted or suppressed KC, ignoring the fact that it is not possible to make a judgment on suppression unless there is a long follow-up period. Meanwhile, knowing the fact that the fellow eye has obvious keratoconus automatically puts this eye into the high-risk category without the additional need for a separate designation. Regarding these facts and the lack of clinical benefits, we, as well as some opinion leaders, recommend avoiding the use of this terminology.[34]

Keratoconus Suspect

This term is more commonly used for patients who have no clinical signs or symptoms of keratoconus, but where topography and/or tomography show some suspicious or borderline data and patterns resembling KC, while some other parameters are within normal limits and the autodetection software of the instrument by which the image was acquired fails to identify it as keratoconus.[35] The parameters can be qualitative, such as color patterns, or quantitative, such as curvature, thickness, elevation, and other calculated indices. These indices include inferior-superior asymmetry represented as inferior and, less commonly, superior steepening, central steepening, truncated or asymmetric bowtie pattern with or without skewed radial axis, oblique or against-the-rule

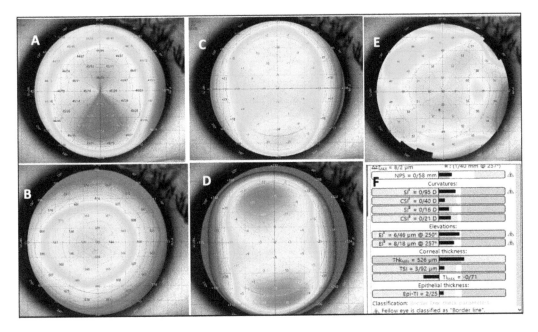

Figure 2.3 Axial (A), thickness (B), anterior elevation (C), posterior elevation (D), epithelial thickness (E), and keratoconus screening display (F) of a 36-year-old female showing inferior steepening of around 2 diopters. Other maps are not suggestive of keratoconus, but a KC screening program suggests a borderline case. The patient has no clinical risk factors. Based on our KRASP system (discussed later in this chapter), she is classified as moderately suspect and needs close follow-up.

astigmatism, subnormal or borderline topographic, tomographic, and biomechanical indices, and some degrees of asymmetry between the two eyes.[30,35]

In recent years, with the advent of new topography and tomography instruments and the ability to measure corneal biomechanics and epithelial thickness, as well as the availability of some sophisticated and highly efficient algorithms based on artificial intelligence, the accuracy of KC screening has improved drastically (Figure 2.3); however, there is still a substantial number of cases that are not successfully classified by these means and it is left to the clinical judgment of the physician to assess the risk of developing frank keratoconus or ectasia, either spontaneously or following corneal refractive surgery. So, it is risk assessment and not an exact diagnosis that works in this situation. Regarding the importance of this issue, we will discuss it more in the following paragraphs.

Subclinical Keratoconus

There is no clear-cut definition of this term and it has been used interchangeably with other terms that were mentioned earlier.[30,36] As implied by this composite term, the patients exhibit all or at least most of the imaging criteria to be listed as mild keratoconus but have no clinical findings at the time of examination. So, we suggest reserving the term for this situation only.

False and Pseudo-Keratoconus

False keratoconus was first described by Doyle and his colleagues in 1996.[37] They reported a series of cases with abnormal topographic patterns such as inferior steepening and/or skewed radial axis which lacked the criteria to be categorized as true keratoconus. They attributed this abnormality to high-angle kappa and proposed the term "displaced apex" or false keratoconus for this situation. No further studies supported this finding and this term is not commonly used anymore.

Pseudo-keratoconus has not been well defined in the literature, but may be applied to cases that have localized steepening which is induced by elevated anterior corneal opacity or localized epithelial thickening. Hyperopic ablation may also simulate this condition. In our experience, a higher value of anterior elevation compared with posterior elevation on the elevation maps is a pathognomonic finding in these cases, but history and slit-lamp examination are more reliable

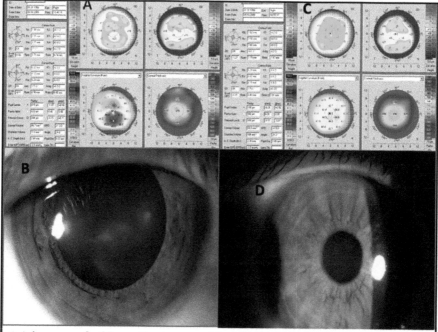

Axial map of this patient resembles keratoconus (A). But slit lamp examination showed corneal opacity due to epithelial dystrophy (B). Epithelial debridement resulted in normal topography (C), clear cornea (D) and improved vision. This pattern can be considered as pseudo-keratoconus.

Figure 2.4 Pseudo-keratoconus.

clues for the diagnosis (Figure 2.4). Contact lens-induced corneal warpage can resemble keratoconus and has been named pseudo-keratoconus by some authors;[38] the best way to differentiate this situation from true KC is to instruct the patient to discontinue contact lens wear for a set period of time. Improvement of the curvature of the suspected area indicates a case of pseudo-keratoconus; otherwise, the level of suspicion of keratoconus increases.

Role of the Epithelial Thickness Map

Measurement and clinical applications of corneal epithelium were first introduced by Reinstein and his colleagues.[39,40] This imaging technique is used to classify keratoconus suspects into either being or not being true keratoconus. We refer the readers to the chapter 6 "Epithelial Thickness Mapping for Keratoconus Screening by VHF Digital Ultrasound or Anterior Segment OCT" in this book which covers this subject in more detail.

Keratoconus Susceptibility and Risk Assessment

As was mentioned earlier, employing multidevice and multimodal approaches by using the rotating Scheimpflug camera system, optical coherence tomography (OCT), Placido, and biomechanical technologies and analyzing the data by means of artificial intelligence has improved the sensitivity and accuracy of screening and has increased the probability of more accurately distinguishing and classifying these cases. However, despite the emergence of these new technologies and software, unequivocal diagnosis of keratoconus may still not be possible in some abnormal and keratoconus-like patterns. So, risk assessment is the way to go, rather than designating a specific diagnosis.[41,42] Susceptibility and risk assessment help us to make the right decision in suspicious cases.

Several software and indices had been introduced to detect KC based on corneal topography parameters,[43,44] but Randleman and his colleagues were the first groups to design an ectasia risk scoring system (ERSS) based on a retrospective case–control study, which included Placido disc-based corneal topography findings and some other clinical parameters.[42,45] This system was validated by further studies and has been widely accepted as a reliable tool for risk assessment.[45] However, with the advent of advanced technologies, such as Scheimpflug- and OCT-based imaging, and the introduction of a wide range of new parameters and indices, there has been a demand for more comprehensive and inclusive systems. Thereafter, a variety of keratoconus screening indices and software have been proposed by investigators and have been incorporated into different imaging devices. Some of them were mentioned earlier in this chapter.[16,46,47]

To enhance the overall strategy and reach the desired outcome, additional elements must be considered. These elements include clinical predisposing factors and risk factors. We have to revise our classification and transform it into a new system based on the integration of imaging and other risk factors. For this purpose, we primarily include all these cases in the "keratoconus suspect" category, based on the imaging characteristics, and then recategorize them with respect to added clinical risk factors. The term "keratoconus suspect" is more appropriate because it is a familiar and commonly used term. It covers a spectrum of cases that can be classified as neither keratoconus nor normal. However, not all cases in this category are at the same level of suspicion. Some of them have a mild abnormality with few abnormal parameters, while others may have a more severe abnormality and a higher number of abnormal indices. So, we have to subclassify these cases, based on the severity of abnormality, into mildly, moderately, and highly suspect.

By combining clinical and topographical findings, we propose a new system, called keratoconus risk assessment spectrum and pyramid (KRASP), which is shown in Figure 2.5.

Based on this system, if the patient is mildly keratoconus suspect based on topography findings or by having one or more additional risk factors, such as family history, eye rubbing, and/or biomechanical impairment, they will be considered to be highly suspect and highly susceptible and will be managed accordingly. In this pyramid, determining the degree of suspicion has been left to the judgment and impression of an experienced clinician to fit the cases into the spectrum based on the frequency and severity of abnormal patterns and parameters, but we hope that this approach becomes validated by further studies, and that investigators provide clear-cut clues

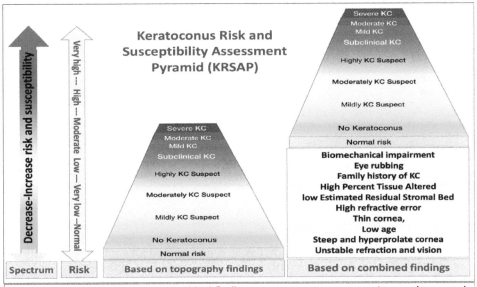

By combining clinical and topographical findings, we propose a new system and approach called keratoconus risk assessment spectrum and pyramid (KRASP) which is shown in this figure. Severity of the disease, risk and susceptibility of the case increases from button to the top as shown by the pyramid at the left side of the image. These are cases that only have topographic and/or tomographic finding with no additional risk factors. The right part of the image is specified for the cases that have additional clinical findings and risk factors. Adding every risk factor moves the risk one level up or even more, depending on the weight of that factor and increases susceptibility score accordingly.

Figure 2.5 Keratoconus risk assessment spectrum and pyramid (KRASP).

to subclassify KC suspect cases by more objective parameters derived from different diagnostic devices.

In conclusion, the classification systems for keratoconus have evolved with the progress in development of imaging techniques, image analysis technologies, and treatment developments. Newer classification systems have included more clinical and imaging parameters. Although classification for obvious keratoconus does not have many challenges, there are controversies and confusion in using terminology and classifying the cases that are borderline and suspect. We have tried to review the different opinions, to propose a new approach for classifying this group of patients.

REFERENCES

1. Krachmer JH, Feder RS, Belin MW. Keratoconus and related noninflammatory corneal thinning disorders. *Surv Ophthalmol.* 1984;28:293–322.

2. Seiler T, Koufala K, Richter G. Iatrogenic keratectasia after laser in situ keratomileusis. *J Refract Surg.* 1998;14:312–317.

3. Ambrósio R, Dawson DG, Salomão M, et al. Corneal ectasia after LASIK despite low preoperative risk: tomographic and biomechanical findings in the unoperated, stable, fellow eye. *J Refract Surg.* 2010;26:906–911.

4. Wollensak G, Spoerl E, Seiler T. Riboflavin/ultraviolet-A-induced collagen cross-linking for treating keratoconus. *Am J Ophthalmol.* 2003;135:620–627.

5. Gomes JA, Tan D, Rapuano CJ, et al. Global consensus on keratoconus and ectatic diseases. *Cornea.* 2015;34:359–369.

6. Amsler M. "The forme fruste" of keratoconus. *Wiener Klinische Wochenschrift.* 1961;73:842–843.

7. Perry HD, Buxton JN, Fine BS. Round and oval cones in keratoconus. *Ophthalmology.* 1980;87:905–909.

8. Vega Estrada A, Sanz Díez P, Aliό JL. Keratoconus grading and its therapeutic implications. In: Aliό J. (eds) *Keratoconus. Essentials in ophthalmology,* 2017, pp. 177–184. https://doi.org/10.1007/978-3-319-43881-8_15.

9. Rabinowitz YS. Keratoconus. *Surv Ophthalmol.* 1998;42:297–319.

10. Fernandez-Vega Cueto L, Lisa C, Poo-Lopez A, Madrid-Costa D, Merayo-Lloves J, Alfonso JF. Intrastromal corneal ring segment implantation in 409 paracentral keratoconic eyes. *Cornea.* 2016;35(11):1421–1426.

11. Aliό JL, Shabayek MH. Corneal higher order aberrations: A method to grade keratoconus. *J Refract Surg.* 2006;22:539–545.

12. McMahon TT, Szczotka-Flynn L, Barr JT, et al. A new method for grading the severity of keratoconus: The Keratoconus Severity Score (KSS). *Cornea.* 2006;25:794–800.

13. Aliό JL, Piñero DP, Alesón A, et al. Keratoconus-integrated characterization considering anterior corneal aberrations, internal astigmatism, and corneal biomechanics. *J Cataract Refract Surg.* 2011;37:552–568.

14. Belin MW, Duncan JK. Keratoconus: The ABCD grading system. *Klin Monbl Augenheilkd.* 2016;233:701–707.

15. Smolek MK, Klyce SD. Current keratoconus detection methods compared with a neural network approach. *Invest Ophthalmol Vis Sci.* 1997;38: 2290–2299.

16. Villavicencio OF, Gilani F, Henriquez MA, et al. Independent population validation of the belin/ambrósio enhanced ectasia display: implications for keratoconus studies and screening. *Int J Keratoconus Ectatic Corneal Dis.* 2014;3:1–8.

17. Saad A. Validation of a new scoring system for the detection of early forme of keratoconus. *Int J Keratoconus Ectatic Corneal Dis.* 2012;1:100–108.

18. Doctor K, Vunnava KP, Shroff R, et al. Simplifying and understanding various topographic indices for keratoconus using Scheimpflug based topographers. *Indian J Ophthalmol.* 2020;68:2732–2743.

19. Moshirfar M, Motlagh MN, Murri MS, et al. Galilei corneal tomography for screening of refractive surgery candidates: a review of the literature, part II. *Med Hypothesis Discov Innov Ophthalmol.* 2019;8:204–218.

20. Gokul A, Vellara HR, Patel DV. Advanced anterior segment imaging in keratoconus: a review. *Clin Exp Ophthalmol.* 2018;46:122–132.

21. Gao HB, Pan ZG, Shen MX, Lu F, Li H, Zhang XQ. KeratoScreen: Early keratoconus classification with zernike polynomial using deep learning. *Cornea.* 2022;41(9):1158–1165.

22. O'Brart DP, Chan E, Samaras K, Patel P, Shah SP. A randomised, prospective study to investigate the efficacy of riboflavin/ultraviolet A (370 nm) corneal collagen cross-linkage to halt the progression of keratoconus. *Br J Ophthalmol.* 2011;95(11):1519–1524.

23. Guber I, McAlinden C, Majo F, Bergin C. Identifying more reliable parameters for the detection of change during the follow-up of mild to moderate keratoconus patients. *Eye Vis. (Lond).* 2017;4:24.

24. Rubinfeld RS, Littner R, Trattler WB, et al. Pentacam HR criteria for curvature change in keratoconus and postoperative LASIK ectasia. *J Refract Surg.* 2013;29(10):666.

25. Mahmoud AM, Nuñez MX, Blanco C, et al. Expanding the cone location and magnitude index to include corneal thickness and posterior surface information for the detection of keratoconus. *Am J Ophthalmol.* 2013;156(6):1102–1111.

26. Duncan JK, Belin MW, Borgstrom M. Assessing progression of keratoconus: novel tomographic determinants. *Eye Vis (Lond).* 2016;3:6.

27. Belin MW, Alizadeh R, Torres-Netto EA, et al. Determining progression in ectatic corneal disease. *Asia Pac J Ophthalmol (Phila).* 9;2020:541–548.

28. Vinciguerra R, Belin MW, Borgia A, et al. Evaluating keratoconus progression prior to crosslinking: maximum keratometry vs the ABCD grading system. *J Cataract Refract Surg.* 2021;47:33–39.

29. Dubinsky-Pertzov B, Reinhardt O, Gazit I, et al. The ABCD keratoconus grading system–a useful tool to estimate keratoconus progression in the pediatric population. *Cornea.* 2020;00:1

30. Klyce DS. Chasing the suspect: Keratoconus. *Br J Ophthalmol.* 2009;93(7):845–857.

31. Henriquez MA, Hadid M. A systematic review of subclinical keratoconus and forme fruste keratoconus. *J Refract Surg.* 2020;36(4):270–279.

32. Hick S, Laliberte JF. Effects of misalignment during corneal topography. *J Cataract Refract Surg.* 2007;33(9):1522–1529.

33. Klyce SD. Chasing the suspect: keratoconus. *Br J Ophthalmol.* 2009;93:845–847.

34. Carlson AN, Ambrósio Jr R, Belin MW, Trattler WB. Does-this-patient-have-keratoconus? J Crstoday. 2019.

35. Klyce SD. Can You spot the Keratoconus Suspect?. *International Journal of Keratoconus and Ectatic Corneal Diseases.* 2013;1(3):0–1

36. Shetty R, Rao H, Khamar P, et al. Keratoconus screening indices and their diagnostic ability to distinguish normal from ectatic. *Am J Ophthalmol.* 2017;181:140–148.

37. Doyle SJ, Hynes E. PRK in patients with a keratoconic topography picture. The concept of a physiological 'displaced apex syndrome. *Br J Ophthalmol.* 1996; 80:25–28.

38. Eghbali F. Keratoconus Suspect or Pseudokeratoconus? *Contact Lens Spectrum.* 1997;12:30–2

39. Reinstein DZ, Silverman RH, Coleman DJ. High-frequency ultrasound measurement of the thickness of the corneal epithelium. *Refract Corneal Surg.* 1993;9(5):385–387.

40. Reinstein DZ, Archer TJ, Gobbe M. Stability of LASIK in topographically suspect keratoconus confirmed non-keratoconic by Artemis VHF digital ultrasound epithelial thickness mapping: 1-year follow-up. *J Refract Surg.* 2009;25(7):569–577.

41. McMonnies CW. Screening for keratoconus suspects among candidates for refractive. *Clin Exp Optom.* 2014;97:6.

42. Randleman JB, Woodward M, Lynn MJ, Stulting RD. Risk assessment for ectasia after corneal refractive surgery. *Ophthalmology.* 2008;115:37–50.

43. Rabinowitz YS, Rasheed K. KISA% index: a quantitative videokeratography algorithm embodying minimal topographic criteria for diagnosing. Keratoconus. *J Cataract Refract Surg.* 1999;25:1327–1335.

44. Maeda N, Klyce SD, Smolek MK, Thompson HW. Automated keratoconus screening with corneal topography analysis. *Invest Ophthalmol Vis Sci.* 1994;35:2749–2757.

45. Randleman JB, Trattler WB, Stulting RD. Validation of the Ectasia risk score system for pre-operative laser in situ keratomileusis screening. *Am J Ophthalmol.* 2008;145(5):813–818.

46. Vinciguerra R, Ambrósio R, Elsheikh A, et al. Detection of keratoconus with a new biome-chanical index. *J Refract Surg.* 2016;32(12):803–810.

47. Ambrosio Jr R, Machado AP, Leao E, et al. Optimized artificial intelligence for enhanced ectasia detection using Scheimpflug-based corneal tomography and biomechanical data. *Am J Ophthalmol.* 2023;251:126–42.

3 Updates on Keratoconus Diagnosis

Mehrdad Mohammadpour and Zahra Heidari

INTRODUCTION

Keratoconus (KC) is a progressive and asymmetric ectatic corneal disease that commonly occurs in adolescents and progresses dramatically in the absence of treatment.[1] It is characterized by progressive central corneal thinning, irregular astigmatism, increased higher-order aberrations, and decreased visual acuity. The prevalence of KC shows large variations in different general populations, with 0.15% in the United States,[2] 4% in the rural population of Iran,[3] 37.4% in South Korea,[4] and 192.1 per 100,000 in Norway.[5] KC is more common in males (odds ratio (OR) = 2.30, $P<0.05$) and researchers have reported its aggregation in families.[3]

Corneal imaging is commonly used by ophthalmologists to inform the shape and curvature of the cornea. Corneal topography assesses the front surface of the cornea and shows different data by using a color-coded map. Furthermore, corneal tomography evaluates the thickness of the cornea, which can elucidate the posterior surface of the cornea.[6] In the early stages, the visual acuity may not be decreased, and slit-lamp examination may not show any characteristics of KC, then corneal topography/tomography could be a gold standard test for the detection of corneal ectasia in the initial stages.

The ability of different corneal imaging techniques to monitor disease progression, and patient selection for specific surgical procedures, makes them one of the most important imaging studies in ophthalmology. This chapter aims to identify the current corneal imaging modalities for better interpretation of the results in KC detection.

TOPOGRAPHY

Corneal topography is non-contact imaging that provides front surface information of the cornea.[7] The corneal topography methods include Placido and slit-scanning techniques. There are different types of Placido topographers based on the projection of consequence rings on the cornea, such as the Magellan Mapper (Nidek), Medmont E300 (Medmont), Scout and Keratron (EyeQuip), ReSeeVit (Veatch Ophthalmic Instruments), ATLAS 995 and 9000 (CarlZeiss Meditec), and Tomey (Computed Anatomy TMS-1). Most topographic corneal tools are based on a Placido disc which analyzes the reflected rings on the corneal surface and cannot assess the posterior parts of the cornea.

Slit-scanning technology is based on measuring the slit-scanning beam that is projected into the cornea. Orbscan I is the slit-scanning corneal topographer that could evaluate the posterior corneal surface and measure the corneal thickness as well as the curvature of the both anterior and posterior surfaces of the cornea. Orbscan II has integrated a Placido disc to obtain curvature measurements directly, while the Orbscan IIz has combined the Shack–Hartmann aberrometer into the Zyoptix workstation. The reflection of the illuminated Placido disc on the cornea is preserved, followed by the projection of 40 slits (each slit is 12.5 mm high and 0.30 mm wide) of 20 left and right at an angle of 45 degrees to the axis of the instrument. Backscatter images are captured by the available video camera in the device. The third generation of Orbscan (Orbscan III) provides anterior and posterior corneal information by calculating 23,000 points on the whole of the cornea.[8]

Maps
Axial Map

The axial or sagittal map is the most common map and indicates the curvature of the anterior corneal surface in relation to the visual axis (Figure 3.1). The anterior surface shape is mainly used for screening because it can be correlated with the subject's refractive status and gives an average picture of the anterior corneal curvature. The distance between a defined point and the visual axis shows the radius of curvature of the cornea. The axial map cannot determine the subtle changes in the corneal curvature at the periphery.

Tangential Map

The tangential provides more detail about the corneal shape, especially at the peripheral parts of the cornea (Figure 3.2). The tangential map could determine small curvature changes of the anterior surface of the cornea in corneal pathology such as subclinical KC (SKC). These data can

DOI: 10.1201/9781003371601-3

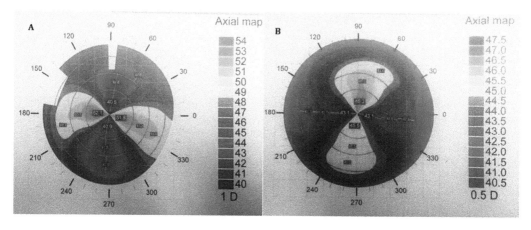

Figure 3.1 Axial map with symmetric bow-tie pattern in against (A) and with the rule astigmatism (B) in eyes with astigmatism.

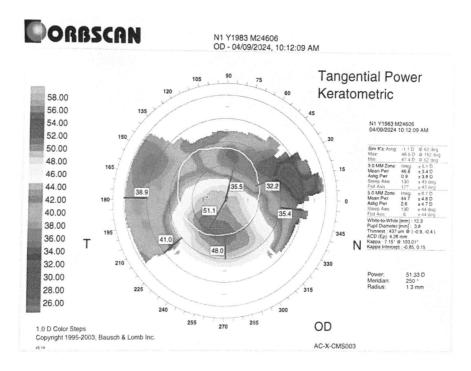

Figure 3.2 Tangential map of keratoconus cornea.

be used to choose the proper treatment plan, such as implanting an intracorneal ring or placing a different lens design.

Refractive Power Map

A refractive power map is a tangent projection map and can measure the power and curvature of individual points on the cornea with the greatest accuracy (Figure 3.3). This display provides the most accurate peripheral data and is very useful for fitting special lenses. In addition, it is very useful for understanding the power of corneal imaging and analyzing the effects of surgery. However, the refractive map cannot provide more information about the shape of the anterior surface of the cornea.

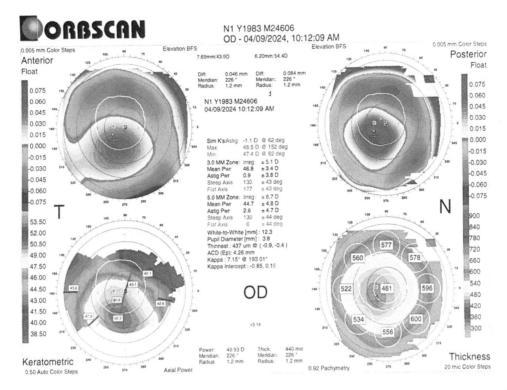

Figure 3.3 Orbscan refractive maps include elevation maps of the anterior/posterior surfaces of the cornea, as well as keratometric and pachymetric maps.

Elevation Map

The elevation display map shows the actual shape of the cornea. Placido disc topography systems use complex algorithms to extrapolate elevation data by reconstructing the actual curvature, while Scheimpflug systems measure elevation directly, so the latter systems may provide the most accurate data. Elevation data is measured based on the "best-fit sphere (BFS)" and systems calculate relative elevation or depression areas based on deviations from the proper sphere, and deviation values are shown in microns (Figure 3.3). Blue areas in the elevation map represent negative values and red areas determine positive values. Moreover, points above BFS indicate positive values, and points below BFS indicate negative values, and in corneal astigmatism, one meridian is steeper than the other. Placido systems only measure the front surface of the cornea, while Scheimpflug systems measure both the front and posterior elevation parts.

Pachymetry Map

Pachymetry measurement capabilities are only available on slit-scan topographs and Scheimpflug cameras, as these instruments measure the posterior and anterior surfaces of the cornea. The pachymetry map can be used to assess disease progression (i.e., KC) by monitoring changes in corneal thickness due to the extent of corneal ectasia (Figure 3.3). Orbscan can measure the thickness of the entire cornea, although, it may overestimate the corneal pachymetry compared with ultrasound pachymetry.[3]

Statistical Indices in Topography

Corneal topography provides several indices that can be used for screening the keratoconic corneas by quantitative values. Some of them are simple keratometric indices and some of them are computed from several indices by artificial intelligence (AI) methods.

Simple indices: surface asymmetry index (SAI), surface regularity index (SRI), predicted visual acuity (PVA), inferior-superior (I-S) value, irregular astigmatism index (IAI), opposite sector index (OSI), differential sector index (DSI), central/comprehensive index (CSI), average central diopter

Table 3.1 Diagnostic Criteria for Normal, Keratoconus Suspect (SKC), and Definite Keratoconus (KC) for Orbscan[8]

Criteria	Normal	SKC	KC
Anterior corneal curvature (D)	< 47.2	47.2–49	>49
Anterior BFS (D)	<47.8	47.8–50	>50
Posterior BFS (D)	< 50	50–52	>52
Ratio of anterior/posterior curvature (Efkarpides)	< 1.21	1.21–1.27	> 1.27
Difference most anterior elevated point to BFS (μm)	<25	25–30	> 30
Difference most posterior elevated point to BFS (μm)	< 35	35-50	>50
Axial anterior corneal curvature (D)	< 47.2	47.2–48.7	> 48.7
Difference of mean K of two eyes (D)	< 1	1 - 2	> 2
Skewed steepest radial axis (SRAX)	<10	10-20	>21
Inferior-superior difference (IS value) at 3 mm (D)	<1.4	1.4–1.9	>1.9
Inferior-superior difference (IS value) at 5 mm (D)	<1.4	1.4–2.5	>2.5
Irregularity difference in central 3 mm	<1.5	1.5–3	>3
Thinnest point (μm)	>500	470–500	<470

power (ACP), and analyzed area (AA). Orbscan indices and the suggested values for diagnosing KC, SKC, and normal eyes are presented in Table 3.1.

Integrated indices: keratoconus severity index (KSI), keratoconus prediction index (KPI), and KISA.

The KISA index is expressed in terms of keratometry (K), inferior superior (IS), astigmatism (A) and skewed radial axes (SRAX) according to the following formula:

$$\text{KISA\% index} = \left[\frac{(K) \times (I-S) \times (AST) \times (SRAX) \times 100}{300} \right].$$

TOMOGRAPHY

Tomography is a three-dimensional image of the anterior and posterior surfaces of the cornea, and corneal thickness is measured, unlike topography where only the anterior surface of the cornea is mapped. Topography gives a complete assessment of the entire cornea and improves the detection of corneal ectasia in the early stages. The main goal of any tomography tool is to perform appropriate screening and create better refractive outcomes after surgery. Early diagnosis of ectasia allows the surgeon to initiate protective treatment, such as collagen cross-linking, which may slow down or stop KC progression in an ideal corneal state. In this section, we review the popular tomographers and discuss their diagnostic abilities in KC detection.

Pentacam

The Pentacam® (Oculus Optikgeräte GmbH, Wetzlar, Germany) has a Scheimpflug camera, which has been known since 2002 as a perfect non-invasive device for corneal topography. Various studies have shown that the Pentacam system can fully maintain repeatability and reproducibility.[9,10] Pentacam has excellent intra-observed accuracy compared with other tomographic devices, such as Galilei.[11] Pentacam provides different maps for comprehensive evaluation of both the anterior and posterior surfaces of the cornea. Each map contains curvature-based, elevation-based, pachymetric, and various simple or integrated indices.[12]

Refractive Map

Four Maps Refractive is the most commonly used display, which includes an axial or sagittal map, similar to the Placido display, a pachymetry map, and two maps of anterior and posterior corneal elevation (Figure 3.4). Anterior and posterior elevation maps are based on the best-fit sphere (BFS), best-fit ellipse (BFE), or best-fit toric ellipsoid (BFTE) standard references. Our proposed diagnostic criteria for normal, SKC, and definite KC based on Pentacam indices are shown in Table 3.2.

The Belin–Ambrósio Enhanced Ectasia Display

This display combines the following parameters: anterior elevation at the minimum thickness point, posterior elevation at the minimum thickness point, change in anterior elevation, change in

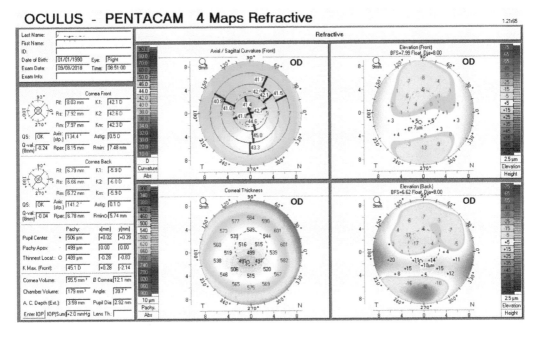

Figure 3.4 Refractive maps of Pentacam.

Table 3.2 Diagnostic Criteria for Normal, Keratoconus Suspect (SKC) and Definite Keratoconus (KC) for Pentacam[12]

	Normal	SKC	KC
Kmax (D)	<47.2	47.2–49	> 49
Against the rule astigmatism (D)	<1	1–2	>2
Corneal astigmatism (D)	<6	6–7	>7
Thinnest point (μm)	>500	470–500	< 470
Difference between pachymetry apex and thinnest location (μm)	< 10	10–20	>20
Difference central thickness between two eyes (μm)	<10	10–30	>30
Displacement of the thinnest point from the center (mm)	<0.5	0.5– 1	>1
Skewed steepest radial axis (SRAX) (degrees)	<10	10–20	>21
IS value (inferior–superior difference at the 3 mm) (D)	<1.4	1.4–1.9	>1.9
IS value (inferior–superior difference at the 5 mm) (D)	<1.4	1.4–2.5	>2.5
Anterior elevation (μm)	<10	10–12	>12
Posterior elevation (μm)	<15	15–17	>17

posterior elevation, corneal thickness at minimum thickness point, location of the thinnest point, pachymetric progression (PPI), Ambrósio relational thickness (ART), and K_{max} (Figure 3.5). The third version of the Belin–Ambrósio enhanced ectasia display (BAD III) index provides individual information on each parameter and then performs a discriminant analysis along with these indexes that allow the distinction between healthy and KC eyes. Progression of corneal thickness (PTI), and the corneal thickness spatial profile (CTSP) are significant profiles for the analysis of corneal thickness. An average value of more than 1.2 in the red line indicates KC. Our proposed pachymetric values for diagnosing normal, SKC, and definite KC using the BAD display are shown in Table 3.3.

The Fast Screening Report Maps

This is an important display for rapid evaluation of the cornea. This map shows typical quad maps data from the anterior and posterior surface of the cornea, as well as corneal densitometry. The

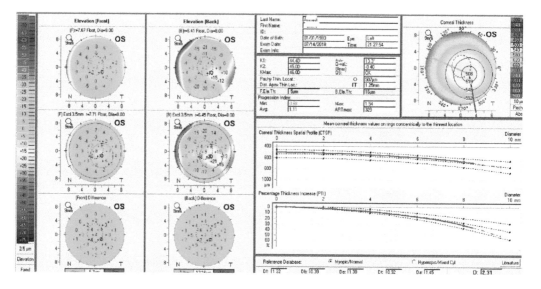

Figure 3.5 The Belin–Ambrósio enhanced ectasia display of Pentacam.

Table 3.3 Pachymetry Indices for Diagnosis of Normal, Keratoconus Suspect (SKC), and Definite Keratoconus (KC)[12]

	Normal	SKC	KC
Pachymetric Progression Index average (PPI-Ave)	<1.0	1.0–1.2	>1.2
Maximum Pachymetric Progression Index (PPI-Max)	<1.2	1.2–1.4	> 1.4
Ambrosio relational thickness average (ART-Ave)	>430	400–430	<400
Maximum Ambrósio relational thickness (ART-Max)	>340	300–340	< 300
Belin/Ambrosio enhanced ectasia total deviation value (BAD)	<1.6	1.6–2.6	> 2.6

green color indicates the normal state and the red color determines the pathological distribution. This map shows the index of the grade of disease using topographic keratoconus classification (TKC), Belin–Ambrósio (BAD), and the grade of the nuclear opacity using the Pentacam Nucleus Staging (PNS) classification (Figure 3.6).

Topometric KC Staging Map

The sagittal and tangential curvature of the radius and refractive power of the cornea are shown in this map. However, different elevation maps can be selected based on reference levels. True net power with respect to the posterior surface of the cornea, the four maps, and the comparative different examinations are specified in this map. The TKC display is used for the diagnosis of ectasia. All parameters related to KC classification are shown at a glance. KC indices and their normal/abnormal values are presented in Table 3.4 and Figure 3.7.

We evaluated 70 patients with clinical KC, 79 patients with subclinical KC, and 68 normal subjects, and found that Pentacam random forest index (PRFI) and index of height decentration(IHD) in KC eyes and inferior-superior (IS) difference value in SKC eyes had the highest diagnostic ability.[13] However, Huseynli et al.[14] showed that IHD and index of height asymmetry (IHA) were accurate items for KC detection,[15] even though IHD was more sensitive than BAD for diagnosing KC.

There are different management strategies for the treatment of KC. We have developed a simple and practical algorithm for the management of KC based on its progression (Figure 3.8).

Belin ABCD Progression Display

The new Belin ABCD progression display is based on the ABCD classification of KC by Professor Belin, MD, USA. This system uses four parameters to determine KC progression: anterior ("A") and posterior ("B") radius of curvature from a 3.0-mm optical zone centered on the thinnest point, "C"

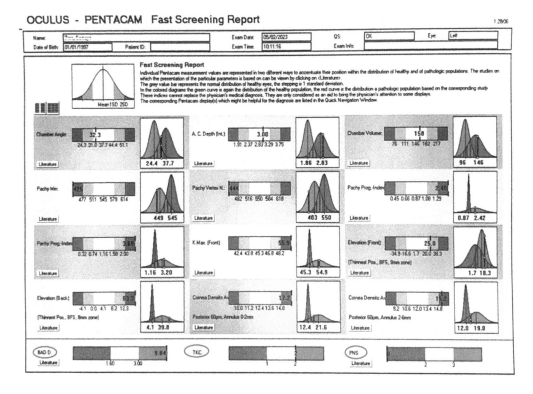

Figure 3.6 The fast report map of Pentacam.

Table 3.4 Keratoconus Screening Values[1,14]

Indices	Abnormal	Pathological
Topographic keratoconus classification (TKC)	≥ 1.00	≥2.00
Index of surface variance (ISV)	≥37	≥41
Index of vertical asymmetry (IVA)	≥0.28	≥0.32
Keratoconus index (KI)	-	>1.07
Central keratoconus index (CKI)	-	≥1.03
Minimum sagittal curvature (Rmin)	-	<6.71
Index of height asymmetry (IHA)	≥19	>21
Index of height decentration (IHD)	≥0.014	≥0.016
Inferior-superior difference (IS) value	1.4–1.9	>1.9
Keratoconus percentage index (KISA)	60%–100%	>100%

is the minimum corneal thickness, and "D" the best distance visual acuity with spectacles (Figure 3.9). The ABCD progression display represents each parameter graphically and uses color-coded maps to indicate the statistical changes in measurement.

The Zernike Maps

The wavefront parameters are derived from the height data of Pentacam using Zernike coefficient polynomials. These parameters are presented as lower-order (tilt and defocus) and higher-order (coma, trefoil), spherical aberration, higher- (fourth-) order astigmatism, four-lobed defects, higher- (fifth-) order coma, higher- (fifth-) order trefoil, five-lobed defect, higher- (sixth-) order spherical aberration, higher- (sixth-) order astigmatism, higher (sixth-) order four-lobed defect, six-lobed defect) aberrations (Figure 3.10). We found that front vertical coma (Z^3_{-1}) with 75% sensitivity, 100% specificity, and AUC = 0.857 had the highest accuracy for SKC detection compared with other Pentacam aberration parameters.[16]

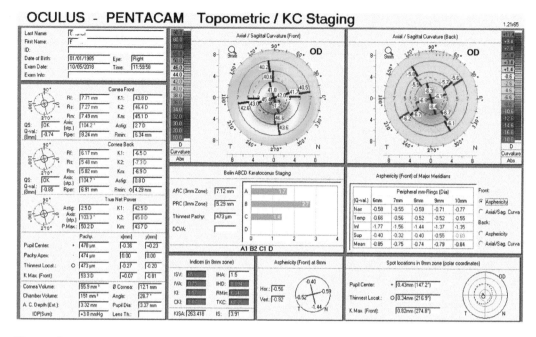

Figure 3.7   Topometric KC staging map of Pentacam.

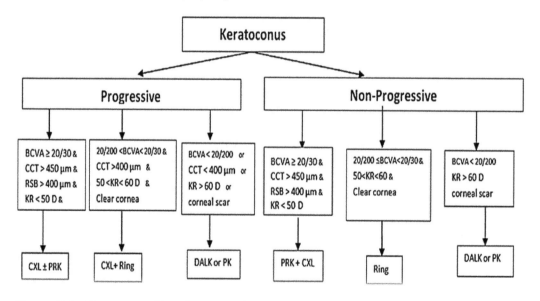

Figure 3.8   Keratoconus Classification and Surgical Management Algorithm.

Surgical algorithm for management of keratoconus. Age 25 years and in conjunction with corneal crosslinking (CXL).
BCVA: Best corrected visual acuity; CCT: Central corneal thickness; RSB: Residual stromal bed; KR:
Keratometry reading; D: Diopter; CXL: Cross-linking; PRK: Photorefractive keratectomy; DALK: Deep
anterior lamellar keratoplasty; PK: Penetrating keratoplasty.
Adapted from: Mohammadpour M, Heidari Z, Hashemi H. Updates on Managements for Keratoconus. J Curr
Ophthalmol, 2018. 30:110–124.[17]

■ **Sirius**

Sirius (Costruzione Strumenti Oftalmici, Florence, Italy) is a corneal tomographer with both
Placido and Scheimpflug technology and advanced neural network software (Phoenix). This
artificial intelligence-based software provides an accurate 3-dimensional (3D) evaluation of the
cornea on the anterior and posterior surfaces. The keratoconus screening report is presented on

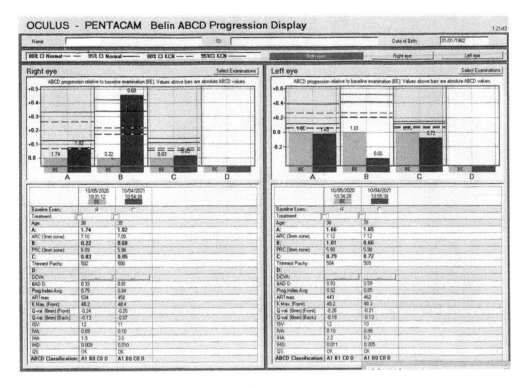

Figure 3.9   Belin ABCD progression map of Pentacam.

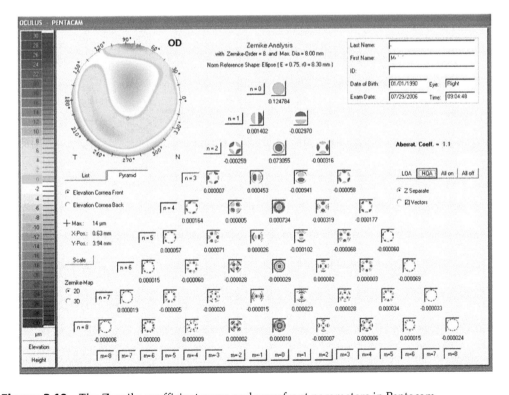

Figure 3.10   The Zernike coefficient maps and wavefront parameters in Pentacam.

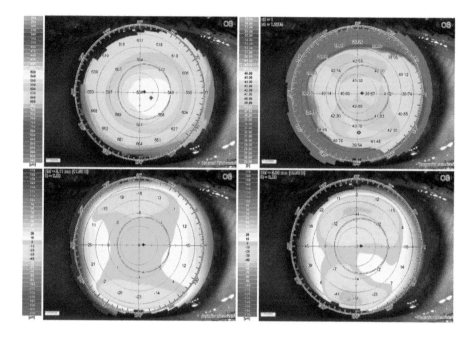

Acquisition quality		Coverage(SC.) = 99%		Not edited(SC.) = 100%	
		Coverage(P.) = 85%		Centration(P.) = 98%	

Summary indices	K readings	Shape indices	Refractive analysis
HVID = 12.96 mm	Sim-k: K1 = 40.98 D @ 177°	Anterior Ø=4.5mm: rf = 40.91 D Ax 171°	Ø=4.5mm: Cyl = -0.76 D Ax = 3°
+ Pupil (Topographic)	K2 = 42.00 D @ 87°	rs = 41.71 D	MPP = 41.12 D
x = 0.36 mm, y = 0.05 mm	Avg = 41.48 D	Q = 0.23	⚠ LSA = 1.44 D
Ø = 4.26 mm	Cyl = -1.03 D Ax 177°	RMS/A = 0.03 µm/mm²	
◈ Thinnest location	Anterior Ø=3mm: K1 = 40.66 D @ 179°	Posterior Ø=4.5mm: rf = -5.73 D Ax 165°	Keratoconus screening
x = 0.91 mm, y = -0.41 mm	K2 = 41.68 D @ 89°	rs = -6.08 D	SIf = 0.51 D
Thk = 528 µm	Avg = 41.16 D	Q = 0.09	⊞ KVf = 5 µm
✪ Apex	Cyl = -1.02 D Ax 179°	⚠ RMS/A=0.17µm/mm²	BCVf = 0.02 D @ 290°
x = 0.15 mm, y = -3.00 mm	Anterior Ø=5mm: K1 = 40.80 D @ 178°	Anterior Ø=8.0mm: rf = 40.81 D Ax 179°	⚠ SIb = 0.32 D
Curv = 43.97 D	K2 = 41.88 D @ 88°	rs = 42.11 D	◈ KVb = 21 µm
Anterior chamber	Avg = 41.34 D	Q = 0.08	⚠ BCVb = 0.84 D @ 306°
CCT + AD =	Cyl = -1.08 D Ax 178°	RMS/A = 0.04 µm/mm²	
0.534 + 3.02 = 3.55 mm	Anterior Ø=7mm: K1 = 40.83 D @ 178°	Posterior Ø=8.0mm: rf = -5.85 D Ax 171°	Thk = 528 µm
Volume = 168 mm³	K2 = 42.08 D @ 88°	rs = -6.14 D	Class:
Iridocorneal angle = 43°	Avg = 41.44 D	Q = -0.46	- Borderline - check parameters
HACD = 12.49 mm	Cyl = -1.25 D Ax 178°	RMS/A = 0.20 µm/mm²	
Corneal volume (Ø=10mm)			
Volume = 54.5 mm³			

Figure 3.11 Summary index map for a subclinical keratoconus case.

the keratoconus summary map. This map includes axial, elevation, and thickness maps along with summary indices.[18]

The Symmetry Index of the anterior curvature (SIf), the Symmetry Index of the posterior curvature (SIb), the highest point of ectasia on the anterior corneal surface (KVf), the highest point of ectasia on the anterior corneal surface (KVb), the Baiocchi–Calossi–Versaci at the front and back surfaces of the cornea (BCVf/b), and the thinnest point of the cornea (ThkMin) are important parameters for KC screening (Figure 3.11). In addition, horizontal visible iris diameter (HVID) size, topographic pupil size, thinnest point of the cornea, location and pachymetry of the thinnest point, location, pachymetry, and curvature of the steepest point of the cornea (apex), anterior chamber depth, and central corneal thickness with aqueous depth (CCT + AD) are shown in the summary index display. We found that KVb with AUC = 0.999 in the KC eyes and SIb with area under curve (AUC) = 0.908 in the SKC eyes had the best diagnostic ability,[13] whereas another study reported KVb with AUC = 0.970 had the highest discriminative ability for KC detection.[19]

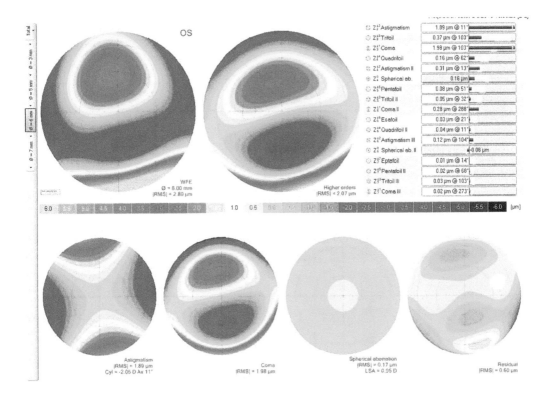

Z₁²Astigmatism	1.89 µm @ 11°	
Z₃³Trifoil	0.37 µm @ 103°	
Z₃¹Coma	1.98 µm @ 103°	
Z₄⁴Quadrifoil	0.16 µm @ 62°	
Z₄²Astigmatism II	0.31 µm @ 13°	
Z₄⁰Spherical ab.	0.16 µm	
Z₅⁵Pentafoil	0.08 µm @ 51°	
Z₅³Trifoil II	0.05 µm @ 32°	
Z₅¹Coma II	0.28 µm @ 288°	
Z₆⁶Esafoil	0.03 µm @ 21°	
Z₆⁴Quadrifoil II	0.04 µm @ 11°	
Z₆²Astigmatism III	0.12 µm @ 104°	
Z₆⁰Spherical ab. II	-0.06 µm	
Z₇⁷Eptafoil	0.01 µm @ 14°	
Z₇⁵Pentafoil II	0.02 µm @ 68°	
Z₇³Trifoil III	0.03 µm @ 103°	
Z₇¹Coma III	0.02 µm @ 273°	

Figure 3.12 Aberrometry map of Sirius.

Aberration Map

The analysis of corneal aberration is presented in the corneal aberrometric map. It displays wavefront parameters in anterior, posterior, or total aberrometry with different selectable pupil diameters (Figure 3.12). A comprehensive evaluation of the quality of vision is obtained by wavefront error (WFE) parameters. We found that BCVf in Sirius, with 87.7% sensitivity, 83% specificity, and AUC = 0.887 for SKCN, and front root mean square values per unit area (RMS/A), higher-order aberrations (HOAs), residual HOA, BCV, RMS trefoil, and RMS coma, with 100% sensitivity and specificity, had the highest accuracy for KC detection.[17]

Galilei

The Galilei (Ziemer Ophthalmic Systems AG, Port, Switzerland) is a dual Scheimpflug analyzer with two diagnostic methods, namely the Placido system for evaluating curvature data and the Scheimpflug system for accurate assessment of the elevation data. The combination of these systems improves imaging methods with a high evaluation of the central cornea based on 3D analysis. Galilei has two opposing Scheimpflug cameras, each rotating 180 degrees apart. Thus, the device captures slit images from opposite sides and the correlation of the dual views allows easy averaging of corresponding pachymetry values and elevation data in a short time. The refraction, keratoconus, and wavefront maps are important reports in the Galileo output.[20]

Refractive Map

The refractive map is the common report for the axial, elevation, and thickness of the cornea. Several indices, such as simulated keratometry (SimK) values, SimK steep, SimK flat, and steeper astigmatism with the angle from the anterior axial curvature map, K steep, K flat, and steeper astigmatism with the angle from the posterior axial curvature, total corneal power (TCP) by ray tracing, and eccentricity are presented in the refractive map (Figure 3.13). The cutoff values for central and steep TCP are reported as 45.55 µm and 46.29 µm, respectively.[21]

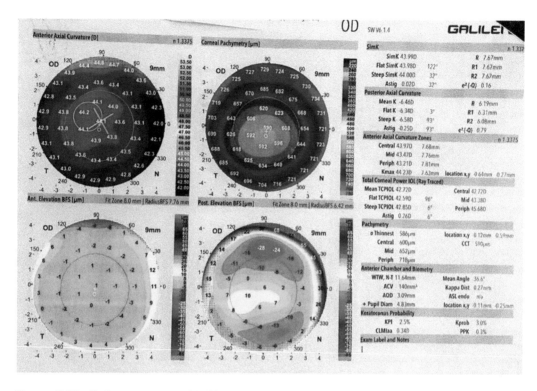

Figure 3.13 Refractive report of Galilei.

Keratoconus Report

The average corneal power difference is determined by the surface asymmetry index (SAI), with SAI greater than 0.50 being considered abnormal. The surface regularity index (SRI) indicates local irregularities of the cornea, and SRI less than 1.0 is a normal value. In spherical surfaces, SRI=0, and any irregularity in the cornea increases this index. The difference between inferior and superior hemispheres is determined by the inferior-superior (IS) index, with a IS greater than 1.4 D being suspicious of a KC cornea. The irregular astigmatism index (IAI) abnormal value is more than 0.50. The asymmetry of asphericity over the corneal surface is defined by the asphericity asymmetry index (AAI). The difference in corneal power between the central 3.0-mm diameter of the cornea and 3.0–6.0 mm around the center of the cornea is defined as the center/periphery index (CSI), and a CSI lower than 1.0 being accepted as a normal value. The differential sector index (DSI) refers to the amount of corneal asymmetry, and it increases in irregular astigmatism. The difference between two opposite 45° sectors is indicated in the opposite sector index (OSI). The cone location and magnitude index (CLMI), the keratoconus prediction index (KPI), and the percentage probability of keratoconus (PPK) are also important parameters for KC detection in Galilei. The abnormal values of these parameters are shown in Table 3.5.

Wavefront Map

The Galilei device automatically calculates spherical aberration, quatrefoil, secondary astigmatism, and total root mean square (RMS) for third-, fourth-, fifth-, sixth-, and total higher-order aberrations. Researchers were shown that several wavefront parameters in Galilei could detect the KC corneas; moreover, the RMS for third-order to sixth-order, and total higher-order RMS were significantly different between normal eyes and SKC eyes.[22]

ABERROMETRY

Aberration is the difference between the ideal image of refracted rays in a perfect optical system (Snell's Law) and what is truly obtained. These differences can affect the quality of the optical system and are related to monochromatic (not chromatic) aberrations. Low-order aberrations (LOA) consist of zero- to second-order aberrations, and the aberrations greater than third-order

Table 3.5 Accepted Abnormality Thresholds of Keratoconus Indices for Galilei[21]

Variables	Abnormal Values
Asphericity asymmetry index (AAI)	> 25
The center/surround index (CSI)	> 1.00
Differential sector index (DSI)	> 3.50
Irregular astigmatism index (IAI)	> 0.50
Inferior-superior difference (IS) value	> 1.4
Keratoconus prediction index (KPI)	> 30
Opposite sector index (OSI)	> 2.10
Percentage probability of keratoconus (PPK)	> 45
Deviation of Corneal Power (SDP)	> 2.00
Surface asymmetry index (SAI)	> 0.50

are referred to as HOAs. The modulation transfer function (MTF), point spread function (PSF), and root mean square (RMS) are important parameters to define aberrations and image quality. Aberrations can be measured with aberrometer devices using Zernike polynomials (C^n_m) based on the shape of the wavefront. Hartmann–Shack (HS) is an outgoing refractive aberrometry technique and is the most common aberrometer.

Retinal imaging aberrometry (Tscherning), incoming adjustable refractometry (Scheiner), combination of Scheimpflug and Placido, retinal ray tracing, and double pass aberrometry (Slit Skiascopy) are other types of aberrometer, with Zywave, Schwind Aberrometer, Sirius, iTrace, and OPD scan III are examples of the afore-mentioned aberrometers, respectively (Figure 3.14).

In the evaluation of the correlation between manifest and corneal astigmatism and HOAs in 375 eyes of 188 refractive surgery candidates, we found a positive significant correlation between the amount of astigmatism and HOAs.[23] In another study, we compared the accuracy of the aberration parameters in Scheimpflug, Placido, and HS aberrometer with Sirius, Pentacam, and OPD Scan III. We found corneal wavefront indices have acceptable validity for discrimination of normal corneas from SKC (AUC > 0.80) and KC (AUC = 1.00) eyes, and this can be very useful for screening purposes prior to refractive surgery.[17]

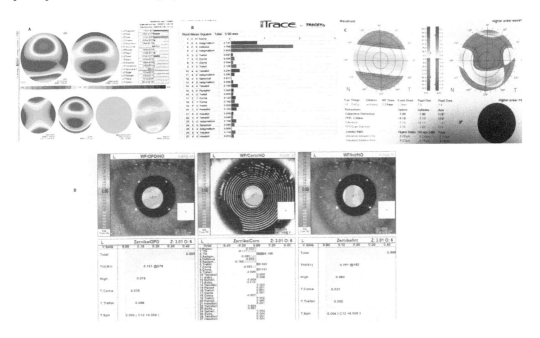

Figure 3.14 A) Sirius and B) iTrace (raytracing), C) Zywave, and D) OPD scan III (Slit Skiascopy) aberrometers.

BIOMECHANICS

Corneal biomechanics are related to the behavior of the biological structure of the cornea. The cornea requires enough flexibility to bulge out in an aspheric half-sphere, but it needs enough stiffness to hold its shape and resist the intraocular pressure (IOP). Due to the variation in collagen orientation and density, each layer of the cornea contributes to the overall biomechanical resistance to a different extent. However, the stroma, as the largest part of the cornea, is the main layer which defines the biomechanical properties of the cornea.

Like most biological tissues, the cornea has viscoelastic properties. Corneal elasticity refers to the static properties of a material and is derived from the tensile properties of the collagen microstructure. Viscosity refers to the deformation response of dynamic properties and is fully reversible with time. In a keratoconic cornea, degeneration of corneal extracellular matrix (ECM) components leads to a loss of collagen fibril orientation, weakness of the biomechanics, and cone-shaped corneal protrusion.

Ocular Response Analyzer (ORA) and Corvis ST are important non-contact tonometer tools that can assess biomechanical properties. Corneal hysteresis (CH), and corneal resistance factor (CRF) in ORA and dynamic corneal response (DCR) in Corvis ST, such as corneal length, time, and velocity applanation, deformation amplitude, deflection parameters, Ambrósio relational thickness to the horizontal profile (ARTh), stiffness parameter, and corneal biomechanical index (CBI), are important biomechanical parameters (Figure 3.15).

Today, Corvis ST integrated with Pentacam creates a new topographic and biomechanical index (TBI) (Figure 3.16). The CH and CRF parameters in ORA can be useful in differentiating KC from normal eyes. However, they may not be helpful for SKC diagnosing, which is a major concern of refractive surgeons.[24] Several studies have shown that the TBI in the Corvis is the most sensitive parameter for SKC and KC differentiation from the normal cornea.[13,25,26]

ANTERIOR SEGMENT OPTICAL COHERENCE TOMOGRAPHY

Optical coherence tomography (OCT) is a high-resolution cross-sectional corneal imaging process that was identified for anterior segment evaluation in 1994.[27] Anterior segment (AS)-OCT offers a longer wavelength (1050–1310 nm) than retinal OCT (800–900 nm) due to minimized scatter and greater penetration.[28] AS-OCT with an axial resolution of 1–5 is superior to ultrasound biomicroscopy with a resolution of 35–70 μm.[29]

AS-OCT can be classified into the time domain (TD) and spectral domain (SD)-OCT. The TD-OCT like Visante OCT (Carl Zeiss Meditec, Oberkochen, Germany) with a wavelength of

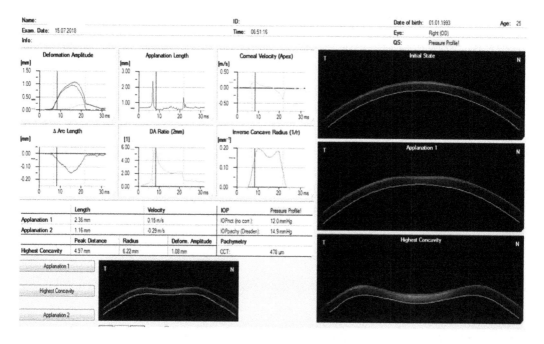

Figure 3.15 Dynamic corneal response parameters in Corvis ST.

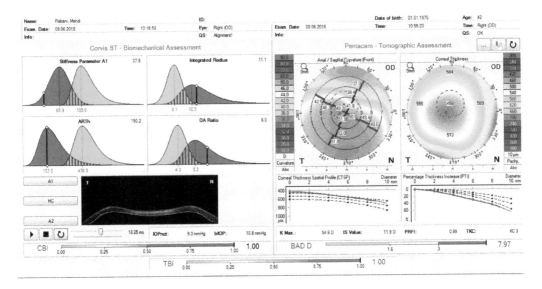

Figure 3.16 Topographic and biomechanical index developed by Corvis ST and Pentacam devices.

1310 nm, a 16-mm scan width, and a 6-mm scan depth for scanning the tissue plane limits the time taken of the reference mirror.[30] Otherwise, in SD-OCT, such as the Spectralis (Heidelberg Engineering GmbH, Heidelberg, Germany), RTVue (Optovue, Inc., Fremont, CA, USA), and Cirrus OCT (Carl Zeiss Meditec, Jena, Germany), taking the image is not limited and higher image acquisition also increases image resolution and reduces motion error.[31]

SD-OCT, such as RTVue, with a wavelength of 830 nm and a high axial resolution of 4–7 μm and a camera recording speed of 26,000 A-scans per second, is 13 times faster than the Visante.[32] MS-39 (Costruzione Strumenti Oftalmici, Florence, Italy) is an SD-OCT with 22 rings of Placido disk with an axial resolution of 3.5 nm that provides excellent tomography.[33] A new form of SD-OCT is the swept-source OCT, which uses a narrowband source to sweep across a wide optical bandwidth. DRI Triton swept-source OCT (Topcon, Tokyo, Japan), with an axial resolution of 5 μm, has a speed scan of 100,000 per second and 1050 nm wavelength.

There are several applications of AS-OCT for the diagnosis of corneal pathology, especially for the early detection of KC. Evaluation of several corneal layers with AS-OCT is extremely useful for the detection and management of anterior surface diseases. The assessment of epithelium and stromal layers is an important application of OCT for patients with KC; in these cases, the epithelial thickness increases and stromal thinning occurs at the corneal cone. AS-OCT can allow the comprehensive assessment of corneal thickness with epithelial and stromal thickness maps with several parameters: I–S (average difference between inferior corneal thickness and superior thickness); IT–SN (difference between inferotemporal thickness and superonasal thickness); minimum thickness; minimum-maximum thickness; and thinnest point of the cornea at the central 2 mm (Figure 3.17).

Studies have shown that monitoring the progression of KC by epithelial thickness mapping (ETM) can be very useful and valuable. In addition, early changes in corneal thickness that are not evident in topography have been identified in AS-OCT corneal maps.[34,35] Elkitkat et al. reported that MS-39 AS-OCT with AUC> 0.90 has a high accuracy for KC detection.[36] In the evaluation of the 45 mild KC, and 44 moderate-to-severe KC eyes, we found the inferior and IT sectors of the cornea are the most common thinning parts of the cornea in KC eyes.[37] Thinner central corneal thickness (CCT), lower min thickness, more negative min–max, min–med, and higher I–S and SN–IT were found in KC eyes compared with the control group ($P < 0.001$). CCT had the greatest diagnostic ability to differentiate between mild KC (AUC, sensitivity, and specificity: 0.822, 87.0%, 60.37%, respectively) and moderate-to-severe KC (0.902, 87.82%, 73.08%, respectively) from normal corneas. Similarly, Temset et al.[38] found form fruste keratoconus (FFKC) had a lower epithelial thickness in the thinnest corneal zone compared with normal corneas, and greater epithelial thickness in the thinnest corneal zone compared to keratoconic corneas ($P < .005$). They reported that epithelial thickness in the thinnest corneal point in forme fruste corneas was placed inferiorly

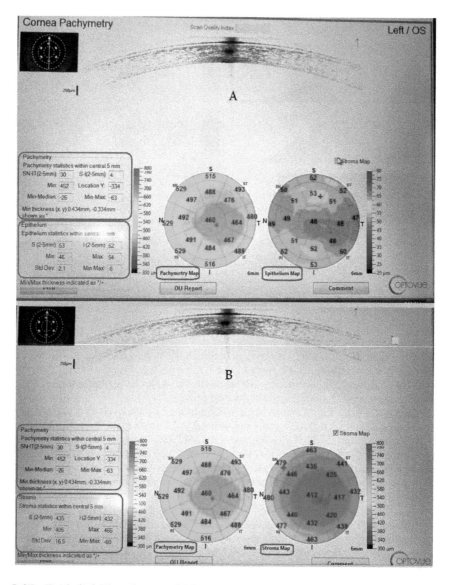

Figure 3.17 Epithelial (A) and stromal (B) maps with their associated parameters on AS-OCT in a case of subclinical keratoconus. Thinning of the stroma seems to be the main pathology for the development of keratoconus.

($P < 0.005$). Furthermore, I–S > 31 μm; IT–SN > 48 μm; min thickness < 492 μm; min–max thickness < −63 μm was reported by Li et al.[39] as the cutoff point for KC detection. In addition, stromal thickness compared to other corneal layers has a higher diagnostic ability to differentiate normal eyes from KC (sensitivity 81.7%, specificity 73.6%, AUC 0.871) and SKC (sensitivity 80.70, specificity 56.6%, AUC 0.751) eyes.[40] Thus, assessment of stromal thickness using AS-OCT may be useful for the early detection of KC (Figure 3.17).

ARTIFICIAL INTELLIGENCE

Artificial intelligence (AI) is a branch of computer science that imitates human behavior and plays crucial roles in clinical translation.[41] Artificial intelligence is classified into two modes including machine learning (ML) and deep learning (DL).[42] Today, teleophthalmology has been developed and has played an important role in maintaining visual acuity.[43] In the future, diagnostic methods based on AI methods can be a reliable tool for the diagnosis and management of anterior segment diseases in remote areas.[44]

Timely diagnosis and appropriate treatment are the important roles of artificial intelligence to prevent vision loss.[45] In the early stages of KC, routine clinical procedures can be time-consuming and lead to poor decision-making. Therefore, the early detection of subclinical KC by corneal indices that are generated based on AI algorithms can be done more accurately at the lowest cost.

The diagnostic accuracy of corneal imaging modalities based on AI models has been reported in various studies. Neural network models such as feed-forward neural networks, convolutional neural networks (CNN), support vector machine learning (SVM), multilayer perceptron (MLP), and decision tree classification (DT) have shown high accuracy in distinguishing KC eyes from normal eyes.[46] Various advanced corneal imaging systems with AI-based classifiers are available to detect corneas at risk of ectasia. CNN with six color-coded maps of AS-OCT had greater than 99% accuracy for KC detection.[47,48]

In Placido disc-based topography, such as OPD Scan III (Nidek Co. Ltd, Gamagori, Japan), there is a corneal navigator function based on neural network processing.[49] In Scheimpflug-based systems, such as Pentacam (Oculus Optikgeräte GmbH, Wetzlar, Germany), tomographic information from the rotating Scheimpflug camera is calculated from the anterior and posterior surfaces of the cornea. Belin–Ambrósio (BAD) and topographic keratoconus classification (TKC) are two

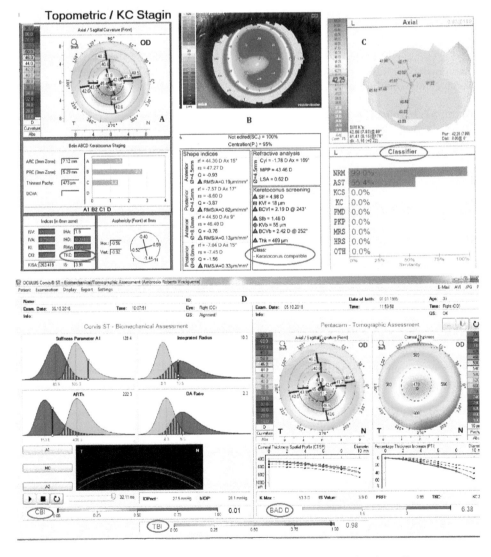

Figure 3.18 Tomographic and biomechanical indexes based on artificial intelligence in Pentacam (A), Sirius (B), OPD scan, and Corvis ST (D) devices.

Pentacam diagnostic indices derived from AI methods.[50] In combined systems of both the Placido and Scheimpflug technologies, such as Sirius (Costruzione Strumenti Oftalmici, Florence, Italy), Scheimpflug with Placido images in less than one second are analyzed with Phoenix software through a neural network process.[51] Some of the most important tomographic and biomechanical indices that developed from AI models are shown in Figure 3.18. In our study, 212 eyes were examined based on clinical findings by three independent expert ophthalmologists and classified into 92 normal eyes, 52 SKC eyes, and 68 KC eyes.[52] We found that the previously mentioned AI-based classifiers can be very useful for the diagnosis of KC, although they cannot replace clinical decision-making, especially before refractive surgery. We found that Phoenix had the highest agreement with the clinical expert with sensitivity, specificity, and κ of 84.62%, 90.0%, and 0.70, respectively, for SKC eyes and 80.02%, 96.60%, and 0.79, respectively, for KC eyes.

Recently, we conducted a comparative analysis of different corneal imaging modalities using AI models to diagnose KC, SKC, and FFKC.[53] Our systematic search across various scientific databases yielded valuable insights. Meta-analysis calculated pooled estimated accuracy (PEA) and the results showed that the Scheimpflug system (PEA: 92.25, 95% confidence interval (CI): 94.76–97.51) and a combination of Scheimpflug and Placido (PEA: 96.44, 95% CI: 93.13–98.19) exhibited the highest diagnostic accuracy for detecting SKC and FFKC, respectively. Moreover, simultaneous Scheimpflug and Placido corneal imaging demonstrated high diagnostic accuracy for the early detection of KC.

REFERENCES

1. Rabinowitz YS, Nesburn AB, McDonnell PJ. Videokeratography of the fellow eye in unilateral keratoconus. *Ophthalmology*. 1993;100:181–6.

2. Munir SZ, Munir WM, Albrecht J. Estimated prevalence of keratoconus in the United States from a large vision insurance database. *Eye Contact Lens*. 2021;47:505–10.

3. Hashemi H, Heydarian S, Yekta A, Ostadimoghaddam H, Aghamirsalim M, Derakhshan A, et al. High prevalence and familial aggregation of keratoconus in an Iranian rural population: a population-based study. *Ophthalmic Physiol Opt*. 2018;38:447–55.

4. Hwang S, Lim DH, Chung TY. Prevalence and incidence of keratoconus in South Korea: a Nationwide Population-based Study. *Am J Ophthalmol*. 2018;192:56–64.

5. Kristianslund O, Hagem AM, Thorsrud A, Drolsum L. Prevalence and incidence of keratoconus in Norway: a nationwide register study. *Acta Ophthalmol*. 2021;99:e694–e9.

6. Fan R, Chan TC, Prakash G, Jhanji V. Applications of corneal topography and tomography: a review. *Clin Exp Ophthalmol*. 2018;46:133–46.

7. Missotten L. Corneal topography. *Curr Opin Ophthalmol*. 1994;5:68–74.

8. Mohammadpour M, Heidari Z. Orbscan. In: Mohammadpour M (ed) *Diagnostics in ocular imaging*. Springer, Cham. 2021:23–63.

9. McAlinden C, Khadka J, Pesudovs K. A comprehensive evaluation of the precision (repeatability and reproducibility) of the Oculus Pentacam HR. *Invest Ophthalmol Vis Sci*. 2011;52:7731–7.

10. Meyer JJ, Gokul A, Vellara HR, Prime Z, McGhee CN. Repeatability and agreement of Orbscan II, Pentacam HR, and Galilei Tomography systems in Corneas with keratoconus. *Am J Ophthalmol*. 2017;175:122–8.

11. Hernández-Camarena JC, Chirinos-Saldaña P, Navas A, Ramirez-Miranda A, de la Mota A, Jimenez-Corona A, et al. Repeatability, reproducibility, and agreement between three different Scheimpflug systems in measuring corneal and anterior segment biometry. *J Refract Surg*. 2014;30:616–21.

12. Mohammadpour M, Heidari Z. Pentacam. In: Mohammadpour M (ed) *Diagnostics in ocular imaging*. Springer, Cham. 2021:65–162.

13. Heidari Z, Hashemi H, Mohammadpour M, Amanzadeh K, Fotouhi A. Evaluation of corneal topographic, tomographic and biomechanical indices for detecting clinical and subclinical keratoconus: a comprehensive three-device study. *Int J Ophthalmol*. 2021;14:228–39.

14. Huseynli S, Abdulaliyeva F. Evaluation of scheimpflug tomography parameters in sub-clinical keratoconus, clinical keratoconus and normal caucasian eyes. *Turk J Ophthalmol*. 2018;48:99–108.

15. Kovács I, Miháltz K, Kránitz K, Juhász É, Takács Á, Dienes L, et al. Accuracy of machine learning classifiers using bilateral data from a Scheimpflug camera for identifying eyes with preclinical signs of keratoconus. *J Cataract Refract Surg*. 2016;42:275–83.

16. Heidari Z, Mohammadpour M, Hashemi H, Jafarzadehpur E, Moghaddasi A, Yaseri M, et al. Early diagnosis of subclinical keratoconus by wavefront parameters using Scheimpflug, Placido and Hartmann-Shack based devices. *Int Ophthalmol*. 2020;40:1659–71.

17. Mohammadpour M, Heidari Z, Hashemi H. Updates on managements for keratoconus. *J Curr Ophthalmol*. 2018;30:110–24.

18. Mohammadpour M, Heidari Z. SIRIUS® In: Mohammadpour M (ed) *Diagnostics in ocular imaging*. Springer, Cham. 2021:183–264.

19. Vega-Estrada A, Alio JL. Keratoconus corneal posterior surface characterization according to the degree of visual limitation. *Cornea*. 2019;38:730–6.

20. Feizi S. Galilei dual scheimpflug analyzer. In: Mohammadpour M (ed) *Diagnostics in ocular imaging*. Springer, Cham. 2021:163–82.

21. Moshirfar M, Motlagh MN, Murri MS, Momeni-Moghaddam H, Ronquillo YC, Hoopes PC. Galilei corneal tomography for screening of refractive surgery candidates: a review of the literature, part II. *Med Hypothesis Discov Innov Ophthalmol*. 2019;8:204.

22. Reddy JC, Rapuano CJ, Cater JR, Suri K, Nagra PK, Hammersmith KM. Comparative evaluation of dual Scheimpflug imaging parameters in keratoconus, early keratoconus, and normal eyes. *J Cataract Refract Surg*. 2014;40:582–92.

23. Mohammadpour M, Heidari Z, Mohammad-Rabei H, Jafarzadehpur E, Jabbarvand M, Hashemi H, et al. Correlation of higher order aberrations and components of astigmatism in myopic refractive surgery candidates. *J Curr Ophthalmol*. 2016;28:112–6.

24. Mohammadpour M, Etesami I, Yavari Z, Naderan M, Abdollahinia F, Jabbarvand M. Ocular response analyzer parameters in healthy, keratoconus suspect and manifest keratoconus eyes. *Oman J Ophthalmol*. 2015;8:102–6.

25. Ambrósio Jr R, Lopes BT, Faria-Correia F, Salomão MQ, Bühren J, Roberts CJ, et al. Integration of scheimpflug-based corneal tomography and biomechanical assessments for enhancing ectasia detection. *J Refract Surg*. 2017;33:434–43.

26. Steinberg J, Siebert M, Katz T, Frings A, Mehlan J, Druchkiv V, et al. Tomographic and bio-mechanical scheimpflug imaging for keratoconus characterization: a validation of current indices. *J Refract Surg*. 2018;34:840–7.

27. Izatt JA, Hee MR, Swanson EA, Lin CP, Huang D, Schuman JS, et al. Micrometer-scale resolution imaging of the anterior eye in vivo with optical coherence tomography. *Arch Ophthal*. 1994;112:1584–9.

28. Lim SH. Clinical applications of anterior segment optical coherence tomography. *J Ophthalmol.* 2015;2015:605729.

29. Smith SD, Singh K, Lin SC, Chen PP, Chen TC, Francis BA, et al. Evaluation of the anterior chamber angle in glaucoma: a report by the American Academy of Ophthalmology. *Ophthalmology.* 2013;120:1985–97.

30. Ramos JL, Li Y, Huang D. Clinical and research applications of anterior segment optical coherence tomography: a review. *Clin Exp Ophthalmol.* 2009;37:81–9.

31. Bald M, Li Y, Huang D. Anterior chamber angle evaluation with fourier-domain optical coherence tomography. *J Ophthalmol.* 2012;2012:103704.

32. Kiernan DF, Mieler WF, Hariprasad SM. Spectral-domain optical coherence tomography: a comparison of modern high-resolution retinal imaging systems. *Am J Ophthalmol.* 2010;149:18–31.

33. Mohammadpour M, Heidari Z. MS-39® In: Mohammadpour M (ed) *Diagnostics in ocular imaging.* Springer, Cham. 2021:265–84.

34. de Toledo MC, Gonçalves BV. Corneal epithelial thickness mapping in keratoconus. In: Almodin E, Nassaralla BA, Sandes J, (eds) *Keratoconus: a comprehensive guide to diagnosis and treatment.* Springer, Cham. 2022:979–87.

35. Serrao S, Lombardo G, Calì C, Lombardo M. Role of corneal epithelial thickness mapping in the evaluation of keratoconus. *Cont Lens Anterior Eye.* 2019;42:662–5.

36. Elkitkat RS, Rifay Y, Gharieb HM, Ziada HEA. Accuracy of the indices of MS-39 anterior segment optical coherence tomography in the diagnosis of keratoconic corneas. *Eur J Ophthalmol.* 2022;32:2116–24.

37. Hashemi H, Heidari Z, Mohammadpour M, Momeni-Moghaddam H, Khabazkhoob M. Distribution pattern of total corneal thickness in keratoconus versus normal eyes using an optical coherence tomography. *J Curr Ophthalmol.* 2022;34:216–22.

38. Temstet C, Sandali O, Bouheraoua N, Hamiche T, Galan A, El Sanharawi M, et al. Corneal epithelial thickness mapping using Fourier-domain optical coherence tomography for detection of form fruste keratoconus. *J Cataract Refract Surg.* 2015;41:812–20.

39. Li Y, Meisler DM, Tang M, Lu AT, Thakrar V, Reiser BJ, et al. Keratoconus diagnosis with optical coherence tomography pachymetry mapping. *Ophthalmology.* 2008;115:2159–66.

40. Heidari Z, Mohammadpour M, Hajizadeh F, Fotouhi A, Hashemi H. Corneal layer thickness in keratoconus using optical coherence tomography. *Clin Exp Optom.* 2024;107:32–39.

41. Rampat R, Deshmukh R, Chen X, Ting DSW, Said DG, Dua HS, et al. Artificial intelligence in cornea, refractive surgery, and cataract: basic principles, clinical applications, and future directions. *Asia Pac J Ophthalmol (Phila).* 2021;10:268–81.

42. Sidey-Gibbons JAM, Sidey-Gibbons CJ. Machine learning in medicine: a practical introduction. *BMC Med Res Methodol.* 2019;19:64.

43. Mohammadpour M, Heidari Z, Mirghorbani M, Hashemi H. Smartphones, tele-ophthalmology, and VISION 2020. *Int J Ophthalmol.* 2017;10:1909–18.

44. Heidari Z, Baharinia M, Ebrahimi-Besheli K, Ahmadi H. A review of artificial intelligence applications in anterior segment ocular diseases. *Med Hypothesis Discov Innov Optom.* 2022;3:22–33.

45. Balyen L, Peto T. Promising artificial intelligence-machine learning-deep learning algorithms in ophthalmology. *Asia Pac J Ophthalmol (Phila)*. 2019;8:264–72.

46. Ting DSJ, Foo VH, Yang LWY, Sia JT, Ang M, Lin H, et al. Artificial intelligence for anterior segment diseases: emerging applications in ophthalmology. *Br J Ophthalmol*. 2021;105:158–68.

47. Kamiya K, Ayatsuka Y, Kato Y, Fujimura F, Takahashi M, Shoji N, et al. Keratoconus detection using deep learning of colour-coded maps with anterior segment optical coherence tomography: a diagnostic accuracy study. *BMJ Open*. 2019;9:e031313.

48. Lavric A, Valentin P. KeratoDetect: keratoconus detection algorithm using convolutional neural networks. *Comput Intell Neurosci*. 2019;2019:8162567.

49. Klyce SD, Karon MD, Smolek MK. Screening patients with the corneal navigator. *J Refract Surg*. 2005;21:617–22.

50. Belin MW, Khachikian SS. Keratoconus/ectasia detection with the oculus pentacam: Belin/Ambrósio enhanced ectasia display. *Highlights Ophthalmol*. 2007;35:5–12.

51. Belin MW, Villavicencio OF, Ambrósio RR, Jr. Tomographic parameters for the detection of keratoconus: suggestions for screening and treatment parameters. *Eye Contact Lens*. 2014;40:326–30.

52. Mohammadpour M, Heidari Z, Hashemi H, Yaseri M, Fotouhi A. Comparison of artificial intelligence-based machine learning classifiers for early detection of keratoconus. *Eur J Ophthalmol*. 2022;32:1352–60.

53. Hashemi H, Doroodgar F, Niazi S, Khabazkhoob M, Heidari Z. Comparison of different corneal imaging modalities using artificial intelligence for diagnosis of keratoconus: a systematic review and meta-analysis. *Graefes Arch Clin Exp Ophthalmol*. 2024;262(4):1017–39.

4 Role of Artificial Intelligence in Detecting Keratoconus and Assessing Ectasia Risk before Laser Vision Correction

Aydano P Machado and Renato Ambrósio Jr.

INTRODUCTION

The emergence of artificial intelligence has brought about significant advancements in technology and society. Machines can now perform tasks and solve problems that were once exclusive to humans, marking the beginning of a new era that we are privileged to be a part of.

One of the areas which has been most receptive to artificial intelligence and machine learning algorithms is healthcare. Nowadays, it is not easy to find a health professional who has yet to hear about these terms or attend a conference where they are not discussed in numerous speeches and presentations.

When it comes to discussing keratoconus, the same scenario arises.

ARTIFICIAL INTELLIGENCE AND MACHINE LEARNING

Artificial intelligence (AI) is a branch of computer Science encompassing a range of computational processes which would be considered intelligent if performed by a human being. The concept is broad and receives as many definitions as the different meanings of the word "intelligence".

The discussion regarding the intelligence of machines has been ongoing ever since modern computers came into existence. In 1950, Alan Turing wrote an article entitled "Computing Machine and Intelligence" and introduced his widely known test.[1]

In 1956, Dartmouth College hosted a conference, led by John McCarthy, that brought together esteemed researchers such as Minsky, McCarthy, Newell, and Simon to study what they called Artificial Intelligence. AI is an expression used to designate a type of intelligence built by man to endow machines with intelligent behavior.

Several efforts have been made to simulate and perform intelligent behaviors on computers through AI techniques. Because of different understandings of intelligence, researchers have historically pursued many versions of AI. To facilitate comprehension, Russell and Norvig[2] have classified the explanations of AI in literature into four categories. This was done based on two viewpoints: *human* vs. *purely rational* and *thought* vs. *behavior*. Therefore, there are four potential goals or perspectives regarding AI: behaving like a human, thinking like a human, behaving rationally, and thinking rationally.

Most AI solutions for the health domain focus on behaving like humans, and some must act rationally as their central core. After several years of researching, working, and giving classes in the AI domain, mainly applying it to health and ophthalmology, instead of forcing a definition, I prefer to understand AI as a field of study that aims to endow the machine with the ability to _____. And you can freely fill in the space however you like, or even introduce the human word into the definition if you want to bring it closer to the human context. For example, providing the machine with the human ability to speak, write, read, see, paint, recognize an object, make decisions, drive, etc.

Following this perspective, what has gained prominence in recent years is to endow the machine with the ability to learn and, given its importance, this has become a sub-area of AI called machine learning (ML). This area of research aims to study and develop computational methods to obtain systems capable of automatically acquiring knowledge. The main challenge of machine learning algorithms is to maximize the generalization ability of its learner.

In the field of machine learning, learning involves enhancing performance through experience. This means that machines are not simply programmed to perform a task but are designed to endlessly improve their performance by optimization through repetition in performing that task.

This can be useful in two situations: when a task is so complex that we do not know how to build an algorithm to solve it or when the machine needs to adapt to each case or work in a dynamic situation. Preparing the machine to find its own algorithm and adapt to environmental changes would be better.

There are three main categories of machine learning algorithms.[2] These categories play a significant role in determining the problems that machine learning can address. They are supervised learning, unsupervised learning, and reinforcement learning.

DOI: 10.1201/9781003371601-4

Supervised learning is applied in predictive tasks. In this scenario, machine learning algorithms utilize labeled training datasets to create a predictive model. For future instances, the model can then predict a target attribute's value based on its features' importance, which consists of paired inputs and outputs (e.g., an eye tomography correctly labeled as "keratoconus"). The goal is to discover a universal formula or rules to associate new data inputs with the appropriate outcomes. Supervised learning is typically utilized for classification or regression issues. When forecasting or assessing detached and unordered results, such as keratoconus or normal eyes, this is seen as a classification problem. When attempting to predict or estimate a numerical index for keratoconus stage or ectasia susceptibility, this can be addressed as a regression problem.

For each type of problem in machine learning, there are various algorithms available that can be used. One such algorithm for supervised learning is artificial neural networks (ANNs), which were developed in the 1950s and mimic the behavior of biological neurons. A new type of neural network, called deep learning, has emerged as a significant subfield of machine learning. With today's advanced computational power, deep learning constructs intricate ANNs with multiple layers of neurons. The first layers of the neural network extract features, which human engineers previously carried out. The most significant aspect of deep learning is that these features are learned from data using a general-purpose learning procedure instead of relying on instructions from human engineers.[3]

Unsupervised learning is a type of machine learning that deals with unlabeled data, meaning that there are no input–output pairs. Instead, computers are tasked with finding patterns and structures within the data. Clustering is a common task performed by unsupervised learning algorithms, where inputs are grouped based on their similarities or differences. For instance, one might want to cluster keratoconus eyes based on their topography or tomography examinations to understand how phenotype profiles are expressed. Unlike supervised learning, no predetermined grouping exists, and different algorithms or similarity measures can yield different results.

Reinforcement learning is a type of learning that involves trial and error. An agent, or computer program, is instructed to achieve a goal in a dynamic environment. The program learns how to act to maximize the rewards it receives from the environment. Reinforcement learning has been successfully used in game-playing and robotic control. For instance, this machine-learning algorithm can be used to train robots to assist in intrastromal ring implant surgery.

Understanding these primary categories of problems helps us comprehend the different types and techniques of machine learning and how they can be applied in our daily lives.

ROLE OF PHYSICIANS IN AI SOLUTION DEVELOPMENT USING MACHINE LEARNING

Even though AI allows machines to learn and perform activities they are not explicitly programmed for, they still require programming. Despite the mystical tone sometimes associated with machine learning, it results from a lot of programming and human work that creates a structure capable of extracting, representing, and storing knowledge from experience.

The constant advances in information technology have enabled the storage of the most diverse types of experience in large and multiple databases, and these are generally the sources for the process of automatic knowledge discovery. This process comes with theories and tools, and it is classically known as knowledge discovery in databases (KDD), the nontrivial, interactive, and iterative process of identifying valid, novel, potentially useful, and ultimately understandable patterns in data.[4]

The concept of KDD involves various significant steps, including data preparation (selection, cleaning, enrichment, and transformation), pattern search (machine learning algorithm), knowledge evaluation, and refinement. These steps are repeated in multiple iterations, as shown in Figure 4.1.[4]

When the KDD definition says "nontrivial," it refers to a scenario requiring a search or inference process. It is not simply a matter of calculating predefined quantities, such as finding the average value of a set of numbers. At this stage, the presence of a domain specialist is crucial. The physician should be involved right from the start of the KDD process, comprehending and directing the entire process alongside the knowledge engineer or machine learning specialist.

The user's role in driving KDD applications is vital, as it helps to extract valuable, innovative, practical, engaging, and understandable patterns. In a KDD process, the user plays a crucial role in accurately formulating the objectives and selecting the appropriate data pre-processing methods to produce applicable models for clinical practice.

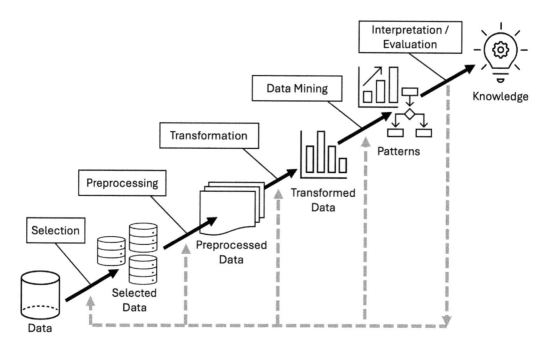

Figure 4.1   An overview of the steps that compose the KDD process.

ROLE OF AI IN KERATOCONUS AND ECTATIC DISEASES

Given the characteristics and usefulness of artificial intelligence and machine learning presented in the previous section, it is easy to imagine its application as a support tool in diagnosing, managing, and treating keratoconus.

This is already occurring, as demonstrated by various publications and works released in recent years.[5] The level of scientific production has advanced significantly, resulting in the availability of articles that offer comprehensive summaries, presentations, and valuable comparisons of research findings.[6,7]

The following subsections will present some of these works.

Role of AI in Keratoconus and Topography

The pioneering work on utilizing AI and neural networks for keratoconus detection via videokeratography with Placido disks was documented in 1995 by Maeda, Klyce, and Smolek.[8] Human experts classified corneal topography into seven categories: normal, with-the-rule astigmatism, keratoconus (mild, moderate, advanced), post-photorefractive keratectomy, and post-keratoplasty. A trained neural network accurately classified all 108 maps in the training sample and 80% of the maps in the test set. The accuracy and specificity for each category exceeded 90%, while sensitivity ranged from 44% to 100%. The model was helpful in automated pattern interpretation for corneal topography.

In 1997, Smolek and Klyce[9] demonstrated a neural network classification for detecting keratoconus (KC) and keratoconus suspects (KCS) using TMS-1 examinations (Tomey). The network also graded the severity of cone-like topography patterns consistent with KC or KCS.

More recently, using a convolutional neural network (CNN), the KeratoDetect algorithm accurately detects keratoconus in the test set with an impressive 99.33% accuracy rate by analyzing corneal topography.[10]

Role of AI in Keratoconus and Tomography

Corneal tomography, including pachymetric mapping and posterior surface evaluation through 3D corneal characterization, is crucial for understanding corneal structure. However, interpreting the available parameters can be highly challenging. That's where machine learning techniques, such as pattern recognition, come in. They can help process large amounts of data, especially in cases of fruste keratoconus, where keratoconus is only evident in one eye but not the other. This is known as VAE-NT (normal topography in very asymmetric ectasia).[11] The detection of VAE-NT was accomplished by authors utilizing various AI methods.

Saad and Gatinel[11] described a linear discriminant-based model, for instance, combined topographic and tomographic indices, resulting in an Area Under the Receiver Operating Characteristic curve (AUROC) of 0.98, coupled with a 93% sensitivity, 92% specificity, and 92% accuracy in differentiating VAE-NT from normal cases.

In 2018, Lopes et al.[12] successfully utilized AI and tomographic data to enhance the detection of corneal ectasia susceptibility. Their random forest machine-learning algorithm, PRFI, was trained to achieve a remarkable sensitivity of 85.2% and a specificity of 96.6% in identifying normal topographic eyes in highly asymmetrical cases (VAE-NT) while only considering the independent test set. The previous best tomographic index, BAD-D, had only a 55.3% accuracy in classifying post-LASIK ectasia, while PRFI had an 80% accuracy.

Kovács et al.[13] used neural networks and bilateral patient data to approach the VAE-NT detection problem two years earlier. They achieved an AUC of 0.96, with a sensitivity of 92% and specificity of 85%, similar to that obtained with the PRFI (AUC=0.968).

In 2022, Almeida et al.[14] developed the Boosted Ectasia Susceptibility Tomography Index (BESTi) using multiple logistic regression analysis. The dataset included 187 eyes with very asymmetric ectasia and typical corneal topography and tomography (VAE-NTT) in the VAE-NTT group, 2296 eyes with healthy corneas in the control group (CG), and 410 eyes with ectasia in the ectasia group. BESTi achieved an AUC of 0.91, with 86.02% sensitivity and 83.97% specificity when used in groups CG and VAE-NTT.

Although accuracy has improved, more research is needed to better understand the corneal structure, including the epithelial thickness data seen in segmental tomography. Additionally, analyzing the biomechanical status of the cornea could add significant value.[11,14]

Role of AI in Keratoconus and Biomechanics

AI has been used to detect keratoconus by analyzing corneal biomechanics. The first study to utilize AI, machine learning, and corneal biomechanics in keratoconus detection was published by Machado et al. in 2011.[15] This study was followed by Ventura et al., who released an article utilizing machine learning and an ocular response analyzer (ORA) to improve the accuracy of detecting keratoconus grades I and II.[16]

A 2015 paper combines image processing, AI, and biomechanics to analyze corneal vibration parameters. The study includes 493 normal eyes and 279 eyes with keratoconus. The CART algorithm achieved 98% specificity, 85% sensitivity, and 92% accuracy.[17]

A significant milestone in the study of corneal biomechanics was achieved with the development of the Corvis Biomechanical Index (CBI) by Vinciguerra et al. (2016).[18] The index is calculated using a logistic regression equation based on Corvis biomechanical parameters, including the Ambrósio Relational Thickness for the horizontal meridian (ARTh), which measures corneal thickness. The CBI presented results for normal eyes and keratoconus: AUC 0.983, accuracy 98.2%, specificity 100%, and sensitivity 94.1%.

Mercer et al. (2017) proposed a logistic regression model based exclusively on Corvis biomechanical parameters to differentiate between keratoconus and normal eyes. The model achieved a sensitivity of 92.9%, specificity of 95.7%, accuracy of 94.4%, and AUC of 98.5.[19] The same year, Vinciguerra et al. studied 12 subclinical keratoconus cases without topographic or tomographic changes and found abnormalities in biomechanics.[20]

In 2019, Leão et al. used image processing and machine learning to evaluate the effect of intraocular pressure on Corvi's images. They proposed a new classification method based on biomechanical information, using 195 normal eyes and 136 eyes with keratoconus. The improved approach achieved an AUC of 0.960 in distinguishing the two groups.[21]

Role of AI in Keratoconus Treatment

AI and machine learning algorithms predicted asphericity and mean keratometry following Ferrara ICRS (Intra Corneal Rings Segments) implantation in patients with keratoconus. This was the first study to use predictive models based on machine learning and corneal tomography data. The study found that using machine learning models improved predictability and reduced errors in post-operative asphericity and mean keratometry for keratoconus patients who received intrastromal corneal ring segments compared to the reference nomogram.[22]

ROLE OF AI IN KERATOCONUS AND MULTIMODAL ANALYSIS

Artificial intelligence also shows its role when the complexity of the task is increased by having data and information from different sources, and the multimodal analysis needs to be performed by a specialist.

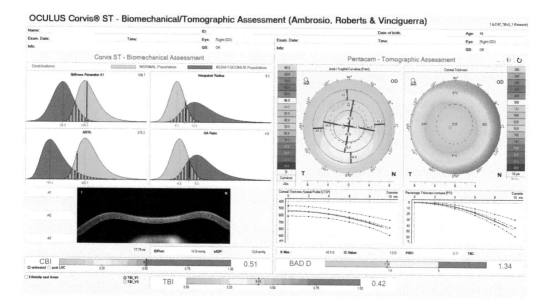

Figure 4.2 Tomographic-biomechanical display of a patient with CBI, BAD-D, and TBI indexes.

The Tomographic and Biomechanical Index (TBI), published by Ambrósio et al., took this path.[23] TBI uses the machine-learning random forest algorithm with leave-one-out cross-validation (RF/LOOCV) to create a predictive model that combines tomographic and biomechanical information. This study utilized a dataset containing 480 normal eyes, 204 eyes with keratoconus, 72 cases of

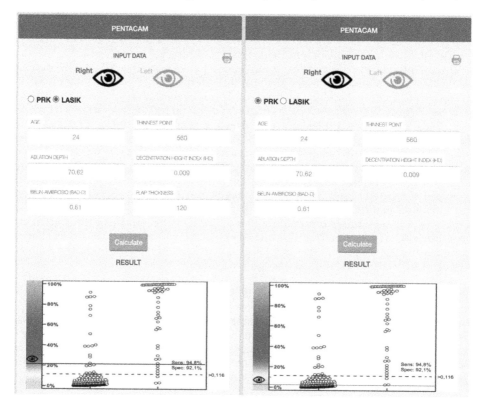

Figure 4.3 BrAIN Cornea model calculating ectasia susceptibility in a single patient's eye using LASIK and PRK procedures.

Very Asymmetric Ectasia (VAE-E), and 94 cases of Very Asymmetric Ectasia with normal topography (VAE-NT). When considering all four groups, the classification performance metrics were: AUC of 0.996, accuracy of 97.5%, specificity of 98.8%, and sensitivity of 96.2%, with a cutoff point of 0.48. These results were compared to BAD-D (AUC of 0.956) and CBI (AUC of 0.936) and showed improved performance. These indices can be viewed on the Tomographic-Biomechanical Display shown in Figure 4.2, and a new version of this index called BrAIN-TBI or TBIv2 was developed.[24]

In addition, to accurately detect ectatic or susceptible cases and assess ectasia risk before laser vision correction, it is essential to integrate data that resemble the biomechanical impact of the clinical information.[25]

In 2016, the group BrAIN (Brazilian Artificial Intelligence Network in Medicine) developed a predictive model using the machine-learning algorithm RBF neural network to integrate clinical data (age), type of surgery (PRK/LASIK), ablation depth, central corneal thickness, and tomography (BAD-D and IHD). This support tool helps select candidates for refractive surgery by considering a sample of 2,980 stable post-LASIK eyes and 65 ectasia cases. It correlates clinical, tomographic, and surgical data to determine ectasia susceptibility and is freely accessible at brain-cornea.com.[26] The utilization of this concept is shown in Figure 4.3.

CONCLUSION

There is a growing interest in applying artificial intelligence to medicine and ophthalmology. However, implementing these studies into clinical practice is progressing rather slowly. An essential aspect of creating useful tools for clinical practice is the participation of physicians in defining objectives and all stages of the knowledge discovery process, starting with understanding artificial intelligence and machine learning. It would be wise for us to actively participate in driving during the trip rather than solely relying on being passengers in the backseat.

REFERENCES

1. Turing AM. I.—Computing machinery and intelligence. *Mind*. 1950 Oct 1;LIX(236):433–60.

2. Russell SJ, Norvig P. *Artificial intelligence: a modern approach*. Fourth edition. Hoboken: Pearson; 2021. (Pearson series in artificial intelligence).

3. LeCun Y, Bengio Y, Hinton G. Deep learning. *Nature*. 2015 May 28;521(7553):436–44.

4. Fayyad U, Piatetsky-Shapiro G, Smyth P. From data mining to knowledge discovery in databases. *AIMag*. 1996 Mar 15;17(3):37.

5. Grzybowski A, editor. Artificial intelligence in ophthalmology [Internet]. Springer, Cham. International Publishing; 2021 [cited 2023 Aug 13]. Available from: https://link.springer.com /10.1007/978-3-030-78601-4

6. Mohammadpour M, Heidari Z, Hashemi H, Yaseri M, Fotouhi A. Comparison of artificial intelligence-based machine learning classifiers for early detection of keratoconus. *Euro J Ophthalmol*. 2022 May;32(3):1352–60.

7. Heidari Z, Mohammadpour M, Amanzadeh K, Fotouhi A. Evaluation of corneal topographic, tomographic and biomechanical indices for detecting clinical and subclinical keratoconus: a comprehensive three-device study. *Int J Ophthalmol*. 2021 Feb 18;14(2):228–39.

8. Maeda N, Klyce SD, Smolek MK. Neural network classification of corneal topography. Preliminary demonstration. *Invest Ophthalmol Vis Sci*. 1995 Jun;36(7):1327–35.

9. Smolek MK, Klyce SD. Current keratoconus detection methods compared with a neural network approach. *Invest Ophthalmol Vis Sci*. 1997 Oct;38(11):2290–9.

10. Lavric A, Valentin P. KeratoDetect: Keratoconus detection algorithm using convolutional neural networks. *Comput Intell Neurosci*. 2019;2019:8162567.

11. Saad A, Gatinel D. Topographic and tomographic properties of forme fruste keratoconus corneas. *Invest Ophthalmol Vis Sci.* 2010 Nov 1;51(11):5546.

12. Lopes BT, Ramos IC, Salomão MQ, Guerra FP, Schallhorn SC, Schallhorn JM, Vinciguerra R, Vinciguerra P, Price FW, Price MO, Reinstein DZ, Archer TJ, Belin MW, Machado AP, Ambrósio R. Enhanced tomographic assessment to detect corneal ectasia based on artificial intelligence. *Am J Ophthalmol.* 2018 Nov;195:223–32.

13. Kovács I, Miháltz K, Kránitz K, Juhász É, Takács Á, Dienes L, Gergely R, Nagy ZZ. Accuracy of machine learning classifiers using bilateral data from a Scheimpflug camera for identifying eyes with preclinical signs of keratoconus. *Journal of Cataract and Refractive Surgery.* 2016 Feb;42(2):275–83.

14. Almeida Jr GC, Guido RC, Balarin Silva HM, Brandão CC, de Mattos LC, Lopes BT, Machado AP, Ambrósio R. New artificial intelligence index based on Scheimpflug corneal tomography to distinguish subclinical keratoconus from healthy corneas. *J Cataract Refract Surg.* 2022 Oct;48(10):1168–74.

15. Machado AP, Lyra JM, Ambrósio R, Ribeiro G, Araújo LPN, Xavier C, Costa E. Comparing machine-learning classifiers in keratoconus diagnosis from ORA examinations. In: Peleg M, Lavrač N, Combi C, editors. *Artificial Intelligence in Medicine* [Internet]. Berlin, Heidelberg: Springer Berlin Heidelberg; 2011 [cited 2021 Mar 18]. p. 90–5. (Lecture Notes in Computer Science; vol. 6747). Available from: http://link.springer.com/10.1007/978-3-642-22218-4_12

16. Ventura BV, Machado AP, Ambrósio R, Ribeiro G, Araújo LN, Luz A, Lyra JM. Analysis of waveform-derived ORA parameters in early forms of keratoconus and normal corneas. *J Refract Surg.* 2013 Sep;29(9):637–43.

17. Koprowski R, Ambrósio R. Quantitative assessment of corneal vibrations during intraocular pressure measurement with the air-puff method in patients with keratoconus. *Comput Biol Med.* 2015 Nov;66:170–8.

18. Vinciguerra R, Ambrósio R, Elsheikh A, Roberts CJ, Lopes B, Morenghi E, Azzolini C, Vinciguerra P. Detection of keratoconus with a new biomechanical index. *J Refract Surg.* 2016 Dec 1;32(12):803–10.

19. Mercer RN, Waring GO, Roberts CJ, Jhanji V, Wang Y, Filho JS, Hemings RA, Rocha KM. Comparison of corneal deformation parameters in keratoconic and normal eyes using a non-contact tonometer with a dynamic ultra-high-speed scheimpflug camera. *J Refract Surg.* 2017 Sep;33(9):625–31.

20. Vinciguerra R, Ambrósio R, Roberts CJ, Azzolini C, Vinciguerra P. Biomechanical characterization of subclinical keratoconus without topographic or tomographic abnormalities. *J Refract Surg.* 2017 Jun;33(6):399–407.

21. Leão E, Ing Ren T, Lyra JM, Machado A, Koprowski R, Lopes B, Vinciguerra R, Vinciguerra P, Roberts CJ, Elsheikh A, Krysik K, Ambrósio R. Corneal deformation amplitude analysis for keratoconus detection through compensation for intraocular pressure and integration with horizontal thickness profile. *Comput Bio Med.* 2019 Jun;109:263–71.

22. Lyra D, Ribeiro G, Torquetti L, Ferrara P, Machado A, Lyra JM. Computational models for optimization of the intrastromal corneal ring choice in patients with keratoconus using corneal tomography data. *J Refract Surg.* 2018 Aug 1;34(8):547–50.

23. Ambrósio R, Lopes BT, Faria-Correia F, Salomão MQ, Bühren J, Roberts CJ, Elsheikh A, Vinciguerra R, Vinciguerra P. Integration of scheimpflug-based corneal tomography and biomechanical assessments for enhancing ectasia detection. *J Refract Surg.* 2017 Jul 1;33(7):434–43.

24. Ambrósio R, Machado AP, Leão E, Lyra JMG, Salomão MQ, Esporcatte LGP, Filho JBR da F, Ferreira-Meneses E, Sena NB, Haddad JS, Neto AC, Castelo de Almeida G, Roberts CJ, Elsheikh A, Vinciguerra R, Vinciguerra P, Bühren J, Kohnen T, Kezirian GM, Hafezi F, Hafezi NL, Torres-Netto EA, Lu N, Kang DSY, Kermani O, Koh S, Padmanabhan P, Taneri S, Trattler W, Gualdi L, Salgado-Borges J, Faria-Correia F, Flockerzi E, Seitz B, Jhanji V, Chan TCY, Baptista PM, Reinstein DZ, Archer TJ, Rocha KM, Waring GO, Krueger RR, Dupps WJ, Khoramnia R, Hashemi H, Asgari S, Momeni-Moghaddam H, Zarei-Ghanavati S, Shetty R, Khamar P, Belin MW, Lopes B. Optimized artificial intelligence for enhanced ectasia detection using Scheimpflug-based corneal tomography and biomechanical data. *Am J Ophthalmol.* 2022 Dec;S0002939422005062.

25. Ambrósio Jr R, Ramos I, Lopes B, Canedo ALC, Correa R, Guerra F, Luz A, Price Jr FW, Price MO, Schallhor S, Belin MW. Assessing ectasia susceptibility prior to LASIK: the role of age and residual stromal bed (RSB) in conjunction to Belin-Ambrósio deviation index (BAD-D). *Revista Brasileira de Oftalmologia* [Internet]. 2014 [cited 2021 Feb 18];73(2). Available from: http://www.gnresearch.org/doi/10.5935/0034-7280.20140018

26. Data Integration: Key to Improving Decision-Making in Refractive Surgery Screening [Internet]. ASCRS; (Refractive/Cornea Surgery - Runner-Up). Available from: http://ascrs2017.conferencefilms.com/acover.wcs?entryid=0178&bp=1

5 Oxidative Stress in Keratoconus

Parisa Abdi and Mehdi Aminizadeh

OXIDATIVE STRESS

Free radicals are by-products of normal cellular processes and are a mandatory component in normal physiological activities. These oxidants include reactive oxygen species (ROS) and reactive nitrogen species (RNS).[1,2] In the normal redox state, ROS are involved in cellular growth and proliferation, signal transduction, gene expression, immune defence mechanisms, and apoptosis.[3–5] Mitochondria is the major source of endogenous ROS through an oxidative phosphorylation chain which takes place in the inner membrane. Other endogenous sources include peroxisomes and microsomes, NADPH oxidase, cytochrome P450, xanthine oxidase, and nitric oxide synthase (NOS). ROS and RNS may also be produced exogenously after exposure to ultraviolet (UV) and ionizing radiation, and chemical agents. In the presence of iron, hydroxide and hydroxyl radicals are produced through Fenton and Haber–Weiss reactions.[6–8]

During normal homeostasis, antioxidant mechanisms reduce ROS and RNS burden and create an equilibrium between oxidant and antioxidant agents. When this balance is demolished and the oxidative burden is increased, free radicals violate their normally limited functions and start to damage intra- and extracellular components, causing so-called oxidative stress. Oxidative stress can be described by the oxidative stress index (OSI), which is the ratio between total oxidative status and total antioxidative status. OSI increases under oxidative stress.[9,10] Oxidative stress, which specifically occurs in age-related conditions, causes lipid peroxidation of membranes, oxidative alteration in proteins, and also oxidative damage to DNA.[11] Accumulation of these injuries is known to be a pathophysiological factor in certain conditions, such as cataract, uveitis, retinopathy of prematurity, age-related macular degeneration, and primary open-angle glaucoma.[12–20]

OXIDATIVE STRESS IN CORNEA

In normal healthy cornea oxidants and antioxidants create a physiological balance. During the oxidative stress, the level of ROS increases which, in turn, induces inflammatory cytokines. These cytokines trigger production and activation of proteolytic enzymes, such as metalloproteinases, which degrade corneal stroma and cause increased light absorption and corneal hydration.[21–24]

Cornea, as the outermost layer of the globe, is constantly exposed to UV radiation. Shorter wavelength UV (295–320 nm), so-called UV-B, is predominantly absorbed by the cornea. UV-A, with longer wavelength (320–400 nm), is also absorbed by the cornea, albeit to a lower extent.[6,25] This exposure puts the cornea at risk of increased oxidative stress by inducing free radicals such as peroxidic aldehydes produced during UV-induced lipid peroxidation.[1] In normal cornea, both tissue components (especially corneal epithelium) and detoxifying molecules are present to prevent UV-associated increased oxidative stress. Ascorbic acid (vitamin C) and α-tocopherol (vitamin E) serve as low-molecular-weight ROS scavengers in the cornea. In addition to these molecules, the cornea possesses antioxidant enzymes, such as superoxide dismutase (detoxifying the superoxide radical), catalase and glutathione peroxidase (both detoxifying hydrogen peroxide), and aldehyde dehydrogenase (detoxifying peroxidic aldehydes).[26–31]

Oxidative stress is a known factor in the pathophysiology of some corneal diseases such as dry eye disease, keratoconus, pinguecula and pterygia, Fuchs' endothelial corneal dystrophy, and bullous keratopathy.[6,21,32–37]

OXIDATIVE STRESS IN PATHOPHYSIOLOGY OF KERATOCONUS

Keratoconus is an ectatic disorder in which progressive thinning of the corneal stroma causes conical alteration to the corneal structure. These changes lead to irregular astigmatism, myopia, and subsequent decreased vision. Both eyes are affected in keratoconus but disease severity is often more prominent in one eye. Histopathological hallmarks of keratoconus consist of corneal stromal thinning, breaks in Bowman's layer, and iron deposition in the basal layers of the corneal epithelium.[38]

Keratoconus was classically known as a non-inflammatory disease. However, this belief has been criticized after the detection of inflammatory cytokines (IL-1, IL-6, TNF-α, and TGF-β),

DOI: 10.1201/9781003371601-5

metalloproteinases (e.g., MMP-2 and MMP-9).[39] Several factors have been proposed to be involved in the pathogenesis of keratoconus. Similar to other multifactorial diseases, it is difficult to explain the pathophysiology of the disease clearly. Environmental factors, such as eye rubbing, atopy, and contact lens use, and genetic predisposition are underlying factors. Oxidative stress as a central pathophysiological mechanism is involved in all of the mentioned underlying factors.[40–45] It has been shown that oxidative stress is increased in cases of keratoconus. Oxidative stress markers are increased in the tear film, aqueous humour, cornea, and the blood of keratoconus patients.[46] ROS and RNS are significantly increased in these patients. Some of the increased oxidative stress markers include malondialdehyde (MDA), lactate, pyruvate, citrate, and nicotinamide adenine dinucleotide (NAD). On the other hand, total antioxidant capacity is decreased compared with healthy controls, which, in turn, causes greater disturbance of the oxidative balance and escalation of oxidative stress. Superoxide dismutase (SOD), glutathione (GSH), aldehyde (ALDH) and NADPH dehydrogenase, lactoferrin, transferrin, albumin, selenium, and zinc are among antioxidant markers.[39]

Disruption in redox homeostasis in tears, cornea, aqueous humour, and even the systemic blood circulation of keratoconic patients has been shown. Elevation of oxidative stress markers is more distinct in the tears and the cornea than in the aqueous humour. On the other hand, antioxidants are decreased in tears, aqueous humour, and blood. With more attention being paid to different layers of the cornea in patients with keratoconus, an increase in free radicals is more obvious in stromal cells and a decrease in antioxidants is more evident in endothelial cells.[39] *In vitro* production of ROS and RNS is increased in keratoconus fibroblasts, when compared with normal fibroblasts.[47] At the site of breaks of the Bowman's layer, endothelial nitric oxide synthase (eNOS) level is revealed to be elevated. This signifies that the production of nitric oxide (NO) is increased in this area of the cornea. NO and peroxynitrite, in turn, are involved in multiple adverse effects including DNA damage, enhancement of apoptotic pathways, and degradation of tissue inhibitors of matrix metalloproteinases (TIMP).[48–50] Mitochondrial DNA damage has also been witnessed in keratoconic corneas. DNA damage in mitochondria, which are the site of the oxidative phosphorylation chain and ATP production, can increase cellular free radicals and decrease the cell's ability to confront this enhanced oxidative burden.[51–53]

Disruption of local redox homeostasis of the cornea and increased OSI may lead to degradation and modification of the extracellular matrix in the stroma of a keratoconic cornea, further pushing it towards thinning and ectasia. Keratoconus corneas have decreased levels of TIMP-1, which is a major inhibitor of metalloproteinases 2 (MMP-2) and also an inhibitor of apoptosis of certain cell types. MMPs are a class of proteolytic enzymes responsible for degradation of components of extracellular matrix. Activities of cathepsins, which can induce degradation of collagen and proteoglycans through induction of hydrogen peroxide production, are shown to be elevated in keratoconus corneas. Decreased levels of TIMP-1 in keratoconic corneas and increased MMPs and cathepsins accompanied by lysosomal membrane damage and the release of its proteolytic enzymes during oxidative stress contribute to thinning of the stroma and development of ectasia.[1,50,54,55]

REDUCTION OF OXIDATIVE STRESS IN KERATOCONUS

Antioxidant agents, such as 4-coumaric acid, trehalose (a disaccharide), and hyaluronic acid, are shown to protect normal corneas against free radicals after UV-B radiation.[56–60] Vitamins C and D are two major antioxidants of the human body. Vitamin D is secreted into aqueous humour and tear film and can then be transported into the cornea where it can be activated after UV exposure. A role of vitamin D deficiency in the pathogenesis of keratoconus has been shown. Vitamin C is the major antioxidant of the cornea and plays important roles in collagen synthesis and wound healing.[61–63] Although the antioxidant capacities of vitamin C and vitamin D are known, using these two molecules and other known antioxidants as oral or topical supplementations in keratoconus patients has yet to be investigated. There are ongoing clinical trials in progress to address this issue.

Eye rubbing is a widely known risk factor for the development and progression of keratoconus. One of the suggested mechanisms for this matter is that eye rubbing induces inflammatory mediators such as ILs and MMPs. This gives rise to accumulation of ROS, cellular damage, keratocyte apoptosis, and reduced corneal rigidity.[64–67] Therefore, one way to reduce corneal oxidative stress in keratoconus patients is the prohibition of eye rubbing.

REFERENCES

1. Wojcik K, Kaminska A, Blasiak J, Szaflik J, et al. Oxidative stress in the pathogenesis of keratoconus and fuchs endothelial corneal dystrophy. *Int J Mol Sci.* 2013 Sep; 14(9):19294–19308.

2. Karamichos D, Hutcheon AEK, Rich CB, Trinkaus-Randall V, et al. In vitro model suggests oxidative stress involved in keratoconus disease. *Sci Rep.* 2014;4:4608.

3. Dröge W. Free radicals in the physiological control of cell function. *Physiol Rev.* 2002;82:47–95.

4. Finkel T, Holbrook NJ. Oxidants, oxidative stress and the biology of ageing. *Nature* 2000;408:239–247.

5. Birben E, Sahiner UM, Sackesen C, Erzurum S, et al. Oxidative stress and antioxidant defense. *World Allergy Organ J.* 2012;5:9–19.

6. Cejka C, Cejkova J. Oxidative stress to the cornea, changes in corneal optical properties, and advances in treatment of corneal oxidative injuries. *Oxid Med Cell Longev.* 2015;2015:591530.

7. Wilkinson-Berka JL, Rana I, Armani R, Agrotis A, Reactive oxygen species, Nox and angiotensin II in angiogenesis: implications for retinopathy. *Clinl Sci.* 2013;124(10):597–615.

8. Kohen R, Nyska A. Oxidation of biological systems: oxidative stress phenomena, antioxidants, redox reactions, and methods for their quantification. *Toxicol Pathol.* 2002;30:620–650.

9. Toprak I, Kucukatay V, Yildirim C, Kilic-Toprak E. Increased systemic oxidative stress in patients with keratoconus. *Eye (Lond).* 2014 Mar;28(3):285–289.

10. Harma M, Harma M, Erel O. Increased oxidative stress in patients with hydatidiform mole. *Swiss Med Wkly* 2003;133:563–566.

11. Wakamatsu TH, Dogru M, Ayakoetal I. Evaluationoflipid oxidative stress status and inflammation in topic ocular surface disease. *Molecular Vision.* 2010;19(16):2465–2475.

12. Spector A. Oxidative stress-induced cataract: mechanism of action. *FASEB J.* 1995;9(12):1173–1182.

13. Yadav UCS, Kalariya NM, Ramana KV. Emerging role of antioxidants in the protection of uveitis complications. *Curr Med Chem.* 2011;18(6):931–942.

14. Ishimoto SI, Wu GS, Hayashi S, Zhang J, et al. Free radical tissue damages in the anterior segment of the eye in experimental autoimmune uveitis. *Invest Ophthalmol Vis Sci.* 1996;37(4):630–636.

15. Gritz D. C, Montes C, Atalla L. R, Wu G S, et al. Histochemical localization of superoxide production in experimental autoimmune uveitis. *Curr Eye Res.* 1991;10(10):927–931.

16. Niesman MR, Johnson KA, Penn JS. Therapeutic effect of liposomal superoxide dismutase in an animal model of retinopathy of prematurity. *Neurochem Res.* 1997;22(5):597–605.

17. Chiras D, Kitsos G, Petersen MB, Skalidakis I, et al. Oxidative stress in dry age-related macular degen- eration and exfoliation syndrome. *Crit Rev Clin Lab Sci.* 2005;52(1):12–27.

18. Ammar DA, Hamweyah KM, Kahook MY. Antioxidants protect trabecular meshwork cells fromhydrogen peroxide-induced cell death. *Transl Vis Sci Technol.* 2012;1(1):4–8.

19. Aslan M, Dogan S, Kucuksayan E. Oxidative stress and potential applications of free radical scavengers in glaucoma. *Redox Rep.* 2013;18(2):76–87.

20. Pinazo-Durán MD, Zanon-Moreno V, Garcia-Medina JJ, Gallego-Pinazo R. Evaluation of presumptive biomarkers of oxidative stress, immune response and apoptosis in primary open-angle glaucoma. *Curr Opin Pharmacol.* 2013;13(1):98–107.

21. Buddi R, Lin B, Atilano SR, Zorapapel NC, et al. Evidence of oxidative stress in human corneal diseases. *J Histochem Cytochem.* 2002;50(3):341–351.

22. Cejkova JC, Ardan T, Cejka C, Kovaceva J, et al. Irradiation of the rabbit cornea with UVB rays stimulates the expression of nitric oxide synthase-generated nitric oxide and the formation of cytotoxic nitrogen-related oxidants. *Histol Histopathol.* 2005;20(2):467–473.

23. Cejkova JC, Tıpek SS, Crkovskaetal J. UV rays, the prooxidant / antioxidant imbalance in the cornea and oxidative eye damage. *Physiol Res.* 2004;53(1):1–10.

24. Zhou T, Zong R, Zhangetal Z. SERPINA3Kprotectsagainst oxidative stress via modulating ROS generation/degradation and KEAP1-NRF2 pathway in the corneal epithelium. *Invest Ophthalmol Vis Sci.* 2012;53(8):5033–5043.

25. Eaton JW. UV-mediated cataractogenesis: a radical perspective. *Doc Ophthalmol.* 1994;88(3):233–242.

26. Ringvold A. The significance of ascorbate in the aqueous humour protection against UV-A and UV-B. *Exp Eye Res.* 1996;62(3):261–264.

27. Ringvold A. In vitro evidence for UV-protection of the eye by the corneal epithelium mediated by the cytoplasmic protein, RNA, and ascorbate. *Acta Ophthalmol Scand.* 1997;75(5):496–498.

28. Brubaker RF, Bourne WM, Bachman LA, McLaren JW. Ascorbic acid content of human corneal epithelium. *Invest Ophthalmol Vis Sci.* 2000;41(7):1681–1683.

29. Bilgihan A, Bilgihan K, Toklu Y, Konuk O, et al. Ascorbic acid levels in human tears after photorefractive keratectomy, transepithelial photorefractive keratectomy, and laser in situ keratomileusis. *J Cataract Refract Surg.* 2001;27(4):585–588.

30. Bilgihan A, Bilgihan K, Yis O, Sezer C, et al. Effects of topical vitamin E on corneal superoxide dismutase, glutathione peroxidase activities and polymorphonuclear leucocyte infiltration after photorefractive kerate- ctomy. *Acta Ophthalmol Scand.* 2003;81(2):177–180.

31. Atalla LR, Sevanian A, Rao NA. Immunohistochemical localization of glutathione peroxidase in ocular tissue. *Curr Eye Res.* 1988;7(10):1023–1027.

32. Alio JL, Ayala MJ, Mulet ME, Artola A, et al. Antioxidant therapy in the treatment of experimental acute corneal inflammation. *Ophthal Res.* 1995;27(3):136–143.

33. Augustin AJ, Spitznas M, Kaviani N, Meller D, et al. Oxidative reactions in the tear fluid of patients suffering from dry eyes. *Graefe's Arch Clin Exp Ophthalmol.* 1995;233(11):694–698.

34. Cejkova J, Ardan T, Simonovaetal Z. Nitricoxidesynthase induction and cytotoxic nitrogen-related oxidant formation in conjunctival epithelium of dry eye (Sjögren's syndrome). *Nitric Oxide—Biol Chem.* 2007;17(1):10–17.

35. Cejkova J, Ardan T, Simonovaetal Z. Decreased expression of antioxidant enzymes in the conjunctival epithelium of dry eye (Sjögren's syndrome) and its possible contribution to the development of ocular surface oxidative injuries. *Histol Histopathol.* 2008;23(12):1477–1483.

36. Cejkova JC, Ardan T, Cejka C, Melec J, et al. Ocular surface injuries in autoimmune dry eye. The severity of microscopical disturbances goes parallel with the severity of symptoms of dryness. *Histol Histopathol.* 2009;24(10):1357–1365.

37. Arnal E, Peris-Martinez C, Menezo JL, Johnsen-Soriano S, et al. Oxidative stress in keratoconus? *Invest Ophthalmol Vis Sci*. 2011;52(12):8592–8597.

38. Rabinowitz YS. Keratoconus. *Surv Ophthalmol*. 1998;42:297–319.

39. Nave V, Malecaze J, Pereira B, Baker JS, et al. Oxidative and antioxidative stress markers in keratoconus: a systematic review and meta-analysis. *Acta Ophthalmol*. 2021;99(6):e777-e794.

40. Romero-Jiménez M, Santodomingo-Rubido J, Wolffsohn JS. Keratoconus: a review. *Cont. Lens Anterior Eye*. 2010;33:157–166.

41. Kim WJ, Rabinowitz YS, Meisler DM, Wilson SE. Keratocyte apoptosis associated with keratoconus. *Exp Eye Res*. 1999;69:475–481.

42. Ahmadi Hosseini SM, Mohidin N, Abolbashari F, Mohd-Ali B, et al. Corneal thickness and volume in subclinical and clinical keratoconus. *Int Ophthalmol*. 2013;33;139–145.

43. Sherwin T, Brookes NH, Morphological changes in keratoconus: pathology or pathogenesis. *Clin Exp Ophthalmol*. 2004;32:211–217.

44. Burdon KP, Vincent AL. Insights into keratoconus from a genetic perspective. *Clin Exp Optom*. 2013;96:146–154.

45. Edwards M, McGhee CN, Dean S. The genetics of keratoconus. *Clin Exp Ophthalmol*. 2001;29:345–351.

46. Zarei-Ghanavati S, Yahaghi B, Hassanzadeh S, Ghayour-Mobarhan M, et al. Serum 25-hydroxyvitamin D, selenium, zinc and copper in patients with keratoconus. *J Curr Ophthalmol*. 2019;32:26–31.

47. Chwa M, Atilano SR, Reddy V, Jordan N, et al. Increased stress-induced generation of reactive oxygen species and apoptosis in human keratoconus fibroblasts. *Invest Ophthalmol Vis Sci*. 2006;47:1902–1910.

48. Buddi R, Lin B, Atilano SR, Zorapapel NC, et al. Evidence of oxidative stress in human corneal diseases. *J Histochem Cytochem*. 2002;50:341–351.

49. Squadrito GL, Pryor WA. Oxidative chemistry of nitric oxide: the roles of superoxide, peroxynitrite, and carbon dioxide. *Free Radic Biol Med*. 1998;25:392–403.

50. Brown DJ, Lin B, Chwa M, Atilano SR, et al. Elements of the nitric oxide pathway can degrade TIMP-1 and increase gelatinase activity. *Mol Vis*. 2004;10:281–288.

51. Atilano SR, Coskun P, Chwa M, Jordan N, et al. Accumulation of mitochondrial DNA damage in keratoconus corneas. *Invest Ophthalmol Vis Sci*. 2005;46:1256–1263.

52. De Grey ADNJ. An introduction to mitochondria. history of the mitochondrial free radical theory of aging, 1954–1995. In *the Mitochondrial Free Radical Theory of Aging*; R.G. Landes Company: Austin, TX, USA, 1999; pp. 20–30, 66–69.

53. Cui H, Kong Y, Zhang H. Oxidative stress, mitochondrial dysfunction, and aging. *J Signal Transduct*. 2012;2012:646354.

54. Collier SA. Is the corneal degradation in keratoconus caused by matrix-metalloproteinases? *Clin Exp Ophthalmol*. 2001;29:340–344.

55. Kenney MC, Chwa M, Atilano SR, Tran A, et al. Increased levels of catalase and cathepsin V/L2 but decreased TIMP-1 in keratoconus corneas: evidence that oxidative stress plays a role in this disorder. *Invest Ophthalmol Vis Sci*. 2005;46:823–832.

56. Cejkova J, Cejka C, Ardan T, Sirc J, et al. Reduced UVB-induced corneal damage caused by reactive oxygen and nitrogen species and decreased changes in corneal optics after trehalose treatment. *Histol Histopathol*. 2010;25(11):1403–1416.

57. Cejkova J, Ardan T, Cejka C, Luyckx J. Favorable effects of trehalose on the development of UVB-mediated antioxidant/pro-oxidant imbalance in the corneal epithelium, proinflammatory cytokine and matrix metalloproteinase induction, and heat shock protein 70 expression. *Graefe's Arch Clin Exp Ophthalmol*. 2011;249(8):1185–1194.

58. Cejkova J, Cejka C, Luyckx J. Trehalose treatment accelerates the healing of UVB-irradiated corneas. Comparative immunohistochemical studies on corneal cryostat sections and corneal impression cytology. *Histol Histopathol*. 2012;27(8):1029–1040.

59. Pauloin T, Dutot M, Joly F, Warnet JM, et al. High molecular weight hyaluronan decreases UVB-induced apop- tosis and inflammation in human epithelial corneal cells. *Mol Vis*. 2009;15:577–583.

60. Li JM, Chou HC, Wang SH. Wu CL, et al. Hyaluronic acid- dependent protection against UVB-damaged human corneal cells. *Environ Mol Mutagen*. 2003;54(6):429–449.

61. Lasagni Vitar RM, Bonelli F, Rama P, Ferrari G. Nutritional and metabolic imbalance in keratoconus. *Nutrients*. 2022;14(4):913.

62. Wimalawansa SJ. Vitamin D deficiency: effects on oxidative stress, epigenetics, gene regulation, and aging. *Biology*. 2019;8:30.

63. Saijyothi AV, Fowjana J, Madhumathi S, Rajeshwari M, et al. Tear fluid small molecular antioxidants profiling shows lowered glutathione in keratoconus. *Exp Eye Res*. 2012;103:41–46.

64. Ben-Eli H, Erdinest N, Solomon A. Pathogenesis and complications of chronic eye rubbing in ocular allergy. *Curr Opin Allergy Clin Immunol*. 2019;19(5):526–534.

65. di Martino E, Ali M, Inglehearn CF. Matrix metalloproteinases in keratoconus - too much of a good thing? *Exp Eye Res*. 2019;182:137–143.

66. McMonnies CW. Mechanisms of rubbing-related corneal trauma in keratoconus. *Cornea*. 2009;28:607–615.

67. Bral N, Termote K. Unilateral keratoconus after chronic eye rubbing by the nondominant hand. *Case Rep Ophthalmol*. 2017;8:558–561.

6 Epithelial Thickness Mapping for Keratoconus Screening by VHF Digital Ultrasound or Anterior Segment OCT

Dan Z. Reinstein and Timothy J. Archer

INTRODUCTION

- Epithelial thickness maps provide a greater sensitivity and specificity in the detection of keratoconus than topography and tomography alone

- Epithelial thickness maps may help *identify* keratoconus in patients that have an otherwise **normal** topography/tomography

- Epithelial thickness maps can be used to help *rule out* keratoconus in some patients with **equivocal** topography/tomography

- Epithelial thickness maps are also essential for evaluating complex corneas in the assessment and therapeutic planning of refractive surgery

- Epithelial thickness map are becoming the gold standard in corneal laser refractive surgery for detecting or excluding keratoconus

Keratoconus screening is the most important safety factor in corneal refractive surgery. It is important to obtain a full clinical picture of the patient including demographic, diagnostic, and examination data. The chapter describes technologies available for detecting early keratoconus. This includes quantitative parameters that are independent of those now obtained by topographic and tomographic analysis, such as corneal epithelial and stromal thickness profiles that may represent such an independent parameter. The differences in epithelial thickness profile between the normal population and the keratoconic population may help to discriminate between normal eyes and keratoconus suspect eyes. Epithelial thickness mapping can exclude the appropriate patients by detecting keratoconus earlier or confirming keratoconus in cases where topographic changes may be clinically judged as being within normal limits. Epithelial maps may also be useful in excluding a diagnosis of keratoconus despite suspect topography. The behaviour of the epithelium in normal and suspect eyes is the main focus of the chapter. With advancements in keratoconus screening to include topography to tomography and now epithelium, we are seeing a shift in the standard of care and we are able to better serve our patients.

Keratoconus is a progressive, corneal dystrophy which manifests as corneal thinning and formation of a cone-shaped protrusion. Because laser refractive surgery may lead to accelerated postoperative ectasia in patients with keratoconus,[1,2] the accurate detection of early keratoconus is a major safety concern. The prevalence of keratoconus in the Caucasian population is approximately 1/2000.[3] The incidence of undiagnosed keratoconus presenting to refractive surgery clinics tends to be much higher than this, as keratoconics develop astigmatism that is more difficult to correct by contact lenses or glasses, leading them to consider refractive surgery.[4] The challenge for keratoconus screening is to have high sensitivity, but for this to be combined with high specificity to minimize the number of atypical normal patients who are denied surgery.

There have been significant efforts made to develop methods for screening of early keratoconus over the past thirty years. In 1984, Klyce[5] introduced color-coded maps derived from computerized front surface Placido topography, which have made the diagnosis of keratoconus easier, as patterns including inferior steepening, asymmetric bow-tie and skew bow-tie typical of keratoconus can be seen early in the progression of the disease.[6,7] Placido-based instruments producing maps of anterior surface topography and curvature became available by the early 1990's and their use in keratoconus screening demonstrated.[7–16] Characterization of corneal thickness and topography of both corneal surfaces using scanning-slit tomography was introduced commercially in the mid 1990s by the Orbscan scanning slit system (Bausch & Lomb, Rochester, NY, USA)[17–19] and later by the Pentacam rotating Scheimpflug-based system (Oculus Optikgeräte, Wetzlar, Germany)[20,21] and other tomography scanners. Wavefront assessment[22] and biomechanical parameter evaluation with the Ocular Response Analyzer (Reichert, Depew, NY, USA)[23] and Corvis ST (Oculus Optikgeräte, Wetzlar, Germany)[24–26] have also been employed as a means for detecting early keratoconus.

DOI: 10.1201/9781003371601-6

Topographic and tomographic evaluation has evolved from qualitative observation[7] to quantitative measurements, and many parameters have been described to aid the differentiation of normal from keratoconus eyes.[7–16] Several statistical and machine-based or computerized learning models have been employed for keratoconus detection, and automated systems for screening based on front and back surface topography and whole corneal tomography and pachymetric profile have been developed.[20,27–34]

Although these approaches have improved the effectiveness of keratoconus screening, there are still equivocal cases where a confident diagnosis cannot be made and undiagnosed keratoconus probably remains the leading cause of corneal ectasia after LASIK.[35–47] The addition of quantitative parameters that are independent of those now obtained by topographic and tomographic analysis could potentially improve screening.

The corneal epithelial and stromal thickness profiles may represent such an independent parameter, and will be the focus of this chapter. As will be described below, the corneal epithelium has the ability to alter its thickness profile to re-establish a smooth, symmetrical optical outer corneal surface and either partially or totally mask the presence of an irregular stromal surface from front surface topography.[48,49] Therefore, the epithelial thickness profile would be expected to follow a distinctive pattern in keratoconus to partially compensate for the cone.

HISTORY OF THE MEASUREMENT OF EPITHELIAL THICKNESS

The first real measurement of the epithelium in vivo was made in 1979 by Brian Holden, using optical pachometry.[50] In 1993,[51] we started measuring epithelial thickness using very high-frequency (VHF) digital ultrasound and published a 3-mm-diameter map in 1994.[52–55] By 2000, we had improved this method to generate a 10-mm map.[48,56–72] VHF digital ultrasound was further developed and is now commercially available as the Artemis Insight 100 VHF digital ultrasound arc-scanner (ArcScan Inc, Golden, CO, USA), which has been previously described in detail.[52,56,59]

During the 1990s, optical pachometry was used for a number of studies measuring epithelial thickness.[73–75] Epithelial thickness was studied using histology from 1992,[76–79] Torben Moller-Pedersen[80–82] started using confocal microscopy in 1997, and OCT was first used for measuring the epithelium in 2001.[83–86] Epithelial thickness maps in an 8-mm diameter using OCT were published by Haque in 2008,[87] followed by David Huang's group in 2012,[88] which are now commercially available using the RTVue/Avanti OCT (Optovue, Fremont, CA, USA). Since then, other OCT devices have been developed that include epithelial thickness mapping, such as the MS-39 OCT (CSO, Florence, Italy) and Cirrus HD OCT (Carl Zeiss Meditec, Jena, Germany).

EPITHELIAL THICKNESS PROFILE IN NORMAL EYES

Before looking at more complicated situations, it is useful to consider the epithelial thickness profile in a population of 110 normal eyes.[59] Somewhat surprisingly, using VHF digital ultrasound, we demonstrated that the epithelium was not a layer of homogeneous thickness, as had previously been thought, but followed a very distinct pattern; on average the epithelium was 5.7 μm thicker inferiorly than superiorly, and 1.2 μm thicker nasally than temporally, with a mean central thickness of 53.4 μm (Figure 6.1). The average central epithelial thickness was 53.4 μm and the standard deviation was only 4.6 μm.[59] This indicated that there was little variation in central epithelial thickness in the population. The thinnest epithelial point within the central 5 mm of the cornea was displaced on average by 0.33 mm (± 1.08) temporally and 0.90 mm (± 0.96) superiorly with reference to the corneal vertex. Studies using OCT have confirmed this superior-inferior and nasal-temporal asymmetric profile for epithelial thickness in normal eyes.[88]

Figure 6.2, Column 1 shows the keratometry, Atlas 995 (Carl Zeiss Meditec, Jena, Germany) corneal topography map and PathFinder™ corneal analysis, Orbscan II (software version 3.00) anterior elevation best-fit sphere (BFS), Orbscan II posterior elevation BFS, and Artemis epithelial thickness profile of a normal eye.

This normal non-uniformity seems to provide evidence that the epithelial thickness is regulated by eyelid mechanics and blinking, as we suggested in 1994.[51] The eyelid might effectively be chafing the surface epithelium during blinking and that the posterior surface of the semi-rigid tarsus provides a template for the outer shape of the epithelial surface. During blinking, which occurs on average between 300 to 1500 times per hour,[89] the vertical traverse of the upper lid is much greater than that of the lower lid. Doane[90] studied the dynamics of eyelid anatomy during blinking and found that during a blink the descent of the upper eyelid reaches its maximum speed at about the time it crosses the visual axis. As a consequence, it is likely that the eyelid applies more force on the superior cornea than on the inferior cornea. Similarly, the friction on the cornea during

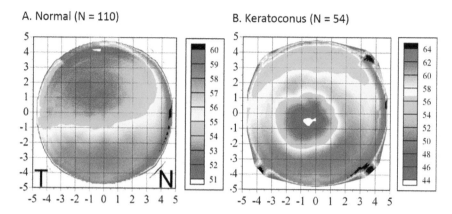

Figure 6.1   Mean epithelial thickness profile for a population of 110 normal eyes (A) and a population of 54 keratoconic eyes (B). The epithelial thickness profiles for all eyes in each population were averaged using mirrored left-eye symmetry. The colour scale represents epithelial thickness in microns. A Cartesian 1-mm grid is superimposed with the origin at the corneal vertex. *Reprinted with permission from SLACK Incorporated: Reinstein, DZ., Gobbe, M., Archer, T., Silverman, R., Coleman, J. (2010). Epithelial, Stromal and Total Corneal Thickness in Keratoconus. Journal or Refractive Surgery, 26, 259–271.*

lid closure is likely to be greater temporally than nasally as the outer canthus is higher than the inner canthus (mean intercanthal angle=3°), and the temporal portion of the lid is higher than the nasal lid (mean upper lid angle=2.7°).[91] Therefore, it seems that the nature of the eyelid completely explains the non-uniform epithelial thickness profile of a normal eye.

Further evidence for this theory is provided by the epithelial thickness changes observed in orthokeratology.[63] In orthokeratology, a shaped contact lens is placed on the cornea overnight that sits tightly on the cornea centrally but leaves a gap in the mid-periphery. Therefore, the natural template provided by the posterior surface of the semi-rigid tarsus of the eyelid is replaced by an artificial contact lens template designed to fit tightly to the centre of the cornea and loosely paracentrally. We found significant epithelial thickness changes with central thinning and mid-peripheral thickening showing that the epithelium had remodelled according to the template provided by the contact lens – i.e., the epithelium is chafed and squashed by the lens centrally while the epithelium is free to thicken paracentrally where the lens is not so tightly fitted.

EPITHELIAL THICKNESS PROFILE IN KERATOCONIC EYES

It is well known that the epithelial thickness changes in keratoconus since extreme steepening leads to epithelial breakdown, as often seen clinically. Epithelial thinning over the cone has been demonstrated using histopathologic analysis of keratoconic corneas by Scroggs et al.[92] and later using custom software and a Humphrey-Zeiss OCT system (Humphrey Systems, Dublin, CA, USA) by Haque et al.[93]

We have characterized the *in-vivo* epithelial thickness profile in a population of 54 eyes with keratoconus.[64] The average epithelial thickness profile in keratoconus revealed that there was significantly more irregularity compared with a normal population. The epithelium was thinnest at the apex of the cone and this thin epithelial zone was surrounded by an annulus of thickened epithelium (see Figure 6.1). While all eyes exhibited the same epithelial doughnut pattern, characterized by a localized central zone of thinning surrounded by an annulus of thick epithelium, the thickness values of the thinnest point and the thickest point as well as the difference in thickness between the thinnest and thickest epithelium varied greatly between eyes. There was a statistically significant negative correlation between the thinnest epithelium and the steepest keratometry (D), indicating that as the cornea became steeper, the epithelial thickness minimum became thinner. In addition, there was a statistically significant correlation between the thickness of the thinnest epithelium and the difference in thickness between the thinnest and thickest epithelium. This indicated that, as the epithelium thinned, there was an increase in the irregularity of the epithelial thickness profile – i.e., that there was an increase in the severity of the keratoconus. The location of the thinnest epithelium within the central 5-mm of the cornea was displaced on

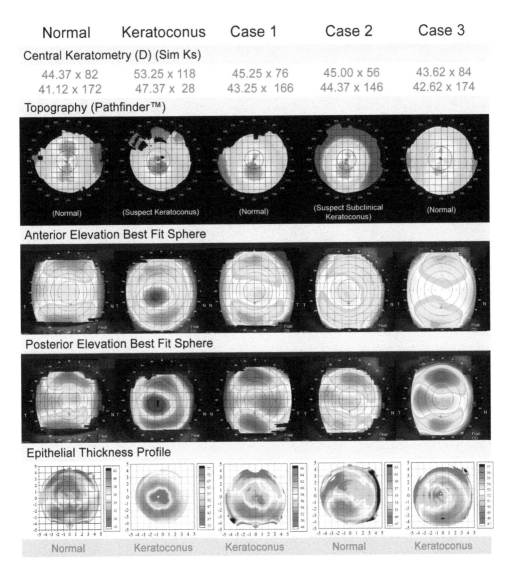

Figure 6.2 Central keratometry, Atlas corneal topography, and PathFinder™ corneal analysis, Orbscan anterior and posterior elevation BFS, and Artemis epithelial thickness profile for one normal eye, one keratoconic eye, and three sample eyes where the diagnosis of keratoconus might be misleading from topography. The final diagnosis based on the epithelial thickness profile is shown at the bottom of each example. *Reprinted with permission from SLACK Incorporated: Reinstein, DZ., Gobbe, M., Archer, T., Silverman, R., Coleman, J. (2010). "Epithelial, Stromal and Total Corneal Thickness in Keratoconus. Journal or Refractive Surgery, 26, 259–271.*

average by 0.48 mm (± 0.66 mm) temporally and by 0.32 mm (± 0.67 mm) inferiorly with reference to the corneal vertex. The mean epithelial thickness for all eyes was 45.7 ± 5.9 μm (range: 33.1 to 56.3 μm) at the corneal vertex, 38.2 ± 5.8 μm (range: 29.6 to 52.4 μm) at the thinnest point and 66.8 ± 7.2 μm (range: 54.1 to 94.4 μm) at the thickest point.[64]

Figure 6.2, Column 2 shows the keratometry, Atlas 995 corneal topography map and PathFinder™ corneal analysis, Orbscan II anterior elevation BFS, Orbscan II posterior elevation BFS, and Artemis epithelial thickness profile of a keratoconic eye. As expected, the front surface topography shows infero-temporal steepening with steep average keratometry and high astigmatism; the anterior and posterior elevation BFS maps demonstrate that the apex of the cone is located infero-temporally and the epithelial thickness profile shows epithelial thinning at the apex of the cone, surrounded by an annulus of thicker epithelium. The steepest cornea coincides with

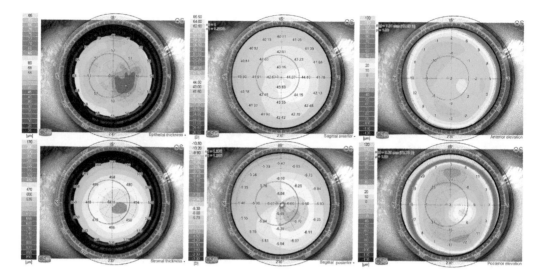

Figure 6.3 MS-39 (CSO, Florence, Italy) 6 map display showing a patient with mild keratoconus showing correspondence between epithelial thinning, pachymetric thinning, curvature, and elevation maps.

the apex of the anterior and posterior elevation BFS as well as with the location of the thinnest epithelium.

Recently, the MS-39 OCT device has been introduced which combines Placido topography with OCT scanning. This enables the MS-39 to simultaneously capture front surface topography and pachymetry data, producing epithelial thickness, corneal thickness, front surface topography, and back surface elevation maps that are all registered to the same measurement location (Figure 6.3). This greatly helps to assess coincidence between these maps.

The epithelial thickness profile for keratoconus as described here has been confirmed by studies using OCT.[88,94-96] The study by Laroche's group[96] elegantly described the different stages of advanced keratoconus demonstrating that as keratoconus moves into its latter stages, a very different epithelial thickness profile becomes apparent. In advanced keratoconus, there is stromal loss often in the location of the cone, for example, due to hydrops. This means that, rather than the cone being elevated relative to the rest of the stroma, this region is now a depression. Therefore, the epithelium changes from thinnest over the cone to thickest in this region, as it compensates for a depression instead of an elevation (see next section). There can be significant stromal loss in such advanced keratoconus, so the epithelium can be as thick as 200 μm in some cases. Examples of this epithelial thickening were also reported by Rocha et al.[94] who concluded that focal central epithelial thinning was suggestive of but not pathognomonic for keratoconus (i.e., the presence of an epithelial doughnut pattern did not prove beyond any doubt that an eye has keratoconus). However, as described by Laroche, these cases only appear in very advanced keratoconus, which means that they are of no interest with respect to keratoconus screening. Eyes with early keratoconus will never present with epithelial thickening in the location of the cone as, by definition, if there has been stromal loss, then the keratoconus must be more advanced and the cornea will be obviously abnormal.

UNDERSTANDING THE PREDICTABLE BEHAVIOUR OF THE CORNEAL EPITHELIUM

Epithelial thickness changes in keratoconus provide another example of the very predictable mechanism of the corneal epithelium to compensate for irregularities on the stromal surface. Epithelial thickness changes have also been described after myopic excimer laser ablation,[60,70,74,97] hyperopic excimer laser ablation,[66] radial keratotomy,[69] intra-corneal ring segments,[57] irregularly irregular astigmatism after corneal refractive surgery,[48,55,72,98-100] and in ectasia.[67]

In all of these cases, the epithelial thickness changes are clearly a compensatory response to the changes to the stromal surface and can all be explained by the theory of eyelid template regulation of epithelial thickness.[49] Compensatory epithelial thickness changes can be summarised by the following rules:

1. The epithelium thickens in areas where tissue has been removed or the curvature has been flattened (e.g., central thickening after myopic ablation[60,70,74] or radial keratotomy[69] and peripheral thickening after hyperopic ablation[66]).

2. The epithelium thins over regions that are relatively elevated or the curvature has been steepened (e.g., central thinning in keratoconus,[64,88,94–96] ectasia,[67] and after hyperopic ablation[66]).

3. The magnitude of epithelial changes correlates to the magnitude of the change in curvature (e.g., more epithelial thickening after higher myopic ablation,[60,74,97] after higher hyperopic ablation,[66] and in more advanced keratoconus[64,88,94–96]).

4. The amount of epithelial remodelling is defined by the rate of change of curvature of an irregularity;[49,101] there will be more epithelial remodelling for a more localized irregularity.[48,72,98,100] The epithelium effectively acts as a low-pass filter, smoothing local changes (high curvature gradient) almost completely, but only partially smoothing global changes (low curvature gradient). For example, there is almost twice as much epithelial thickening after a hyperopic ablation[66] compared with a myopic ablation,[60,74,97] and there is almost total epithelial compensation for small, very localized stromal loss, such as after a corneal ulcer.[66]

DIAGNOSING EARLY KERATOCONUS USING EPITHELIAL THICKNESS PROFILES

Mapping of the epithelial thickness reveals a very distinct thickness profile in keratoconus compared with that of normal corneas, due to the compensatory mechanism of the epithelium for stromal irregularities. The epithelial thickness profile changes with the progression of the disease; as the keratoconus becomes more severe, the epithelium at the apex of the cone becomes thinner and the surrounding annulus of epithelium in the epithelial doughnut pattern becomes thicker. Therefore, the degree of epithelial abnormality in both directions (thinner and thicker than normal) can be used to confirm or exclude a diagnosis of keratoconus in eyes suggestive but not conclusive of a diagnosis of keratoconus on topography at a very early stage in the expression of the disease.[61]

In early keratoconus, we would expect to see the pattern of localized epithelial thinning surrounded by an annulus of thick epithelium coincident with a suspected cone on posterior elevation BFS. The coincidence of epithelial thinning together with an eccentric posterior elevation BFS apex may reveal whether or not to ascribe significance to an eccentric posterior elevation BFS apex occurring *concurrently with* a normal front surface topography. In other words, in the presence of normal or questionable front surface topography, thinning of the epithelium coincident with the location of the posterior elevation BFS apex would represent total masking of or compensation for a sub-surface stromal cone which *does* represent keratoconus (Figure 6.2). Conversely, finding thicker epithelium over an area of topographic steepening or an eccentric posterior elevation BFS apex would imply that the steepening is *not* due to a keratoconic sub-surface stromal cone, but more likely due to localized epithelial thickening.

Evaluation of epithelial thickness profile irregularities provides a very sensitive method of examining ×stromal surface topography – by proxy. Therefore, epithelial thickness mapping provides increased sensitivity and specificity to a diagnosis of keratoconus and, in many cases, before there is any detectable corneal front surface topographic change.

CASE EXAMPLES

Figure 6.2 shows three further selected examples where epithelial thickness profiles helped to interpret and diagnose anterior and posterior elevation BFS abnormalities. In each case, the epithelial thickness profile appears to be able to differentiate cases, where the diagnosis of keratoconus is uncertain, from normal.[61]

Case 1 (OS) represents a 25-year-old male, with a manifest refraction of −1.00 −0.50 × 150 and a best spectacle-corrected visual acuity of 20/16. Atlas corneal topography demonstrated inferior steepening which would traditionally indicate keratoconus. The keratometry was 45.25/43.25 D ×76, and PathFinder™ corneal analysis classified the topography as normal. Orbscan II posterior elevation BFS showed that the posterior elevation BFS apex was decentred infero-temporally. The corneal pachymetry minimum obtained by handheld ultrasound was 479 μm. Contrast sensitivity was slightly below the normal range measured using the CSV-1000 (Vector Vision Inc, Greenville, OH, USA). There was −0.30 μm (OSA notation) of vertical coma on WASCA aberrometry. Corneal hysteresis was 7.5 mmHg and corneal resistance factor was 7.1 mmHg, which are low, but these could be affected by the low corneal thickness. The combination of inferior steepening, an eccentric posterior elevation BFS apex and thin cornea raised the suspicion of keratoconus although there was no suggestion of keratoconus by refraction, keratometry, or PathFinder™ corneal analysis. Artemis epithelial thickness profile showed a pattern typical of keratoconus with an epithelial doughnut shape characterized by a localized zone of epithelial thinning displaced infero-temporally over the eccentric posterior elevation BFS apex, surrounded by an annulus of thick epithelium. The coincidence of an area of epithelial thinning with the apex of the posterior elevation BFS, as well as the increased irregularity of the epithelium confirmed the diagnosis of early keratoconus.

Case 2 (OD) represents a 31-year-old female, with a manifest refraction of −2.25 −0.50 × 88 and a best spectacle-corrected visual acuity of 20/16. Atlas corneal topography demonstrated a very similar pattern to case 1 of inferior steepening, therefore suggesting that the eye could also be keratoconic. The keratometry was 44.12/44.75 D × 148, and PathFinder™ corneal analysis classified the topography as suspect subclinical keratoconus. Orbscan II posterior elevation BFS showed that the apex was slightly decentred nasally. The corneal pachymetry minimum obtained by handheld ultrasound was 538 µm. Contrast sensitivity was in the normal range. There was 0.32 µm (OSA notation) of vertical coma on WASCA aberrometry. Corneal hysteresis was 10.1 mmHg and corneal resistance factor was 9.8 mmHg, which are well within normal range. The combination of inferior steepening, against-the-rule astigmatism, and high degree of vertical coma raised the suspicion of keratoconus, which was also noted by PathFinder™ corneal analysis. Artemis epithelial thickness profile showed a typical normal pattern with thicker epithelium inferiorly and thinner epithelium superiorly. Thicker epithelium inferiorly over the suspected cone (inferior steepening on topography) was inconsistent with an underlying stromal surface cone, and therefore the diagnosis of keratoconus was excluded. This patient would have been rejected for surgery given a documented PathFinder™ corneal analysis warning of suspect subclinical keratoconus, but, given the epithelial thickness profile, this patient was deemed a suitable candidate for LASIK.

The anterior corneal topography in Case 3 (OD) bears no features related to keratoconus. The patient is a 35-year-old female with a manifest refraction of −4.25 −0.50 × 4 and a best spectacle-corrected visual acuity of 20/16. The refraction had been stable for at least ten years and the contrast sensitivity was within normal limits. The keratometry was 43.62/42.62 D × 74 and PathFinder™ analysis classified the topography as normal. Orbscan II posterior elevation BFS showed that the apex was slightly decentred infero-temporally, but the anterior elevation BFS apex was well centred. The corneal pachymetry minimum measured by handheld ultrasound was 484 µm. Pentacam (Oculus, Wetzlar, Germany) keratoconus screening indices were normal. WASCA ocular higher-order aberrations were low (RMS=0.19 µm) as was the level of vertical coma (coma=0.066 µm). Corneal hysteresis was 8.9 mmHg and corneal resistance factor was 8.8 mmHg, both within normal limits. In this case, only the slightly eccentric posterior elevation BFS apex and the low–normal corneal thickness were suspicious for keratoconus, while all other screening methods gave no indication of keratoconus. However, the epithelial thickness profile showed an epithelial doughnut pattern characterized by localized epithelial thinning surrounded by an annulus of thick epithelium, coincident with the eccentric posterior elevation BFS apex. Epithelial thinning with surrounding annular thickening over the eccentric posterior elevation BFS apex indicated the presence of probable sub-surface keratoconus. In this case, it seems that the epithelium had fully compensated for the stromal surface irregularity so that the anterior surface topography of the cornea appeared perfectly regular. Given the regularity of the front surface topography and the normality of nearly all other screening parameters, it is feasible that this patient could have been deemed suitable for corneal refractive surgery and subsequently developed ectasia. As we were able to also consider the epithelial thickness profile, this patient was rejected for corneal refractive surgery. This kind of case may explain some reported cases of ectasia "without a cause."[102]

AUTOMATED ALGORITHM FOR CLASSIFICATION BY EPITHELIUM

Based on this qualitative diagnostic method, we set out to derive an automated classifier to detect keratoconus using epithelial thickness data, together with Ron Silverman and his group at Columbia University.[103] We used stepwise linear discriminant analysis (LDA) and neural network (NN) analysis to develop multivariate models based on combinations of 161 features comparing a population of 130 normal and 74 keratoconic eyes. This process resulted in a six-variable model that provided an area under the receiver operating curve of 100%, indicative of complete separation of keratoconic from normal corneas. Test-set performance, averaged over ten trials, gave a specificity of 99.5 ± 1.5% and sensitivity of 98.9 ± 1.9%. Figure 6.4 shows an example of early keratoconus in which the front surface topography and Pentacam tomography appear normal, although the epithelial thickness profile demonstrates focal thinning which was identified as keratoconus by this automated algorithm. Maps of the average epithelium and LDA function values were also found to be well correlated with keratoconus severity grade. Other groups have also been working on automated classification algorithms based on epithelial thickness data obtained by OCT.[88,104]

Following this study, we then applied the algorithm to a population of ten patients with unilateral keratoconus (clinically and algorithmically topographically normal in the fellow eyes), on the basis that the fellow eye in such patients represents a latent form of keratoconus and, as such, has been considered a gold-standard for studies aimed at early keratoconus detection. These eyes were also analyzed using the Belin–Ambrósio enhanced ectasia display (BAD-D parameter and ART-Max)[20,27,105] and the Orbscan SCORE value as described by Saad and Gatinel.[31–33]

The most interesting finding of this study was that more than 50% of the fellow eyes were classified as normal by all methods. This was similar to the result reported by Bae et al.,[29] who found no difference in the BAD-D or ART-Max values between normal and topographically normal fellow eyes of keratoconus patients. This is in contrast to other studies using unilateral keratoconus populations where a much higher sensitivity was reported; however, these studies often included

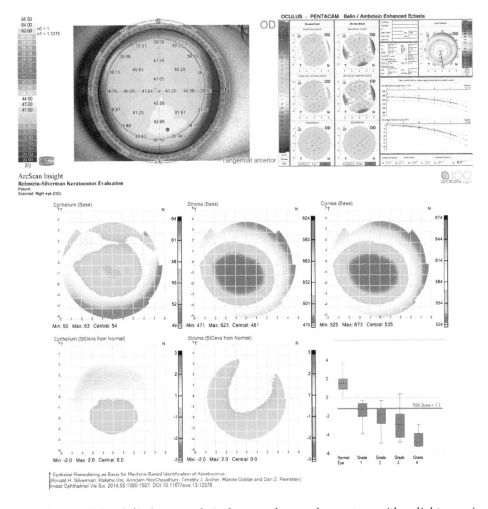

Figure 6.4 MS-39 (top left) shows a relatively normal corneal curvature with a slight superior to inferior difference in keratometry. The corresponding Pentacam Belin–Ambrósia display (top right) shows a normal front and back surface elevation. The AcrScan Insight 100 shows an area of epithelial thinning with surrounding thickening. This is further highlighted in the bottom left map which shows the thickness standard deviations from the normal population. The epithelial map confirms that, despite the topography and tomography findings, the patient has keratoconus.

patients with a suspicious topography in the fellow eye (i.e., some studies use a more rigorous defi-nition of unilateral keratoconus than others).[30] Therefore, the main conclusion from the study was to question the validity of using unilateral keratoconus patients for keratoconus screening studies. The fact that a number of these fellow eyes showed absolutely no indication of keratoconus by any method implies that it is likely that these were truly normal eyes. However, it is generally agreed that keratoconus as a disease must be bilateral,[106] therefore, it appears that these cases are patients who do not have keratoconus, but have induced an ectasia in one eye, for example by eye rubbing or trauma. This means that using "unilateral keratoconus" populations to study kerato-conus screening may be flawed. The significant influence of eye rubbing is becoming increasingly apparent.[107]

The alternative is somewhat more alarming, as this would mean that there are eyes with keratoconus that are literally undetectable by any existing method. This would, however, explain any case of "ectasia without a cause."[102,108] Detection of keratoconus in such cases may require development of new *in-vivo* measurements of corneal biomechanics, although this appears to be outside the scope of current methods, such as the Ocular Response Analyzer[24,25,109] and Corvis,[24,25] due to the wide scatter in the data acquired. Another factor, as has been described using Brillouin microscopy,[110] may be that the biomechanical tensile strength of the cornea may not be different from normal in early keratoconus when measuring the whole cornea globally, but there may be a difference only in the localized region of the cone (or in the location of a future cone). Another potential and final solution would be whether a genotype or other molecular marker for keratoco-nus could be found.[111–113]

Finally, another interpretation of this result is that keratoconus may not necessarily be a disease of abnormal stromal substance. The localization of the reduced corneal biomechanics found in ker-atoconus suggests that this may be caused by a local defect in Bowman's layer due to eye rubbing or other trauma. A break in Bowman's layer would reduce the tension locally and the asymmetric stress concentration would then cause the stroma to bulge in this location. Evidence for changes in Bowman's layer in keratoconus has been reported using ultra-high resolution OCT; Shousha et al.[114] showed that Bowman's layer was thinner inferiorly in keratoconus and described a Bowman's ectasia index (BEI) to use for keratoconus screening. Yadav et al.[115] also described differences in the thickness of Bowman's layer in keratoconus, as well as a difference in light scatter.

FACTORS INFLUENCING THE EPITHELIUM

Although the epithelium is the most sensitive method for detecting very early keratoconus, it is important to recognize there are some other factors that may affect the epithelial pattern. Epithelial changes associated with anterior basement membrane dystrophy (ABMD) may cause focal areas of thickening that can be identified on clinical slit-lamp examination. These clinical findings will often have corresponding changes in the epithelial thickness map (Figure 6.5). If there is paracentral thickening, the epithelial thickness profile can resemble a keratoconus pat-tern as can be seen in Figure 6.6. In addition to ABMD, dry eye can also affect the epithelium. Kannelopolous et al.[116] found the central epithelial thickness in dry eye patients to be 59.5 ± 4.2

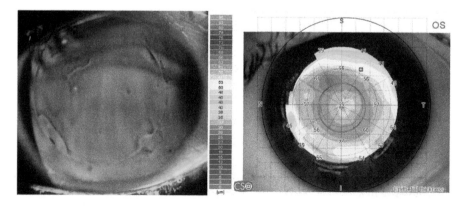

Figure 6.5 Slit-lamp photograph under heavy fluorescein staining showing focal anterior base-ment membrane dystrophy (left) and the associated thickening seen on the MS-39 epithelial map (right).

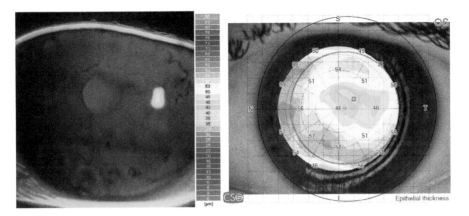

Figure 6.6 Slit-lamp photography under heavy fluorescein staining showing diffuse anterior basement membrane dystrophy (left) and the associated thickening seen on the MS-39 epithelial map (right). The epithelial pattern mimics that seen in keratoconus with an area of central thinning, surrounding by thickening.

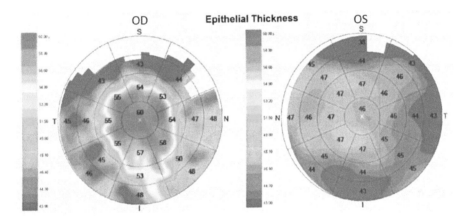

Figure 6.7 Cirrus HD OCT epithelial thickness map showing thickening in the right eye due to decreased blinking ability during a Bell's palsy episode. The left eye epithelial thickness is normal.

μm compared with 53.0 ± 2.7 μm in the control group. Figure 6.7 shows an extreme example of this in a patient who had an episode of Bell's palsy resulting in an incomplete blink. The right eye epithelium thickened by 14 μm centrally during the episode and subsequently returned to normal to match the left eye once the blinking function recovered.

CONCLUSION

Keratoconus detection is ever-evolving. We have demonstrated that the epithelial thickness profile was significantly different between normal eyes and keratoconic eyes. Whereas the epithelium in normal eyes was relatively homogeneous in thickness with a pattern of slightly thicker epithelium inferiorly than superiorly, the epithelium in keratoconic eyes was irregular showing a doughnut-shaped pattern, and a marked difference in thickness between the thin epithelium at the centre of the doughnut and the surrounding annulus of thick epithelium. We have shown that the epithelial thickness profile progresses along with the evolution of keratoconus. More advanced keratoconus produces more irregularity in the epithelial thickness profile. We have found that the distinctive epithelial doughnut pattern associated with keratoconus can be used to confirm or exclude the presence of an underlying stromal surface cone in cases with normal or suspect front surface topography as well as being a "qualifier" for the finding of an eccentric posterior elevation BFS apex.

Knowledge of the differences in epithelial thickness profile between the normal population and the keratoconic population allowed us to identify several features of the epithelial thickness profile that might help to discriminate between normal eyes and keratoconus suspect eyes.

Randleman, in his paper assessing risk factors for ectasia, reported that ectasia might still occur after uncomplicated surgery in appropriately screened candidates.[36] Mapping of epithelial thickness profiles might provide an explanation for these cases; it could be that a stromal surface cone was masked by epithelial compensation and the front surface topography appeared normal.

Mapping of the epithelial thickness profile may increase sensitivity and specificity of screening for keratoconus compared with current conventional corneal topographic screening alone and may be useful in clinical practice in two very important ways.

Firstly, epithelial thickness mapping can exclude the appropriate patients by detecting keratoconus earlier or confirming keratoconus in cases where topographic changes may clinically be judged as being "within normal limits." Epithelial information allows an earlier diagnosis of keratoconus as epithelial changes will occur before changes on the front surface of the cornea become apparent. Epithelial thinning coincident with an eccentric posterior elevation BFS apex, and in particular if surrounded by an annulus of thicker epithelium, is consistent with keratoconus. Excluding early keratoconic patients from laser refractive surgery will reduce and potentially eliminate the risk of iatrogenic ectasia of this etiology and therefore increase the safety of laser refractive surgery. From our data, 136 eyes out of 1,532 consecutive myopic eyes screened for refractive surgery demonstrated abnormal topography indicative of keratoconus. All 136 eyes were screened with Artemis VHF digital ultrasound arc-scanning and individual epithelial thickness profiles were mapped. Out of 136 eyes with suspect keratoconus, only 22 eyes (16%) were confirmed as keratoconus.[62]

Secondly, epithelial thickness profiles may be useful in excluding a diagnosis of keratoconus despite suspect topography. Epithelial thickening over an area of topographic steepening implies that the steepening is not due to an underlying ectatic surface. In such cases, excluding keratoconus using epithelial thickness profiles appears to allow patients who otherwise would have been denied treatment due to suspect topography to be deemed suitable for surgery. From our data, out of the 136 eyes with suspect keratoconus screened with Artemis VHF digital ultrasound arc-scanning, 114 eyes (84%) showed normal epithelial thickness profile and were diagnosed as non-keratoconic and deemed suitable for corneal refractive surgery. One-year post-LASIK follow-up data[62] and preliminary two-year follow-up data[117] on these demonstrated equal stability and refractive outcomes as matched control eyes.

In summary, it is important to obtain a full clinical picture for the patient including demographic, diagnostic, and examination data. With advancements in keratoconus screening to include topography to tomography and now epithelium, we are seeing a shift in the standard of care and we are able to better serve our patients. In the future, advancements in algorithms and deep machine learning may prove to be yet another tool to aid in the early detection of keratoconus.

Financial Disclosure: Dr Reinstein is a consultant for Carl Zeiss Meditec (Carl Zeiss Meditec AG, Jena, Germany). Dr Reinstein is also a consultant for CSO Italia (Florence, Italy) and has a proprietary interest in the Artemis Insight 100 technology (ArcScan Inc, Golden, CO, USA) through patents administered by the Cornell Center for Technology Enterprise and Commercialization (CCTEC), Ithaca, New York. Timothy J Archer *has* no proprietary or financial interest in the materials presented herein.

REFERENCES

1. Ambrosio R, Jr., Wilson SE. Complications of laser in situ keratomileusis: etiology, prevention, and treatment. *J Refract Surg.* 2001;17:350–379.

2. Seiler T, Koufala K, Richter G. Iatrogenic keratectasia after laser in situ keratomileusis. *J Refract Surg.* 1998;14:312–317.

3. Krachmer JH, Feder RF, Belin MW. Keratoconus and related non-inflammatory corneal thinning disorders. *Surv Ophthalmol.* 1984;28:293–322.

4. Wilson SE, Klyce SD. Screening for corneal topographic abnormalities before refractive surgery. *Ophthalmology*. 1994;101:147–152.

5. Klyce SD. Computer-assisted corneal topography. High-resolution graphic presentation and analysis of keratoscopy. *Invest Ophthalmol Vis Sci*. 1984;25:1426–1435.

6. Rabinowitz YS, Yang H, Brickman Y, Akkina J, Riley C, Rotter JI, Elashoff J. Videokeratography database of normal human corneas. *Br J Ophthalmol*. 1996;80:610–616.

7. Rabinowitz YS, McDonnell PJ. Computer-assisted corneal topography in keratoconus. *Refract Corneal Surg*. 1989;5:400–408.

8. Rabinowitz YS. Videokeratographic indices to aid in screening for keratoconus. *J Refract Surg*. 1995;11:371–379.

9. Rabinowitz YS. Tangential vs sagittal videokeratographs in the "early" detection of keratoconus. *Am J Ophthalmol*. 1996;122:887–889.

10. Rabinowitz YS, Rasheed K. KISA% index: a quantitative videokeratography algorithm embodying minimal topographic criteria for diagnosing keratoconus. *J Cataract Refract Surg*. 1999;25:1327–1335.

11. Smolek MK, Klyce SD. Current keratoconus detection methods compared with a neural network approach. *Invest Ophthalmol Vis Sci*. 1997;38:2290–2299.

12. Maeda N, Klyce SD, Smolek MK. Comparison of methods for detecting keratoconus using videokeratography. *Arch Ophthalmol*. 1995;113:870–874.

13. Nesburn AB, Bahri S, Salz J, Rabinowitz YS, Maguen E, Hofbauer J, Berlin M, Macy JI. Keratoconus detected by videokeratography in candidates for photorefractive keratectomy. *J Refract Surg*. 1995;11:194–201.

14. Chastang PJ, Borderie VM, Carvajal-Gonzalez S, Rostene W, Laroche L. Automated keratoconus detection using the EyeSys videokeratoscope. *J Cataract Refract Surg*. 2000;26:675–683.

15. Maeda N, Klyce SD, Smolek MK, Thompson HW. Automated keratoconus screening with corneal topography analysis. *Invest Ophthalmol Vis Sci*. 1994;35:2749–2757.

16. Kalin NS, Maeda N, Klyce SD, Hargrave S, Wilson SE. Automated topographic screening for keratoconus in refractive surgery candidates. *Clao J*. 1996;22:164–167.

17. Auffarth GU, Wang L, Volcker HE. Keratoconus evaluation using the orbscan topography system. *J Cataract Refract Surg*. 2000;26:222–228.

18. Rao SN, Raviv T, Majmudar PA, Epstein RJ. Role of Orbscan II in screening keratoconus suspects before refractive corneal surgery. *Ophthalmology*. 2002;109:1642–1646.

19. Tomidokoro A, Oshika T, Amano S, Higaki S, Maeda N, Miyata K. Changes in anterior and posterior corneal curvatures in keratoconus. *Ophthalmology*. 2000;107:1328–1332.

20. Ambrosio R, Jr., Alonso RS, Luz A, Coca Velarde LG. Corneal-thickness spatial profile and corneal-volume distribution: tomographic indices to detect keratoconus. *J Cataract Refract Surg*. 2006;32:1851–1859.

21. de Sanctis U, Loiacono C, Richiardi L, Turco D, Mutani B, Grignolo FM. Sensitivity and specificity of posterior corneal elevation measured by Pentacam in discriminating keratoconus/subclinical keratoconus. *Ophthalmology*. 2008;115:1534–1539.

22. Saad A, Gatinel D. Evaluation of total and corneal wavefront high order aberrations for the detection of forme fruste keratoconus. *Invest Ophthalmol Vis Sci.* 2012;53:2978–2992.

23. Luce DA. Determining in vivo biomechanical properties of the cornea with an ocular response analyzer. *J Cataract Refract Surg.* 2005;31:156–162.

24. Vellara HR, Patel DV. Biomechanical properties of the keratoconic cornea: a review. *Clin Exp Optom.* 2015;98:31–38.

25. Pinero DP, Alcon N. Corneal biomechanics: a review. *Clin Exp Optom.* 2015;98(2):107–116.

26. Vinciguerra R, Ambrosio R, Jr., Elsheikh A, Roberts CJ, Lopes B, Morenghi E, Azzolini C, Vinciguerra P. Detection of keratoconus with a new biomechanical index. *J Refract Surg.* 2016;32:803–810.

27. Ambrosio R, Jr., Caiado AL, Guerra FP, Louzada R, Roy AS, Luz A, Dupps WJ, Belin MW. Novel pachymetric parameters based on corneal tomography for diagnosing keratoconus. *J Refract Surg.* 2011;27:753–758.

28. Fontes BM, Ambrosio R, Jr., Salomao M, Velarde GC, Nose W. Biomechanical and tomographic analysis of unilateral keratoconus. *J Refract Surg.* 2010;26:677–681.

29. Bae GH, Kim JR, Kim CH, Lim DH, Chung ES, Chung TY. Corneal topographic and tomographic analysis of fellow eyes in unilateral keratoconus patients using Pentacam. *Am J Ophthalmol.* 2014;157:103–109.e101.

30. Muftuoglu O, Ayar O, Ozulken K, Ozyol E, Akinci A. Posterior corneal elevation and back difference corneal elevation in diagnosing forme fruste keratoconus in the fellow eyes of unilateral keratoconus patients. *J Cataract Refract Surg.* 2013;39:1348–1357.

31. Chan C, Ang M, Saad A, Chua D, Mejia M, Lim L, Gatinel D. Validation of an objective scoring system for forme fruste keratoconus detection and post-LASIK Ectasia risk assessment in Asian Eyes. *Cornea.* 2015;34:996–1004.

32. Saad A, Gatinel D. Validation of a new scoring system for the detection of early forme of keratoconus. *Int J Kerat Ect Cor Dis.* 2012;1:100–108.

33. Saad A, Gatinel D. Topographic and tomographic properties of forme fruste keratoconus corneas. *Invest Ophthalmol Vis Sci.* 2010;51:5546–5555.

34. Mahmoud AM, Nunez MX, Blanco C, Koch DD, Wang L, Weikert MP, Frueh BE, Tappeiner C, Twa MD, Roberts CJ. Expanding the cone location and magnitude index to include corneal thickness and posterior surface information for the detection of keratoconus. *Am J Ophthalmol.* 2013;156:1102–1111.

35. Randleman JB, Trattler WB, Stulting RD. Validation of the ectasia risk score system for preoperative laser in situ keratomileusis screening. *Am J Ophthalmol.* 2008;145:813–818.

36. Randleman JB, Woodward M, Lynn MJ, Stulting RD. Risk assessment for ectasia after corneal refractive surgery. *Ophthalmology.* 2008;115:37–50.

37. Seiler T, Quurke AW. Iatrogenic keratectasia after LASIK in a case of forme fruste keratoconus. *J Cataract Refract Surg.* 1998;24:1007–1009.

38. Speicher L, Gottinger W. Progressive corneal ectasia after laser in situ keratomileusis (LASIK). *Klin Monatsbl Augenheilkd.* 1998;213:247–251.

39. Geggel HS, Talley AR. Delayed onset keratectasia following laser in situ keratomileusis. *J Cataract Refract Surg*. 1999;25:582–586.

40. Amoils SP, Deist MB, Gous P, Amoils PM. Iatrogenic keratectasia after laser in situ keratomileusis for less than -4.0 to -7.0 diopters of myopia. *J Cataract Refract Surg*. 2000;26:967–977.

41. McLeod SD, Kisla TA, Caro NC, McMahon TT. Iatrogenic keratoconus: corneal ectasia following laser in situ keratomileusis for myopia. *Arch Ophthalmol*. 2000;118:282–284.

42. Holland SP, Srivannaboon S, Reinstein DZ. Avoiding serious corneal complications of laser assisted in situ keratomileusis and photorefractive keratectomy. *Ophthalmology*. 2000;107:640–652.

43. Schmitt-Bernard CF, Lesage C, Arnaud B. Keratectasia induced by laser in situ keratomileusis in keratoconus. *J Refract Surg*. 2000;16:368–370.

44. Rao SN, Epstein RJ. Early onset ectasia following laser in situ keratomileusus: case report and literature review. *J Refract Surg*. 2002;18:177–184.

45. Malecaze F, Coullet J, Calvas P, Fournie P, Arne JL, Brodaty C. Corneal ectasia after photorefractive keratectomy for low myopia. *Ophthalmology*. 2006;113:742–746.

46. Randleman JB, Russell B, Ward MA, Thompson KP, Stulting RD. Risk factors and prognosis for corneal ectasia after LASIK. *Ophthalmology*. 2003;110:267–275.

47. Leccisotti A. Corneal ectasia after photorefractive keratectomy. *Graefes Arch Clin Exp Ophthalmol*. 2007;245:869–875.

48. Reinstein DZ, Archer T. Combined Artemis very high-frequency digital ultrasound-assisted transepithelial phototherapeutic keratectomy and wavefront-guided treatment following multiple corneal refractive procedures. *J Cataract Refract Surg*. 2006;32:1870–1876.

49. Reinstein DZ, Archer TJ, Gobbe M. Rate of change of curvature of the corneal stromal surface drives epithelial compensatory changes and remodeling. *J Refract Surg*. 2014;30:800–802.

50. Holden BA, Payor S. Changes in thickness in the corneal layers. *Am J Optom*. 1979;56:821.

51. Reinstein DZ, Silverman RH, Coleman DJ. High-frequency ultrasound measurement of the thickness of the corneal epithelium. *Refract Corneal Surg*. 1993;9:385–387.

52. Reinstein DZ, Silverman RH, Trokel SL, Coleman DJ. Corneal pachymetric topography. *Ophthalmology*. 1994;101:432–438.

53. Cusumano A, Coleman DJ, Silverman RH, Reinstein DZ, Rondeau MJ, Ursea R, Daly SM, Lloyd HO. Three-dimensional ultrasound imaging. Clinical applications. *Ophthalmology*. 1998;105:300–306.

54. Silverman RH, Reinstein DZ, Raevsky T, Coleman DJ. Improved system for sonographic imaging and biometry of the cornea. *J Ultrasound Med*. 1997;16:117–124.

55. Reinstein DZ, Silverman RH, Sutton HF, Coleman DJ. Very high-frequency ultrasound corneal analysis identifies anatomic correlates of optical complications of lamellar refractive surgery: anatomic diagnosis in lamellar surgery. *Ophthalmology*. 1999;106:474–482.

56. Reinstein DZ, Silverman RH, Raevsky T, Simoni GJ, Lloyd HO, Najafi DJ, Rondeau MJ, Coleman DJ. Arc-scanning very high-frequency digital ultrasound for 3D pachymetric mapping of the corneal epithelium and stroma in laser in situ keratomileusis. *J Refract Surg*. 2000;16:414–430.

57. Reinstein DZ, Srivannaboon S, Holland SP. Epithelial and stromal changes induced by intacs examined by three-dimensional very high-frequency digital ultrasound. *J Refract Surg*. 2001;17:310–318.

58. Reinstein DZ, Rothman RC, Couch DG, Archer TJ. Artemis very high-frequency digital ultrasound-guided repositioning of a free cap after laser in situ keratomileusis. *J Cataract Refract Surg*. 2006;32:1877–1882.

59. Reinstein DZ, Archer TJ, Gobbe M, Silverman RH, Coleman DJ. Epithelial thickness in the normal cornea: three-dimensional display with Artemis very high-frequency digital ultrasound. *J Refract Surg*. 2008;24:571–581.

60. Reinstein DZ, Srivannaboon S, Gobbe M, Archer TJ, Silverman RH, Sutton H, Coleman DJ. Epithelial thickness profile changes induced by myopic LASIK as measured by Artemis very high-frequency digital ultrasound. *J Refract Surg*. 2009;25:444–450.

61. Reinstein DZ, Archer TJ, Gobbe M. Corneal epithelial thickness profile in the diagnosis of keratoconus. *J Refract Surg*. 2009;25:604–610.

62. Reinstein DZ, Archer TJ, Gobbe M. Stability of LASIK in corneas with topographic suspect keratoconus, with keratoconus excluded by epithelial thickness mapping. *J Refract Surg*. 2009;25:569–577.

63. Reinstein DZ, Gobbe M, Archer TJ, Couch D, Bloom B. Epithelial, stromal, and corneal pachymetry changes during orthokeratology. *Optom Vis Sci*. 2009;86:E1006–1014.

64. Reinstein DZ, Archer TJ, Gobbe M, Silverman RH, Coleman DJ. Epithelial, stromal and corneal thickness in the keratoconic cornea: three-dimensional display with Artemis very high-frequency digital ultrasound. *J Refract Surg*. 2010;26:259–271.

65. Reinstein DZ, Archer TJ, Gobbe M, Silverman RH, Coleman DJ. Repeatability of layered corneal pachymetry with the artemis very high-frequency digital ultrasound arc-scanner. *J Refract Surg*. 2010;26:646–659.

66. Reinstein DZ, Archer TJ, Gobbe M, Silverman RH, Coleman DJ. Epithelial thickness after hyperopic LASIK: three-dimensional display with artemis very high-frequency digital ultrasound. *J Refract Surg*. 2010;26:555–564.

67. Reinstein DZ, Gobbe M, Archer TJ, Couch D. Epithelial thickness profile as a method to evaluate the effectiveness of collagen cross-linking treatment after corneal ectasia. *J Refract Surg*. 2011;27:356–363.

68. Reinstein DZ, Archer TJ, Gobbe M. Very high-frequency digital ultrasound evaluation of topography-wavefront-guided repair after radial keratotomy. *J Cataract Refract Surg*. 2011;37:599–602.

69. Reinstein DZ, Archer TJ, Gobbe M. Epithelial thickness up to 26 years after radial keratotomy: three-dimensional display with artemis very high-frequency digital ultrasound. *J Refract Surg*. 2011;27:618–624.

70. Reinstein DZ, Archer TJ, Gobbe M. Change in epithelial thickness profile 24 hours and longitudinally for 1 year after myopic LASIK: three-dimensional display with artemis very high-frequency digital ultrasound. *J Refract Surg*. 2012;28:195–201.

71. Reinstein DZ, Archer TJ, Gobbe M. Stability of epithelial thickness during 5 minutes immersion in 33 degrees C 0.9% saline using very high-frequency digital ultrasound. *J Refract Surg*. 2012;28:606–607.

72. Reinstein DZ, Archer TJ, Gobbe M. Improved effectiveness of trans-epithelial phototherapeutic keratectomy versus topography-guided ablation degraded by epithelial compensation on irregular stromal surfaces [plus video]. *J Refract Surg.* 2013;29:526–533.

73. Gauthier CA, Holden BA, Epstein D, Tengroth B, Fagerholm P, Hamberg-Nystrom H. Factors affecting epithelial hyperplasia after photorefractive keratectomy. *J Cataract Refract Surg.* 1997;23:1042–1050.

74. Gauthier CA, Holden BA, Epstein D, Tengroth B, Fagerholm P, Hamberg-Nystrom H. Role of epithelial hyperplasia in regression following photorefractive keratectomy. *Br J Ophthalmol.* 1996;80:545–548.

75. Gauthier CA, Epstein D, Holden BA, Tengroth B, Fagerholm P, Hamberg-Nystrom H, Sievert R. Epithelial alterations following photorefractive keratectomy for myopia. *J Refract Surg.* 1995;11:113–118.

76. Shieh E, Moreira H, D'Arcy J, Clapham TN, McDonnell PJ. Quantitative analysis of wound healing after cylindrical and spherical excimer laser ablations. *Ophthalmology.* 1992;99:1050–1055.

77. Beuerman RW, McDonald MB, Shofner RS, Munnerlyn CR, Clapham TN, Salmeron B, Kaufman HE. Quantitative histological studies of primate corneas after excimer laser photorefractive keratectomy. *Arch Ophthalmol.* 1994;112:1103–1110.

78. Lohmann CP, Patmore A, Reischl U, Marshall J. The importance of the corneal epithelium in excimer-laser photorefractive keratectomy. *Ger J Ophthalmol.* 1996;5:368–372.

79. Lohmann CP, Reischl U, Marshall J. Regression and epithelial hyperplasia after myopic photorefractive keratectomy in a human cornea. *J Cataract Refract Surg.* 1999;25:712–715.

80. Li HF, Petroll WM, Moller-Pedersen T, Maurer JK, Cavanagh HD, Jester JV. Epithelial and corneal thickness measurements by in vivo confocal microscopy through focusing (CMTF). *Curr Eye Res.* 1997;16:214–221.

81. Moller-Pedersen T, Li HF, Petroll WM, Cavanagh HD, Jester JV. Confocal microscopic characterization of wound repair after photorefractive keratectomy. *Invest Ophthalmol Vis Sci.* 1998;39:487–501.

82. Moller-Pedersen T, Vogel M, Li HF, Petroll WM, Cavanagh HD, Jester JV. Quantification of stromal thinning, epithelial thickness, and corneal haze after photorefractive keratectomy using in vivo confocal microscopy. *Ophthalmology.* 1997;104:360–368.

83. Feng Y, Varikooty J, Simpson TL. Diurnal variation of corneal and corneal epithelial thickness measured using optical coherence tomography. *Cornea.* 2001;20:480–483.

84. Wirbelauer C, Pham DT. Monitoring corneal structures with slitlamp-adapted optical coherence tomography in laser in situ keratomileusis. *J Cataract Refract Surg.* 2004;30:1851–1860.

85. Haque S, Fonn D, Simpson T, Jones L. Corneal and epithelial thickness changes after 4 weeks of overnight corneal refractive therapy lens wear, measured with optical coherence tomography. *Eye Contact Lens.* 2004;30:189–193; discussion 205–186.

86. Sin S, Simpson TL. The repeatability of corneal and corneal epithelial thickness measurements using optical coherence tomography. *Optom Vis Sci.* 2006;83:360–365.

87. Haque S, Jones L, Simpson T. Thickness mapping of the cornea and epithelium using optical coherence tomography. *Optom Vis Sci.* 2008;85:E963–976.

88. Li Y, Tan O, Brass R, Weiss JL, Huang D. Corneal epithelial thickness mapping by Fourier-domain optical coherence tomography in normal and keratoconic eyes. *Ophthalmology*. 2012;119:2425–2433.

89. Bentivoglio AR, Bressman SB, Cassetta E, Carretta D, Tonali P, Albanese A. Analysis of blink rate patterns in normal subjects. *Mov Disord*. 1997;12:1028–1034.

90. Doane MG. Interactions of eyelids and tears in corneal wetting and the dynamics of the normal human eyeblink. *Am J Ophthalmol*. 1980;89:507–516.

91. Young G, Hunt C, Covey M. Clinical evaluation of factors influencing toric soft contact lens fit. *Optom Vis Sci*. 2002;79:11–19.

92. Scroggs MW, Proia AD. Histopathological variation in keratoconus. *Cornea*. 1992;11:553–559.

93. Haque S, Simpson T, Jones L. Corneal and epithelial thickness in keratoconus: a comparison of ultrasonic pachymetry, Orbscan II, and optical coherence tomography. *J Refract Surg*. 2006;22:486–493.

94. Rocha KM, Perez-Straziota CE, Stulting RD, Randleman JB. SD-OCT analysis of regional epithelial thickness profiles in keratoconus, postoperative corneal ectasia, and normal eyes. *J Refract Surg*. 2013;29:173–179.

95. Kanellopoulos AJ, Aslanides IM, Asimellis G. Correlation between epithelial thickness in normal corneas, untreated ectatic corneas, and ectatic corneas previously treated with CXL; is overall epithelial thickness a very early ectasia prognostic factor? *Clin Ophthalmol*. 2012;6:789–800.

96. Sandali O, El Sanharawi M, Temstet C, Hamiche T, Galan A, Ghouali W, Goemaere I, Basli E, Borderie V, Laroche L. Fourier-domain optical coherence tomography imaging in keratoconus: a corneal structural classification. *Ophthalmology*. 2013;120:2403–2412.

97. Kanellopoulos AJ, Asimellis G. Longitudinal postoperative lasik epithelial thickness profile changes in correlation with degree of myopia correction. *J Refract Surg*. 2014;30:166–171.

98. Reinstein DZ, Archer TJ, Gobbe M. Refractive and topographic errors in topography-guided ablation produced by epithelial compensation predicted by three-dimensional Artemis very high-frequency digital ultrasound stromal and epithelial thickness mapping. *J Refract Surg*. 2012;28:657–663.

99. Reinstein DZ, Gobbe M, Archer TJ, Youssefi G, Sutton HF. Stromal surface topography-guided custom ablation as a repair tool for corneal irregular astigmatism. *J Refract Surg*. 2015;31:54–59.

100. Reinstein DZ, Archer TJ, Dickeson ZI, Gobbe M. Trans-epithelial phototherapeutic keratectomy protocol for treating irregular astigmatism based on population epithelial thickness measurements by Artemis very high-frequency digital ultrasound. *J Refract Surg*. 2014;30:380–387.

101. Vinciguerra P, Roberts CJ, Albe E, Romano MR, Mahmoud A, Trazza S, Vinciguerra R. Corneal curvature gradient map: a new corneal topography map to predict the corneal healing process. *J Refract Surg*. 2014;30:202–207.

102. Klein SR, Epstein RJ, Randleman JB, Stulting RD. Corneal ectasia after laser in situ keratomileusis in patients without apparent preoperative risk factors. *Cornea*. 2006;25:388–403.

103. Silverman RH, Urs R, Roychoudhury A, Archer TJ, Gobbe M, Reinstein DZ. Epithelial remodeling as basis for machine-based identification of keratoconus. *Invest Ophthalmol Vis Sci.* 2014;55:1580–1587.

104. Temstet C, Sandali O, Bouheraoua N, Hamiche T, Galan A, El Sanharawi M, Basli E, Laroche L, Borderie V. Corneal epithelial thickness mapping using Fourier-domain optical coherence tomography for detection of form fruste keratoconus. *J Cataract Refract Surg.* 2015;41:812–820.

105. Ambrosio R, Jr., Faria-Correia F, Ramos I, Valbon BF, Lopes B, Jardim D, Luz A. Enhanced screening for ectasia susceptibility among refractive candidates: the role of corneal tomography and biomechanics. *Curr Ophthalmol Rep.* 2013;1:28–38.

106. Gomes JA, Tan D, Rapuano CJ, Belin MW, Ambrosio R, Jr., Guell JL, Malecaze F, Nishida K, Sangwan VS. Global consensus on keratoconus and ectatic diseases. *Cornea.* 2015;34:359–369.

107. Najmi H, Mobarki Y, Mania K, Altowairqi B, Basehi M, Mahfouz MS, Elmahdy M. The correlation between keratoconus and eye rubbing: a review. *Int J Ophthalmol.* 2019;12:1775–1781.

108. Ambrosio R, Jr., Dawson DG, Salomao M, Guerra FP, Caiado AL, Belin MW. Corneal ectasia after LASIK despite low preoperative risk: tomographic and biomechanical findings in the unoperated, stable, fellow eye. *J Refract Surg.* 2010;26:906–911.

109. Dupps WJ, Jr., Kohnen T, Mamalis N, Rosen ES, Koch DD, Obstbaum SA, Waring GO, 3rd, Reinstein DZ, Stulting RD. Standardized graphs and terms for refractive surgery results. *J Cataract Refract Surg.* 2011;37:1–3.

110. Scarcelli G, Besner S, Pineda R, Yun SH. Biomechanical characterization of keratoconus corneas ex vivo with Brillouin microscopy. *Invest Ophthalmol Vis Sci.* 2014;55:4490–4495.

111. Abu-Amero KK, Al-Muammar AM, Kondkar AA. Genetics of keratoconus: where do we stand? *J Ophthalmol.* 2014;2014:641708.

112. Burdon KP, Vincent AL. Insights into keratoconus from a genetic perspective. *Clin Exp Optom.* 2013;96:146–154.

113. Rabinowitz YS, Dong L, Wistow G. Gene expression profile studies of human keratoconus cornea for NEIBank: a novel cornea-expressed gene and the absence of transcripts for aquaporin 5. *Invest Ophthalmol Vis Sci.* 2005;46:1239–1246.

114. Abou Shousha M, Perez VL, Fraga Santini Canto AP, Vaddavalli PK, Sayyad FE, Cabot F, Feuer WJ, Wang J, Yoo SH. The use of Bowman's layer vertical topographic thickness map in the diagnosis of keratoconus. *Ophthalmology.* 2014;121:988–993.

115. Yadav R, Kottaiyan R, Ahmad K, Yoon G. Epithelium and Bowman's layer thickness and light scatter in keratoconic cornea evaluated using ultrahigh resolution optical coherence tomography. *J Biomed Opt.* 2012;17:116010.

116. Kanellopoulos AJ, Asimellis G. In vivo 3-dimensional corneal epithelial thickness mapping as an indicator of dry eye: preliminary clinical assessment. *Am J Ophthalmol.* 2014;157:63–68. e62.

117. Reinstein DZ, Archer TJ, Gobbe M. *Stability of LASIK in corneas with topographic suspect keratoconus confirmed non-keratoconic by epithelial thickness mapping: 2-years follow-up.* San Fransisco: AAO, 2009.

7 Prescription of Spectacles in Keratoconus

Elham Azizi

INTRODUCTION

Keratoconus, as a progressive corneal ectasia, leads to the presence of progressive myopia, irregular astigmatism and higher-order aberrations. Visual acuity (VA) is usually affected from the first stages of the condition, such that the patient cannot be corrected to a clear 20/20 VA.[1] As a chronic condition, keratoconus requires long-time care with non-surgical and surgical management options.[2] In the first stages of the condition, i.e., in the mild stage or even when no keratoconus has been diagnosed yet and it may appear as an uncorrected refractive error, the first and simplest option is spectacles correction.[1] As the disease progresses, blur and distortion may exacerbate due to the increase in higher-order aberrations and corneal irregularity. It is estimated that 90% of patients use contact lenses in moderate stages of the disease.[3] In advanced cases, scleral lenses might be a better solution, especially if other contact lens modalities failed to achieve an acceptable fit.[4,5]

In spite of well-known usage of contact lenses in the management of keratoconus, some patients cannot wear their contact lenses for the whole day. The collaborative longitudinal evaluation of keratoconus (CLEK) study showed that 18% of patients could not wear their contact lenses for reading activity at night and 10% did not wear them during leisure time. Accordingly, 64% of keratoconus patients preferred to have a pair of glasses as an adjunct to contact lens wear and 16.1% of patients wore glasses as their primary vision correction.[6] Therefore, it appears that any patient with a history of keratoconus has experienced using spectacles; however, the methods of spectacle prescription are different in keratoconus patients in comparison with the normal patients. Here, in this chapter, we describe the usage of spectacles in keratoconus and will cover methods of spectacles prescription in these groups of patients.

SPECTACLES CORRECTION

In the early stages of the disease, vision can be corrected with spectacles. Studies have shown that between 58% and 71% of patients achieve VA of 20/40 or better with their spectacles.[7,8] However, as the disease progresses, the quality of vision with spectacles may diminish due to presence of higher-order aberrations and irregular astigmatism. In this situation, while vision cannot be corrected to better than 20/30 with spectacles, rigid gas-permeable (RGP) contact lenses are recommended.[7,9,10] RGP lenses, especially scleral lenses, have the advantage that they can conform to the shape of the cornea and cover all the irregularities, providing a functional vision in severe cases. However, it has been shown that patients might not wear contact lenses all the time, for instance, after waking up or at nights when they were intolerant to contact lenses.[9] In addition, patients used spectacles over their RGP lenses to eliminate residual astigmatism or as a reading glasses in forms of single vision or bifocals in presbyopia.[9] In cases of lost contact lenses or if there is an anterior segment disease which needed a stop to the wearing of contact lenses, patients require a pair of glasses as the first solution or as a back-up. Another indication of using spectacles is when visual impairment is detected in keratoconus children under the age of 20 years.[11] While travelling, patients might need a pair of glasses, especially in aircraft when planning to sleep on board. Although there is no definite consensus regarding the actual amount of usage of spectacles in keratoconus patients, considering all of the above-mentioned situations, having a pair of glasses at any stage of the disease seems necessary.

COMBINATION OF SPECTACLES AND OTHER TREATMENT MODALITIES

Spectacles Correction Following Corneal Cross-Linking (CXL)

It is not uncommon in keratoconus patients to be treated with more than one treatment modality. For instance, if there is a progressive keratoconus accompanied with moderate refractive errors, it can be treated by CXL and contact lenses, if the patient can tolerate them. The CXL is an outpatient surgical treatment with riboflavin (vitamin B2) and UV-A which aims to retard or halt disease progression by providing strong corneal collagen cross-linking. However, if the patient is intolerant to contact lenses, spectacles correction following CXL is suggested.[12] Although there is evidence that RGPs can be well tolerated due to the decreased corneal sensitivity and flattening of the cornea following CXL, it has also been shown that it can cause a delay in regeneration of the

DOI: 10.1201/9781003371601-7

corneal sub-basal nerve plexus.[13] Therefore, spectacles prescription would be logical after CXL for residual optical aberrations.

Spectacles Correction over Rigid Contact Lens Wearing

In patients wearing rigid contact lenses, there might be evidence of residual astigmatism which can be corrected with spectacles. In such cases, while they are wearing their contact lenses, a subjective refraction can be performed using ± 0.5 D cross cylinder at 90°, 180°, 45° and 135° and asking the patient if they see better in any direction. Correcting the residual astigmatism using the spectacles can improve VA and visual performance.[14]

Spectacles Correction Following Intrastromal Corneal Ring Segments (ICRS)

ICRS implantation with a femtosecond laser is recognized as a minimally invasive technique to improve VA in patients with keratoconus when there is severe VA reduction and high myopia and astigmatism.[10] Using this technique helps to improve corneal distortions and reshapes the cornea; however, residual refractive error should be corrected with spectacles or contact lenses.[15]

Spectacles Correction Following Penetrating Keratoplasty (PK)

After PK, patients might be intolerant of contact lenses; therefore, they would benefit from spectacles.[16] Asena and Altinurs observed that, in advanced cases who underwent keratoplasty (either lamellar or penetrating), visual stability took about one year after surgery to achieve and 83% of patients corrected with spectacles in comparison to 17% who wore contact lenses in a 24-month follow-up.[17]

DETERMINATION OF REFRACTIVE ERROR IN KERATOCONUS

Retinoscopy

Refracting the patients in the early stages of the keratoconus is performed as routine using a retinoscope and/or autorefractometer and then subjective refraction. However, the presence of irregular astigmatism and corneal deformities, when the severity increases, causes scissor reflex in retinoscopy which makes the refraction challenging and time-consuming. In such cases, use of mydriatic agent might facilitate the refraction by finding some clear area in parts of the pupil and evaluating the conical and apical areas in relation to the pupil. Keratoconus is usually accompanied with myopia and astigmatism except in Down syndrome (hyperopia and astigmatism). As the disease progresses, the amount of myopia and astigmatism increases. If there is a dim retinoscopic reflex initially, the minus power might be added in larger steps of 2 to 3 diopter (D) to facilitate the refraction. In advanced and severe cases, retinoscopy might become impossible. In such cases, corneal astigmatism can be determined using topographic maps.

Autorefractometry and Aberrometry

An autorefractometer might be used in the early stages of the disease; however, it is not recommended when the severity increases. The majority of autorefractometers sample a few small discrete points on the pupil in which the validity and accuracy of the results might decline due to increases in keratoconic distortion and scarring in more advanced cases.[18] Perhaps the new generations of autorefractometers which use the wavefront technology might give a better estimation of the refractive errors in keratoconus eyes, as they are able to detect higher-order aberrations.[18] Corneal higher-order aberrations, such as coma and trefoil, become higher in keratoconus patients as the disease progresses.[19] In keratoconus eyes, using aberrometry to refract the eye rendered a significantly more negative spherical equivalent in comparison with the subjective refraction.[20] Fredrikson and Behndig showed that using a small zone eccentric laser ray-tracing wavefront aberrometry to obtain the refraction of patients with keratoconus provided better spectacle corrected VA than the standard autorefraction. Keratoconus patients in this study ranged from mild to severe cases. The authors suggested eccentric laser ray-tracing data as a valuable tool to conduct a reliable subjective refraction in patients with keratoconus.[21]

Keratometry

Using keratometry to start the subjective refraction might be useful only in preclinical cases of keratoconus or in the early stages when higher-order aberrations do not yet exist. Keratometry only determines the astigmatic condition in the central 3 mm of the cornea and does not provide any information from the peripheral cornea.

Subjective Refraction

Objective findings from retinoscopy, standard autorefractometry or even keratometry might act as a good starting point, especially in the early stages of the disease. However, subjective refraction is a must in subsequent studies. As the disease progresses, the objective findings might be very different from the patient's actual refraction. Therefore, the best way to find the best refractive correction is starting with a subjective refraction. Subjective refraction and provision of the best spectacle-corrected VA in keratoconus patients remains a challenging task and an important part of the visual rehabilitation.

In the first step, minus lenses are added to the phoropter or trial frame in large steps of 1–2 D to obtain the best spherical VA. After that, the examiner should determine the astigmatic portion of the refractive error, using either an astigmatic dial or a stenopic slit in the trial lens box.

Astigmatic Dial Technique

An astigmatic dial, usually available in the VA charts, is a test with radially arranged lines which can help to find the axis of the astigmatism (Figure 7.1). After determining the sphere with the best VA, the astigmatic dial is shown to the patient and they will be asked to find the blackest and sharpest line on the chart. The blackest and sharpest line would be in parallel with the principal meridians of the eye's astigmatism. Figure 7.2 illustrates a case with compound myopic astigmatism. In this case, the vertical meridian would appear as the blackest and sharpest, as it is closer to the retina. In the next step, the examiner should bring the anterior focal line into the posterior focal line using a minus cylinder lens with an axis perpendicular to the blackest and sharpest line. Doing this will bring the focal lines of the Conoid of Sturm cone into one focal point. Now, all the astigmatic dial lines should appear equally black, although still unclear and out of focus. To make it clear, the examiner reduces or increases plus or minus lenses until the best VA is obtained with a VA chart.

Stenopic Slit Technique

Stenopic slit is an elongated pinhole used to find the approximate principal axes of the astigmatism. In cases with small pupils, corneal or lens opacities, keratoconus with scissor reflex in retinoscopy or irregular astigmatism, it can facilitate finding the spherocylindrical correction. At first, the patient's VA is recorded. In young patients, the eye should be fogged, and then the fog decreased until the most positive spherical power is found. Then, the examiner puts the stenopic slit and rotates it in front of the patient's eye until the sharpest meridian is obtained. Now, trial lenses, either plus or minus, are added in the frame to achieve the best vision on that meridian. Then, the stenopic slit is rotated by 90° and the same procedure is repeated by putting plus or minus lenses until the best vision is obtained in this meridian. The obtained results are then converted into sphere-cylindrical form, noting that the axis is at right angles to the obtained meridian.[22] If, for example, the patient reports the sharpest acuity with −2.00 D when the stenopic slit is at 90° and −6.00 D at 180°, the sphere-cylindrical form of his/her refractive error would be

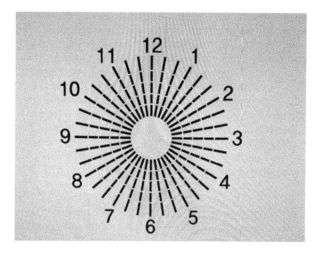

Figure 7.1 Astigmatic dial chart.

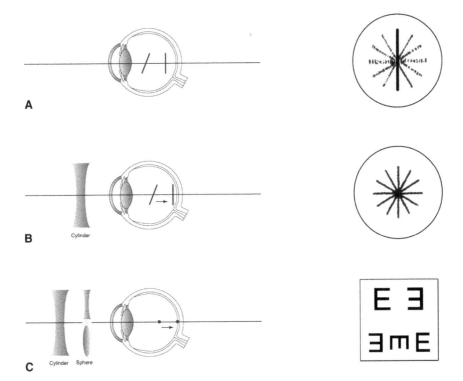

Figure 7.2 Astigmatic dial technique. A. An astigmatic dial as it is seen by a compound myopic astigmatism. B. Using a minus cylinder lens with axis perpendicular to the blackest and sharpest line. Now, all the lines appear equally blurred. C. Using a plus or minus sphere lens until the best VA is attained by using a VA chart.

−2.00– −4.00 ×90. In cases with severe and advanced keratoconus with an irregular astigmatism, the second sharpest meridian might not be perpendicular to the first principal meridian and it can be determined subjectively by rotating the stenopic slit manually until the sharpest view is obtained by the patient.[18]

In general, refraction of the patients with keratoconus, especially in more advanced stages, requires patience and time. Patients' ability to distinguish between the incremental changes in the amount of refractive correction might diminish as the disease progresses. Large steps of change in subjective refraction might be needed to obtain the best corrected VA with spectacles. Methods of binocular balancing in these cases might be meaningless, because in most cases there is not an equal VA between the two eyes.

FRAME SELECTION

After prescription of the spectacles was conducted using one or a combination of the above-mentioned techniques, the next step would be selection of a suitable frame for the patient. The frame selection in these patients in the early stages of the disease would be like normal patients, with no specific criteria, whereas, in advanced and severe cases with higher amounts of myopia and astigmatism, a number of features should be considered. The round or oval frames are better choices in cases with high amounts of astigmatism and myopia, while square-, aviator- or cat's-eye-shaped frames are not suitable. The frame size does not have to be wider than the wearer's face, as it makes the head look narrow in the area behind the frame in comparison with the rest of the face, which is aesthetically unacceptable.[23] The frame should be thick, as the thick rims can cover the thick edges of the high minus prescription and provide an acceptable cosmetic exposure. Flat frames should be selected instead of curved frames to minimize the peripheral distortions and enhance VA. A small lightweight round or oval frame with thick edges, possibly made from plastic material, would be comfortable for long-term wearing by the patient.

LENS MATERIAL

In cases with high levels of astigmatism and myopia, high-index plastic lenses are recommended. The higher index of refraction of a lens material causes a decrease in thickness and a lighter weight. The common CR-39 plastic lenses, used for low to moderate refractive errors have a refractive index of 1.50. High-index plastic lenses are manufactured in different materials such as polycarbonate (refractive index: 1.59), trivex (refractive index: 1.53) and NXT material (refractive index: 1.53). There are other types of lenses with higher refractive indices, such as 1.60, 1.67 and 1.74. Lenses with a refractive index of 1.67 or higher provide less than half of the thickness in comparison to the common CR-39 lenses; however, they are less than 20% thinner than polycarbonate lenses (refractive index: 1.59). High refractive index lenses reflect more light than the regular plastic lenses; therefore, an antireflective coating (AR coating) is essential to maximize light transmission and provide an optimum quality of vision.[23]

SPECTACLES CONTRAINDICATION

Spectacle correction is not able to compensate for irregular astigmatism and higher-order aberrations in advanced and severe cases, especially if the cone is in peripheral.[16] Moreover, in cases of unilateral high refractive errors, anisometropia and aniseokonia, spectacle prescriptions would cause issues for the patients. In such cases, RGP lenses would be an ideal refractive correction, providing a stable VA without fluctuation, especially at night, when there are changes in the pupil size.[24]

CONCLUSION

In conclusion, the prescription of spectacles in patients with keratoconus is a complex yet important part of managing this progressive corneal ectasia. The use of spectacles in keratoconus treatment is highly versatile, serving as primary vision correction in the early stages, an adjunct to contact lens use and a valuable option for visual rehabilitation after surgical interventions such as corneal cross-linking, intrastromal corneal ring segment implantation and penetrating keratoplasty. While contact lenses, particularly RGP lenses and scleral lenses, are commonly used in moderate to severe stages of keratoconus, the need for spectacles remains significant for various reasons, such as intolerance to contact lenses, residual astigmatism and as a backup for lost or temporary contact lens use. The determination of refractive error in keratoconus involves various techniques such as retinoscopy, autorefractometry, aberrometry, keratometry and, most importantly, subjective refraction. The presence of irregular astigmatism and higher-order aberrations, particularly in advanced stages of the disease, necessitates careful and methodical evaluation of the patient's visual needs. In the end, despite the challenges associated with spectacle prescription for keratoconus patients, it is an essential aspect of comprehensive patient care. Considering the prevalence of keratoconus and the significant role that spectacles play in managing this condition, it is crucial for eyecare professionals to understand the strategies and techniques of spectacle prescription in these patients. Future research and technological advancements may further refine these methods, ultimately enhancing the quality of life for individuals living with keratoconus.

REFERENCES

1. Rabinowitz YS. Keratoconus. *Surv Ophthalmol*. 1998;42(4):297–319.

2. Lim L, Lim EWL. Current perspectives in the management of keratoconus with contact lenses. *Eye*. 2020;34(12):2175–2196.

3. Rico-Del-Viejo L, García-Montero M, Hernández-Verdejo JL, et al. Nonsurgical procedures for keratoconus management. *J Ophthalmol*. 2017;2017.

4. Ling J, Mian S, Stein JD, et al. Impact of scleral contact lens use on rate of corneal transplantation for keratoconus. *Cornea*. 2021;40(1):39–42.

5. Koppen C, Kreps EO, Anthonissen L, et al. Scleral lenses reduce the need for corneal transplants in severe keratoconus. *Am J Ophthalmol*. 2018;185:43–47.

6. Wagner H, Barr J, Zadnik K, et al. Collaborative longitudinal evaluation of keratoconus (clek) study: Methods and findings to date. *Cont Lens Anterior Eye*. 2007;30(4):223–232.

7. Weed K, Macewen C, McGhee C. The dundee university scottish keratoconus study ii: A prospective study of optical and surgical correction. *Ophthalmic Physiol Opt*. 2007;27(6):561–567.

8. Zadnik K, Barr JT, Steger-May K, et al. Comparison of flat and steep rigid contact lens fitting methods in keratoconus. *Optom Vis Sci*. 2005;82(12):1014–1021.

9. Zadnik K, Barr JT, Edrington TB, et al. Baseline findings in the collaborative longitudinal evaluation of keratoconus (clek) study. *Invest Ophthalmol Vis Sci*. 1998;39(13):2537–2546.

10. Mohammadpour M, Heidari Z, Hashemi H. Updates on managements for keratoconus. *J Curr Ophthalmol*. 2018;30(2):110–124.

11. Weed K, MacEwen C, Giles T, et al. The dundee university scottish keratoconus study: Demographics, corneal signs, associated diseases, and eye rubbing. *Eye*. 2008;22(4):534–541.

12. Sinjab MM. *Keratoconus: When, why and why not: A step by step systematic approach*. JP Medical Ltd; 2012.

13. Sehra SV, Titiyal JS, Sharma N, et al. Change in corneal microstructure with rigid gas permeable contact lens use following collagen cross-linking: An in vivo confocal microscopy study. *Br J Ophthalmol*. 2014;98(4):442–447.

14. Reynolds A. *Corneal topography: Measuring and modifying the cornea*. Springer Science & Business Media; 2012.

15. Alfonso JF, Lisa C, Fernández-Vega L, et al. Intrastromal corneal ring segments and posterior chamber phakic intraocular lens implantation for keratoconus correction. *J Cataract Refract Surg*. 2011;37(4):706–713.

16. Mazzotta C, Raiskup F, Baiocchi S, et al. *Management of early progressive corneal ectasia: Accelerated crosslinking principles*. Springer; 2017.

17. Asena L, Altınörs DD. Visual rehabilitation after penetrating keratoplasty. *Exp Clin Transplant*. 2016;14(Suppl 3):130–134.

18. Benjamin WJ. *Borish's clinical refraction-e-book*. Elsevier Health Sciences; 2006.

19. Nakagawa T, Maeda N, Kosaki R, et al. Higher-order aberrations due to the posterior corneal surface in patients with keratoconus. *Invest Ophthalmol Vis Sci*. 2009;50(6):2660–2665.

20. Jinabhai A, O'Donnell C, Radhakrishnan H. A comparison between subjective refraction and aberrometry-derived refraction in keratoconus patients and control subjects. *Curr Eye Res*. 2010;35(8):703–714.

21. Fredriksson A, Behndig A. Eccentric small-zone ray tracing wavefront aberrometry for refraction in keratoconus. *Acta Ophthalmol*. 2016;94(7):679–684.

22. Harvey W, Franklin A. *Eye essentials: Routine eye examination*. Elsevier Health Sciences; 2005.

23. Brooks CW, Borish I. *System for ophthalmic dispensing*. Elsevier Health Sciences; 2006.

24. Caporossi A, Mazzotta C, Baiocchi S, et al. Long-term results of riboflavin ultraviolet a corneal collagen cross-linking for keratoconus in italy: The siena eye cross study. *Am J Ophthalmol*. 2010;149(4):585–593.

8 Management of Keratoconus with Contact Lenses

Masoud Khorrami-Nejad and Yasir Adil Shakor

INTRODUCTION

Keratoconus (KCN) is a type of corneal disease that does not involve inflammation but is characterized by the protrusion of a cone-shaped area and gradual thinning of the cornea.[1–3] The thinnest location is usually found at the corneal apex, which is often displaced slightly inferiorly and nasally. Typically, progressive irregular astigmatism can be compensated for with spectacle lenses in the early stages of the disease but requires the fitting of some special types of contact lenses (CLs) as the disease progresses.[4]

CL practitioners can play an essential role in the process of KCN management by providing acceptable vision through different types of contact lenses. Also, this option may preclude or hinder the need for corneal graft surgery. In 1888, Adolf Fick was the first scientist to describe the application of CLs for the optical correction of KCN.[5] Nowadays, there are various CL options with different materials and designs, which can be fitted in KCN patients to provide a satisfactory best corrected distance visual acuity (CDVA), reasonable comfort, and minimum complications. Throughout progression of KCN, these patients can be initially fitted with conventional soft toric CLs.[6] However, more advanced cases should be fitted with specialty contact lenses, including corneal gas-permeable (GP), scleral, hybrid, and piggy-back lenses, to achieve optimum vision.

CL fitting in KCN patients is challenging and requires a certain amount of experience. From the optical point of view, the first corneal GP contact lenses are usually an "amazing experience" for patients with moderate or advanced KCN. At the same time, it is also a tearful event, at least for the first CL attempt. Experienced fitters then note "tolerance normal" in the file, as habituation occurs quickly. A drop of topical anesthetic can be used once before the first trial lenses are worn to make it easier for particularly anxious and sensitive patients to get started.[7,8] If the patient later has an idea of the optimal visual acuity with the determined over-refraction, this usually provides enough motivation to overcome the awkwardness and the initial foreign body sensation. However, it leads to satisfied patients, especially compared with patients with regular refractive anomalies. Patients are usually satisfied with the occasional discomfort, e.g., dust or pollen allergy or tear film disorders, due to the large advances in CDVA and ease of handling, and the drop-out rate tends to be close to zero.

APPLICATION OF CORNEAL GAS-PERMEABLE (GP) CONTACT LENSES IN PATIENTS WITH KERATOCONUS

GP lenses are by far the most commonly used contact lenses for treating KCN patients and improving the visual quality in these cases. These contact lenses are superior to conventional soft contact lenses for patients with KCN.[9] GP lenses are better tolerated in patients with giant papillary conjunctivitis or dry eye.[10] Also, due to the greater tear exchange and oxygen transmissibility, they can preserve corneal health and wettability better than soft contact lenses.[11] Also, because of the material properties of GP lenses, they generally yield better correction of corneal astigmatism and high-order aberrations (HOAs) than spectacles or soft contact lenses in KCN patients.[12] Notably, the risk of contact lens complications, such as microbial keratitis, is considerably less in GP lens wearers.[13–15]

GP lenses are "rigid" lenses that maintain their shape when applied to an irregular cornea. A "tear lens" will be formed between the front surface of the cornea and the back surface of the contact lens, which can smooth the irregular surface of the KCN cornea.[16] By reducing the HOA and covering up both regular and irregular corneal astigmatism, this interaction produces a more even corneal surface and results in vision improvement. However, on some occasions, HOA may persist, particularly coma, and patients with more severe KCN may not be able to obtain 20/20 visual acuity.[17] Despite the marked advantages over soft contact lenses, a poorly fitted GP lens can damage the corneal tissue. For example, a GP lens that is fitted excessively flat on the cornea can bear the central cornea over time and may provoke the development of corneal scarring and progression of the corneal ectasia.[18] The Collaborative Longitudinal Evaluation of Keratoconus (CLEK) study investigated 1209 patients with KCN and found that decreased high- and low-contrast visual acuity in one or both eyes was associated with corneal scarring in 53% of patients with KCN.[19]

DOI: 10.1201/9781003371601-8

Numerous companies manufacture corneal GP lenses, particularly for patients with KCN. For instance, Blanchard, Lens Dynamics, and Acculens produce the CentraCone®, the Dyna Cone®, and the Accukone®, respectively. In addition to these lenses, there are a variety of designs known as Rose K lenses. These kinds of GP lenses are commonly used by contact lens practitioners and are widely available in many countries. The Rose K and Rose K2 designs are suitable for patients with mild to severe KCN, with base curves ranging from 4.30 to 8.60 mm and diameters ranging from 7.9 to 10.4 mm. The Rose K2 has aspheric curves to minimize HOA and a larger optic zone diameter to enhance vision under low-light conditions. Asymmetric Cornea Technology (ACT) is now available in both Rose K and Rose K2. Because of this, the lens's inferior quadrant can be steeper to match the steepest part of the cornea. Moreover, Rose K and Rose K2 are currently manufactured with Asymmetric Cornea Technology (ACT).[20] Because of this technology, the lens's inferior quadrant can be steeper to match the steepest part of the cornea.

The Rose K2 IC model is a corneal GP lens with a larger diameter than conventional Rose K. This lens design is effective for patients with mild to moderate KCN. It is available in diameters of 9.4– 12.0 mm and base curves of 5.70–9.3. Because of its large diameter, the Rose K2 IC typically has good centration on the cornea, resulting in less lens awareness than a decentered lens. In addition, due to its large diameter and less lens movement on the eye, it has less awareness than small GP lenses. Due to these properties, the Rose K IC design causes fewer adaptation symptoms in new wearers. In more severe cases of KCN, this design presents a challenge because, in these patients, the Rose K IC should be fitted with steeper base curves. Therefore, due to the lens's large diameter, the sagittal depth will be increased considerably, making it more likely to result in occasions of lens adherence. Because the epithelium is unable to withstand the pressure of the lens or the decreased oxygen levels resulting from the absence of oxygen-rich tear exchange under the lens. lens adherence is generally regarded as an improper fit. In addition, this design is effective for mild to moderate KCN but not for patients with nipple cones. The Rose K IC lens puts more pressure on the corneal tissue than smaller diameter lenses because of its large diameter. The epithelium can tolerate this pressure because it can be distributed over a larger area by a large cone. The pressure is spread out over a much smaller area of the ectasia by a nipple cone, and epithelial erosions may develop at the apex. Small-diameter corneal GP lenses can be used to successfully fit nipple cones.

From the clinical perspective, several specialty designs for KCN patients can be carved from various GP material buttons. The majority of laboratories utilize conventional GP materials, including Menicon Z® or Boston ES, EO, XO, or XO2. There are differences in some material properties of these materials, such as oxygen permeability (Dk), composition, and wetting angle. Currently, Boston XO2® and Menicon Z® are frequently used to produce GP lenses for KCN.

The corneal GP lenses have the benefits of being relatively easy to fit and being well tolerated by the cornea due to the availability of high Dk materials. In addition, they are relatively inexpensive compared with other options, and the handling and cleaning process are convenient. Furthermore, GP lenses are more deposit resistant than soft lenses and are a more preferable option for patients with atopic symptoms.

Corneal GP lenses have limited success when the cone is decentered in an abnormally inferior position. The visual axis may be outside the optic zone of the GP lens as a result of the lens's tendency to center over the cone's apex. This decentration causes poor vision and glare discomfort.

In patients with very severe KCN, corneal GP lenses typically have poor stability and retention, and their fitting may fail. Additionally, due to the possibility of debris entering under the lens and causing corneal abrasion and discomfort, they are not recommended for patients who work in dusty environments, such as landscaping, construction, or farming.

PRE-CONSIDERATIONS FOR FITTING CORNEAL GAS-PERMEABLE CONTACT LENSES

The visual acuity of patients with KCN can be improved through a variety of contact lens types. When selecting a lens, the most important consideration should be the topographic properties of the cornea, such as the size and location of the cone.[21] However, when selecting the best lens option, the patient's occupation, dexterity, lifestyle, and other ocular health conditions are all essential considerations.

Patients with subclinical or forme fruste KCN can obtain the ideal visual acuity by correcting their refractive error through eyeglasses alone. However, the inferior decentration and abnormal raised curvature of the corneal apex can lead to marked irregular astigmatism and HOAs in patients with moderate to severe KCN. In these situations, spectacles generally cannot provide optimal visual acuity. At these stages, contact lenses are utilized to reduce HOAs and correct irregular astigmatism in order to improve visual acuity.

There is no standard procedure for the fitting of corneal GP contact lenses in patients with KCN.[22,23] In addition to the stage and location of the cone, epithelial condition, tear film, eyelid tension, and corneal measurement data must be considered individually according to clinical practice. After standard measurement of the cornea, "diagnostic fitting" is often the method of choice for fitting GP lenses in KCN patients, i.e., the experimental modification of various lens parameters by the experienced fitter, depending on the fit and behavior of the lens with the fluorescein-stained tear film.[23,24] The static (with the lens being held centrally when required and without eyelid influence) and dynamic fluorescein patterns (with eyelid blink) are assessed.[23,24]

In order to achieve the desired fitting, despite the diversity of KCN designs, corneal GP lenses differ significantly in their structure, the lens design, whereby the back surface determines the fit of a lens to a large extent, while the optical correction of the entire system is then primarily the responsibility of the front surface.

There are six basic lens designs for corneal GP lenses; aspheric, three-curve, four-curve reverse, and aspheric design, KCN design, and quadrant-specific design. Aspheric, three-curve, four-curve, and KCN designs are shown in Figure 8.1:

- Aspheric design (Figure 8.1A): Centrally, a spherical region with posterior surface radius r0 is located, followed by a continuous aspherical region. At 30°, the eccentricity reaches its required flattening value. Eccentricities between 0.4 and 0.9 are possible.[25]

- Three-curve design (Figure 8.1B): In this case, the back surface consists of three radii (r0, r1, and r2) with two different zone diameters (d0 and d1). The peripheral radius r2 is larger than r0, with r1 acting as a link. Radii and zones can be selected individually within certain limits.

- Four-curve reverse design (Figure 8.1C): The posterior surface of this contact lens consists of four radii (r0 to r3) with three zone diameters (d0 to d2). The radius r1 is significantly steeper than r0 (therefore, "reverse"). Subsequently, r2 and r3 are flatter. Again, unique designs of radii and zone diameters are possible.

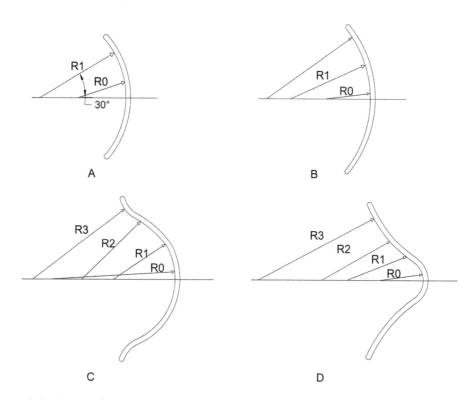

Figure 8.1 Contact lens design. A) Aspherical design; B) three-curve design; C) four-curve reverse design; D) keratoconus design.

- KCN design (Figure 8.1D): The posterior surface consists of four posterior surface radii (r0 to r3) and three zone diameters (d0 to d2). The special keratoconus design has a larger difference between the central radius r0 and r2 compared with the three-curve geometry. The peripheral radius r3 is relatively flat. As in Figures 8.1b and 8.1c, the zones and radii can be customized.

There are three fitting strategies for corneal GP lenses when dealing with KCN patients:[26]

1. *Flat fitting method:* In this method, the central optical zone of the lens bears on the corneal apex. The primary purpose of this fitting philosophy is that the optical zone of the lens flattens the central protruded area of the cornea to correct the ectatic area and provide an ideal vision for the patient. However, this fitting method can result in the development of corneal abrasion and central corneal scar in most cases of KCN.[27]

2. *Steep fitting method:* In this fitting philosophy, the supporting and bearing locations of the GP lens are away from the corneal apex and directed onto the paracentral areas of the cornea. Practically, there is a central clearance area that vaults over the corneal apex. Although this fitting philosophy is associated with the least probability of central corneal abrasion and scarring, it may cause corneal staining at mid-peripheral epithelial areas (3 and 9 o'clock corneal staining), and central cornea steepening.[28–30] They would also probably have a lower visual acuity (although this was not confirmed by the CLEK study, which demonstrated that eyes with mild to moderate KCN wearing steep-fitting lenses typically have higher visual acuity, about half to one line.[30]

3. *Three-point touch method:* In this fitting strategy, the supporting and bearing areas of the lens are divided between the central and mid-peripheral areas of the cornea. Central or peripheral lens bearing can lead to loss of epithelial layers, disturbances of Bowman's membrane and collagen morphology of the anterior corneal stroma, causing likely central corneal opacity, progressive ectasia, and reduction of CDVA.[30,31] Zadnik et al. discovered that the risk of scarring increased by 62% compared with that of eyes without lenses.[30] They also reported that steeper corneal curvature maximized the likelihood of corneal scarring by 26% for each diopter of curvature increase.

When blinking, an optimal fitting of the corneal GP lens should move about 0.5–1.0 mm to allow for tear exchange under the lens.[32] It should also center well to provide a clear vision. With the three-point touch method, the ideal fluorescein pattern should exhibit mid-peripheral touch with feather touch at the apex with surrounding pooling. An edge clearance of 0.5–1.0 mm at the lens edge is also necessary. A bull's eye pattern of concentric rings is the resulting fluorescein pattern. Instead of putting all of the weight of the lens on the cone apex, the mid-peripheral touch helps to spread it out over a larger area. The light apical touch also can reshape the central area resulting in a reduction in HOAs and vision improvement.[33]

Comfort with GP lenses is partly determined by how the upper eyelid and the lens edge interact.[34] Lens comfort is negatively impacted if the edge profile of the lens is poorly contoured or the edge is too thick. Lenses with a flat fitting relationship that decenter either superiorly or inferiorly have a tendency to trigger lid interaction, resulting in more corneal staining and discomfort.[34]

In the CLEK study, the relationship between fitting strategy and comfort was investigated. Patients who were fitted with apical touch or apical clearance reported the same level of comfort.[35] Comparing those with "average" peripheral clearance with those with a rating of "minimal unacceptable," patients with milder KCN were approximately half as likely to report good contact lens comfort.[35]

The most effective method of fitting GP lenses is that the primary lens-cornea bearing touches the corneal apex minimally and covers a large surface area in the middle of the peripheral cornea. There are two reasons why this bearing relationship is considered effective:

1. The thicker peripheral cornea, which supports most of the lens-cornea bearing pressure and has a much larger surface area than the central touch alone,

2. Because epithelial disruption is prevented, minimal contact with the lens preserves the central cornea.

The type and severity of the KCN, as well as the degree of ectasia and the curvature of the healthy peripheral cornea, determine the size and location of bearing area.[36] Because the mid-peripheral cornea is relatively even, this ideal fit is simpler to achieve in early KCN and centrally located nipple cones. However, as the mid-peripheral cornea becomes progressively more asymmetrical and irregular, it becomes more challenging to achieve an ideal fit in more severe cases or inferiorly located oval cones.

TOPOGRAPHY-ASSISTED LENS DESIGN

The fitting of custom GP contact lenses can be simulated using computer software that utilizes corneal topography technology.[37,38] This allows the practitioner to evaluate the quality of the contact lens fit through fluorescein simulation before inserting the lens into the patient's eye.[39] This method has been demonstrated to be safer, more precise, and simpler than conventional empirical trial lens fitting for choosing the initial trial lens.[37,39] This strategy not only reduces patient discomfort, chair time, and cost but also provides more visual improvements and patient satisfaction.[40] Although the initial software-suggested parameters may not be the best fit, they may require further adjustments to the lens parameters. Thereby, clinical expertise is still essential.

SPECIAL FEATURES OF CONTACT LENS FITTING

If the epithelium is in healthy condition, a three-point touch adjustment can be attempted. In this case, the apex of the cone is lightly touched during static fluorescein pattern assessment but flushed with tear fluid during each blink to keep the risk of epithelial erosion to a minimum.[41,42] In an ideal lens fitting for KCN, the apex should be free of irritation even after prolonged lens wear. Therefore, subsequent follow-up examinations are always performed after several hours of lens wear. McMonnies describes a risk of ectasia progression with steep fitting and scarring with flat fitting.[29] However, the longitudinal CLEK study by Zadnik et al. could not prove a causal relationship between flat fitting and scarring.[30] Flat fitting strategy often provides more desirable CDVA and better correction of HOAs than other fitting relationships.[30,33] In patients with KCN who are fitted with corneal GP lenses, routine examinations should be performed frequently because significant complications may be detected late. The reason for this occasion is most often due to the reduced corneal sensitivity in KCN patients who wear GP lenses.[28]

For determining the parameters of the first trial lens, practitioners can make complicated calculations or start with a back surface radius approximately 0.2 mm steeper than the flat corneal meridian, provided the numerical eccentricity is less than 1.0.[43] For higher e-values, it is preferable to choose the CL radius equal to the flat corneal meridian or, in the case of extremely flattened corneas, even somewhat flatter than the flat corneal radius.[24]

Suppose the spherical lens shows a desirable pressure distribution over the corneal area. In that case, it is well tolerated by the patient after adaptation time, and there is no higher cylindrical over-refraction; there is then no reason for a more elaborate design. Low cylindrical values of 0.5 or 0.75 generally require compensation of their spherical equivalent due to diurnal shape variations.

For fitting challenges, the usual procedures for corneal GP lenses can usually be used, e.g., choosing a smaller lens diameter for more movement or a larger one if there is too much movement. However, with large overall diameters, it may often be problematic that the lens shows a completely different pressure distribution in the periphery than in the center. If a peripheral toricity occurs there, for example, which impairs comfort or stabilization, a peripheral toric corneal GP lens can eliminate the problem. If the patient with KCN exceptionally requires a stronger plus effect, the CL will be relatively heavy, especially with larger diameters, and will tend to decenter downward. In this case, an integrated minus carrier helps to bring the lens back up to the center with each blink.[44]

If the patient does not tolerate a corneal GP lens, customized soft KCN lenses are currently available.[45] However, loss of visual acuity must be expected and, due to the extensive coverage of the cornea with moderately oxygen-permeable material, the recommended wearing time should be considered carefully. In addition, more frequent check-ups should be performed.

In most cases with KCN, it is beneficial to work with customized fitting lenses, and a final evaluation (prior to ordering the prescribed lens) regarding fit, visual acuity, and corneal condition should not be performed until the patient has been accustomed to the lenses for at least 14 days.

ALTERNATIVE CONTACT LENSES FOR THE MANAGEMENT OF KERATOCONUS
Piggy-Back System

In some patients, the touch of the center of the GP lens with the apex of the cone may not be tolerated and may lead to the development of superficial punctate keratitis. In patients with subepithelial corneal nodules, a well-fitted GP lens may not be comfortable even with light touch.

To increase lens wearing time and improve comfort, some practitioners may use a piggy-back technique by placing a soft contact lens behind the GP lens.[46] In this method, a soft lens is attached underneath a GP lens in the piggy-back lens complex to provide cushioning for a well-fitting GP lens.[47] According to Barnett and Mannis, this lens complex is especially helpful when GP lenses result in poor comfort, apical epithelial nodules (pip), marked epithelial disruption, or dystrophy of the Bowman layer.[48,49]

Adjusting the power can alter the fitting relationship between the soft lens and the GP lens.[50] A steeper GP lens will be needed if a plus-powered soft lens is utilized. In contrast, a flatter GP lens will be needed if a soft lens with minus power is fitted.

Hydrogel or silicone hydrogel lenses with a daily disposable, 2-week, or monthly wear schedule can be used, with silicone hydrogel providing optimal oxygen transmissibility. In addition, using silicone hydrogel lenses avoids the need for two separate cleaning systems. However, silicone hydrogel soft lenses may cause more epithelial irritation than conventional hydrogel materials.[51,52] In addition, piggy-back lenses are rather inconvenient since their handling is more challenging, their oxygen permeability is reduced, and they involve extra costs.

It is necessary to check the fit of the GP lens with both lenses in place because fitting of the GP lens is different when inserting a piggy-back system.[53] Utilizing fluorescein with a high molecular weight should be performed for the fitting evaluation.

X-Cel's "Flexlens Piggyback®" is comprised of a soft hydrogel lens specifically designed for use with a GP lens and can help keep it centered on the cornea for improved vision and comfort. However, some patients may still require a different lens modality that does not touch the cornea, such as scleral lenses. While piggy-backing may work appropriately for some patients, others may need to be refitted with a different lens type.

Soft Contact Lenses

Patients diagnosed with keratoconus often face difficulty improving their vision quality with soft lenses due to the tendency of the lens to flex over the cornea, failing to create the necessary lacrimal lens to address irregular astigmatism and HOA.[54] However, in patients with subclinical or forme fruste KCN, standard soft lenses, particularly soft toric lenses, may be applicable. Higher-modulus soft lenses with asymmetric design, such as Bausch and Lomb's Kerasoft®, Alden's Novakone®, and X-Cel's Flexlens®, have demonstrated the ability to correct myopia, high regular astigmatism, and certain types of irregular astigmatism.[55,56] In the scientific literature, the term "modulus" is known as the degree of rigidity or stiffness of the lens.[57] A lens with a high modulus will exhibit a slight degree of rigidity, allowing it to maintain its shape effectively over an irregular surface of the cornea. These lenses offer several benefits, including superior patient comfort and suitability for dusty environments. They are particularly useful for treating mild cases of KCN or instances where other treatment options have failed due to poor comfort. In addition, some authors showed a significant improvement of coma and some other HOAs with specialized soft contact lenses similar to corneal GP lenses.[45,58–61] However, there are also some disadvantages to using these lenses, including the potential for poor vision, reduced oxygen supply to the cornea due to low Dk and/or lens thickness, and limited insurance coverage.

Scleral Lenses

Scleral lenses are GP lenses with a large diameter that take their position on the sclera, avoiding contact with the sensitive cornea. They typically feature a central optic zone, limbal clearance area, and haptic zone (edge for scleral lens), which supports the lens's weight (Figure 8.2).[62] Given that the sclera can have significant toricity, a specific haptic design is often necessary. Scleral lenses are being increasingly used to correct regular refractive error and patients with mild or moderate KCN due to their reasonable comfort and less symptoms of dryness or lens intolerance compared with conventional GP lenses.[63] They are also effective in the correction of irregular astigmatism and vision improvements in patients with keratoglobus and pellucid marginal degeneration.[64–66]

Prior to insertion, patients should fill the lens with nonpreserved saline solution to make a lacrimal lens in the space between the lens and cornea, which optically masks regular and irregular astigmatism in the same manner as the lacrimal lens in corneal GP lenses. The benefits of scleral lenses are manifold:

- These lenses can be fitted in patients with advanced KCN that cannot be treated with other lens options because they vault the irregular surface of the cornea.

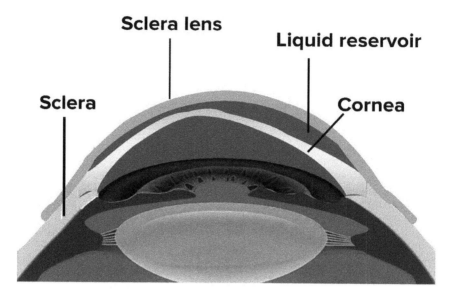

Figure 8.2 Schematic view of a scleral contact lens fitted for an eye with keratoconus.

- They are particularly suitable for patients with nodules at the apex of the cone who cannot tolerate other lens modalities, as well as those with ocular surface diseases like Sjogren Syndrome and ocular Graft Versus Host Disease (GVHD).

- They can be made from high-Dk materials for optimal corneal tolerance, and their large diameter usually ensures optimal centration and improved vision quality through the optic zone.

- Additionally, these lenses tend to be comfortable for several reasons: they rest on the insensitive sclera rather than the cornea, have minimal detectable movement due to their large diameter, and allow for minimal lid interaction because their edge is positioned beyond the palpebral aperture.

One of the drawbacks of scleral lenses is that fitting sessions for these lenses can be lengthy and frequent. They are difficult to fit correctly and require an experienced provider. The improper fitting can result in unusual complications. The two most common problems are: (1) if the sagittal depth is minimal and the back surface of the lens touches the cornea, it can cause a severe corneal abrasion; (2) if the haptic is too tight and causes conjunctival impingement and compression at the edge of the lens, it can lead to conjunctival hypertrophy and corneal neovascularization.Some patients may have difficulty inserting and removing scleral lenses due to their large size and the need for saline solution. After a few hours of wear, the lenses may cause vision to become blurry, which is known as "mid-day fogging" (MDF).[67] This symptom happens because the clear saline in the lens reservoir mixes with the natural tears and metabolic waste from the tear film, leading to turbidity. MDF is more common with scleral lenses, as the lacrimal lens layer is thicker with this modality.[68]

Scleral lenses should not be used in patients with a glaucoma drainage device, as the haptic can increase intraocular pressure.[69] They may also be unsuitable for patients with endothelial disturbance (endothelial cell count less than 1,000 cells/mm^2) because they could cause corneal edema.[70] Additionally, scleral lenses are expensive to fit and replace, and insurance coverage may be limited in some cases.

Hybrid Contact Lenses

Hybrid contact lenses consist of a central GP component and a soft silicone hydrogel or hydrogel surrounding skirt.[71] From the clinical perspective, in cases whose corneal GP lenses do not provide comfort, stability, and optimal centration, hybrid lenses are considered as alternatives.[72] However, Leal et al. could not acknowledge hybrid lenses to be better tolerated.[73] It has been observed that after wearing hybrid lenses, the tolerability of corneal GP lenses increases.[47]

These lenses are currently only produced by SynergEyes® (Carlsbad, CA, USA), which manufactures hybrid lenses with an overall diameter of 14.5mm and a central GP diameter of 8.5 mm.[72]

The first generation of lenses, referred to as the "Legacy Lenses," features a low-Dk hydrogel skirt and a high Dk central GP and is manufactured in two designs known as the "Clearkone®" and "SynergEyes KC®". The latest line of SynergEyes lenses features a high-Dk silicone hydrogel skirt attached around a high-Dk central GP and is manufactured in two designs known as the "Duette®" and the "Ultrahealth®".

The ClearKone is a suitable hybrid lens for treating patients with moderate to severe KCN who have nipple or oval cones. The design of the lens is reverse geometry so that it can completely clear the apex while vaulting over the irregular corneal surface. The lens has a pHEMA skirt and a central GP lens with DK=100.[74] The UltraHealth vaulted design features a hyper Dk GP lens in the center (Dk=130) and a silicone hydrogel skirt (Dk=84) in the periphery. The silicone hydrogel skirt has a 6.50 mm aspheric optic zone with the reverse geometry design, which connects to a steeper reverse geometry lift curve, allowing the GP center to entirely vault the corneal center while the lens rests on the inner soft skirt, which is toric-shaped.[75,76]

For individuals who have mild KCN or pellucid marginal degeneration, there is a tendency for corneal GP lenses to decenter towards the lower part of the cornea, resulting in patient discomfort and poor adaptation. However, hybrid lenses, which have a soft skirt, offer an advantage in that they tend to center more effectively, are better retained, and are generally more comfortable. In contrast to corneal GP lenses, patients using hybrid lenses may experience enhanced visual acuity as a result of their superior centration. Additionally, these lenses have demonstrated good performance in dusty environments, which is comparable to that of scleral lenses.

There are several drawbacks associated with these lenses, namely:

- Limited fitting parameters make it difficult to fit individuals with severe KCN.

- The insertion process can be more challenging compared with corneal GP lenses, as the lens must be filled with saline before insertion.

- Patients may have difficulty removing the lenses due to the silicone hydrogel skirt, particularly those with poor dexterity.

- They can be quite expensive since they are only manufactured by a single company and are occasionally not covered by insurance.

- The junction between the soft skirt and GP center can tear, requiring lens replacement.

Major complications include severe corneal edema,[77] significantly reduced endothelial cell count,[78] intolerance, lens defects, giant papilla formation, and also central corneal neovascularization.[72,79]

PROBLEMS WITH KERATOCONUS LENSES

In general, the following problems can occur with corneal GP lenses:

Infections. Microbial keratitis can be caused by CL wear and lead to serious complications.[80] Bacterial infections caused by *Pseudomonas*, *Serratia*, Gram-negative enterococci, and Gram-positive staphylococci occur mainly in northern regions, while, in southern climates, fungal and mixed infections are more common. *Acanthamoeba keratitis* is rather rare, but most episodes of acanthamoeba keratitis occur in CL wearers.[81,82]

Contact Lens Loss. CL loss is not significantly more common in keratoconus than in "normal" eyes, although CLs are, on average, much smaller in diameter and therefore have less adhesive power. The experienced CL wearer always has the previous set in reserve.

Edge Defects. Small protrusions at the edge of the lens, which usually result from the CL occasionally falling on the edge or being pressed under the fingernail, are not immediately noticed by many KCN patients due to the clear, elevated CL edge and do not necessarily and immediately cause corneal erosion but should be immediately replaced to ensure safety.[83]

Contact Lens Breaks. Because CLs for KCN almost always have minus power, the center thickness is correspondingly low, and the risk of breakage is increased. However, KCN patients are highly experienced lens wearers who can reduce the probability of lens damage.

Surface Deposits. The deposits over the lens surface tend to occur when cleaning is insufficient.[84] Some patients may forget about weekly protein removal in care systems. Therefore, it is often more appropriate to work with abrasive cleaners from the beginning. In the case of particularly steep back surfaces, the use of a cotton swab can help with cleaning.

Surface Scratches. It is quite normal that slight signs of CL use appear on the lens surface over time. These do not cause any problems. More severe scratches reduce wearing comfort and wettability, and the tendency of deposits occurring increases. Depending on the age of the lens, it may be necessary to have the surface polished, ideally by the manufacturer.

Dust Sensitivity. This naturally occurs with relative tear fluid deficiency. A workplace with much dust is not pleasant for any corneal GP lens wearer. However, a patient with KCN usually lacks the possibility to switch to glasses. In extreme cases, workplace alternatives should be considered to protect the corneal epithelium.

Occasional Intolerance. Although many KCN patients are known to suffer from various pollen allergies or neurodermatitis, which at least temporarily reduce the wearing comfort, the CLs are generally worn all year round.[85,86] Apparently, it is possible to resolve this difficult period with the help of antihistamines, tear substitutes, and eyelid sprays.

Foreign Bodies. They are felt more unpleasantly with rigid CLs than with soft lenses. The irritant secretion that occurs is usually sufficient to flush out the foreign body. The professional lens wearer carries his lens box with fresh storage solution or saline solution and can briefly remove the lens and rinse it in the solution if necessary.

Lens Dislocation. Corneal GP lenses are known to be smaller than soft lenses, causing minimized adhesion forces. Decentration due to careless eye rubbing occurs more frequently, especially with beginners or unusual corneal topographies and/or extreme eye movements. After the adaptation period, however, the CL wearer knows how to deal with this and can very easily manually bring the lenses back into position.

CONCLUSION

According to the literature, there are several modalities of lenses for the management of KCN, each with its unique set of benefits and drawbacks. The best corrected visual acuity is achievable with corneal RGP, piggy-back, scleral, or hybrid lenses which are all essentially comparable, as they all employ a rigid surface and lacrimal lens approach. Flexlens®, Novakone®, and Kerasoft® have been shown to produce a better improvement in visual acuity than other soft lenses, but they may not be effective in optimizing acuity in cases of moderate to severe KCN. Choosing the appropriate type of lens should be based on several factors, including corneal topography, cost, history of dry eye/ocular surface disease, history of atopy, hobbies/occupation, and manual dexterity.

It should be emphasized that contact lenses do not have any therapeutic effects on the stage of KCN. Patients need to be informed that using contact lenses does not prevent the progression of KCN and should only be considered when vision with spectacles is poorer than vision achieved with contact lenses.

Both patients and providers should be aware that fitting contact lenses for KCN patients may necessitate several lengthy appointments, and the type of lens used may require to be altered as the KCN advances. Reevaluation should be conducted every 6–12 months and every 12 months for unstable and stable KCN, respectively. If all available lens modalities fail, the situation may necessitate surgical intervention.

To sum up, there are numerous contact lens options employed to enhance vision in patients with KCN. While other designs are becoming more popular, the corneal GP is still the most frequently used and effective option. Familiarity with the different alternatives will facilitate a successful contact lens fitting for the patient.

REFERENCES

1. Romero-Jiménez M, Santodomingo-Rubido J, Wolffsohn JS. Keratoconus: a review. *Contact Lens and Anterior Eye.* 2010;33(4):157–66.

2. Khorrami-Nejad M, Aghili O, Hashemian H, Aghazadeh-Amiri M, Karimi F. Changes in corneal asphericity after MyoRing implantation in moderate and severe keratoconus. *Journal of Ophthalmic & Vision Research.* 2019;14(4):428.

3. Naderi M, Karimi F, Jadidi K, Mosavi SA, Ghobadi M, Tireh H, et al. Long-term results of MyoRing implantation in patients with keratoconus. *Clinical and Experimental Optometry.* 2021;104(4):499–504.

4. Watts A, Colby K. Contact lenses for keratoconus. In Alió, J. (eds), *Keratoconus. Essentials in Ophthalmology.* 2017; Springer, Cham. https://doi.org/10.1007/978-3-319-43881-8_16

5. Fick A. A contact-lens. 1888 (translation). *Archives of Ophthalmology (Chicago, Ill: 1960)*. 1988;106(10):1373–7.

6. Saraç Ö, Kars ME, Temel B, Çağıl N. Clinical evaluation of different types of contact lenses in keratoconus management. *Contact Lens and Anterior Eye*. 2019;42(5):482–6.

7. Bennett ES, Smythe J, Henry VA, Bassi CJ, Morgan BW, Miller W, et al. Effect of topical anesthetic use on initial patient satisfaction and overall success with rigid gas permeable contact lenses. *Optometry and Vision Science*. 1998;75(11):800–5.

8. Gill F, Murphy P, Purslow C. Effect of topical anaesthetic use on rigid gas permeable lens fitting. *Investigative Ophthalmology & Visual Science*. 2009;50(13):6357.

9. Downie LE, Lindsay RG. Contact lens management of keratoconus. *Clinical and Experimental Optometry*. 2015;98(4):299–311.

10. Carracedo G, González-Méijome JM, Martín-Gil A, Carballo J, Pintor J. The influence of rigid gas permeable lens wear on the concentrations of dinucleotides in tears and the effect on dry eye signs and symptoms in keratoconus. *Contact Lens and Anterior Eye*. 2016;39(5):375–9.

11. Carracedo G, Martin-Gil A, Peixoto-de-Matos SC, Abejón-Gil P, Macedo-de-Araújo R, González-Méijome JM. Symptoms and signs in rigid gas permeable lens wearers during adaptation period. *Eye & Contact Lens*. 2016;42(2):108–14.

12. Egorov G, Bobrovskikh N, Savochkina O. Possibilities of compensation of optical aberrations in keratoconus with rigid gas-permeable contact lenses. *Vestnik Oftalmologii*. 2010;126(1):42–6.

13. Morgan PB, Efron N, Hill E, Raynor M, Whiting M, Tullo A. Incidence of keratitis of varying severity among contact lens wearers. *British Journal of Ophthalmology*. 2005;89(4):430–6.

14. Mohammadpour M, Rahimi F, Khorrami-Nejad M. Total necrosis of cornea, iris and crystalline lens with exposure of vitreous hyaloid face in the context of recalcitrant Acanthamoeba keratitis. *Journal of Current Ophthalmology*. 2018;30(4):377–80.

15. Mohammadpour M, Hosseini SS, Khorrami-Nejad M, Bazvand F. Contact lens-related visual loss in the context of microbial keratitis. *Clinical Optometry*. 2019;11:11–4.

16. Gowans M. The lacrimal lens as an assessment factor in hard contact lens fitting. *Ophthalmic and Physiological Optics*. 1995;15(5):499–500.

17. Kosaki R, Maeda N, Bessho K, Hori Y, Nishida K, Suzaki A, et al. Magnitude and orientation of Zernike terms in patients with keratoconus. *Investigative Ophthalmology & Visual Science*. 2007;48(7):3062–8.

18. Macsai MS, Varley GA, Krachmer JH. Development of keratoconus after contact lens wear: patient characteristics. *Archives of Ophthalmology*. 1990;108(4):534–8.

19. Szczotka LB, Barr JT, Zadnik K. A summary of the findings from the Collaborative Longitudinal Evaluation of Keratoconus (CLEK) Study. *CLEK Study Group. Optometry (St Louis, Mo)*. 2001;72(9):574–84.

20. Aggarwal S, Vanathi M, Gupta V, Gupta N, Tandon R. ROSE K2 contact lens rehabilitation in keratoconic corneas. *The Official Scientific Journal of Delhi Ophthalmological Society*. 2022;32(4):28–35.

21. Nejabat M, Khalili MR, Dehghani C. Cone location and correction of keratoconus with rigid gas-permeable contact lenses. *Contact Lens and Anterior Eye*. 2012;35(1):17–21.

22. Edrington TB, Szczotka LB, Barr JT, Achtenberg JF, Burger DS, Janoff AM, et al. Rigid contact lens fitting relationships in keratoconus. *Optometry and Vision Science*. 1999;76(10):692–9.

23. Leung KK. RGP fitting philosophies for keratoconus. *Clinical and Experimental Optometry*. 1999;82(6):230–5.

24. Edrington TB, Barr JT, Zadnik K, Davis LJ, Gundel RE, Libassi DP, et al. Standardized rigid contact lens fitting protocol for keratoconus. *Optometry and Vision Science*. 1996;73(6):369–75.

25. Kok JH. A European fitting philosophy for aspheric, high-Dk RGP contact lenses. *Eye & Contact Lens*. 1992;18(4):232–6.

26. Itoi M, Itoi M. Management of keratoconus with corneal rigid gas-permeable contact lenses. *Eye & Contact Lens*. 2022;48(3):110–4.

27. Korb D, Finnemore V, Herman J. Apical changes and scarring in keratoconus as related to contact lens fitting techniques. *Journal of the American Optometric Association*. 1982;53(3):199–205.

28. McMonnies CW. Keratoconus fittings: apical clearance or apical support? *Eye & Contact Lens*. 2004;30(3):147–55.

29. McMonnies CW. The biomechanics of keratoconus and rigid contact lenses. *Eye & Contact Lens*. 2005;31(2):80–92.

30. Zadnik K, Barr JT, Steger-May K, Edrington TB, McMAHON TT, Gordon MO, et al. Comparison of flat and steep rigid contact lens fitting methods in keratoconus. *Optometry and Vision Science*. 2005;82(12):1014–21.

31. Zadnik K, Barr JT, Edrington TB, Everett DF, Jameson M, McMahon TT, et al. Baseline findings in the Collaborative Longitudinal Evaluation of Keratoconus (CLEK) study. *Investigative Ophthalmology & Visual Science*. 1998;39(13):2537–46.

32. Garcia-Lledo M, Feinbaum C, Alio JL. Contact lens fitting in keratoconus. *Comprehensive Ophthalmology Update*. 2006;7(2):47–52.

33. Jinabhai A, Radhakrishnan H, O'Donnell C. Visual acuity and ocular aberrations with different rigid gas permeable lens fittings in keratoconus. *Eye & Contact Lens*. 2010;36(4):233–7.

34. Sorbara L, Fonn D, Optom D, Optom M, Holden B, Wong R. Centrally fitted versus upper lid-attached rigid gas permeable lenses. Part II. A comparison of the clinical performance. *International Contact Lens Clinic*. 1996;23(4):121–7.

35. Edrington TB, Gundel RE, Libassi DP, Wagner H, Pierce GE, Walline JJ, et al. Variables affecting rigid contact lens comfort in the collaborative longitudinal evaluation of keratoconus (CLEK) study. *Optometry and Vision Science*. 2004;81(3):182–8.

36. Ortiz-Toquero S, Martin R. Fitting gas permeable contact lens in keratoconus; Still a challenge? *Ophthalmol Open J*. 2016;1(2): e9-e12. doi: 10.17140/OOJ1-e004

37. Nosch DS, Ong GL, Mavrikakis I, Morris J. The application of a computerised videokeratography (CVK) based contact lens fitting software programme on irregularly shaped corneal surfaces. *Contact Lens and Anterior Eye*. 2007;30(4):239–48.

38. Rabinowitz YS, Garbus JJ, Garbus C, McDonnell PJ. Contact lens selection for keratoconus using a computer-assisted videophotokeratoscope. *Eye & Contact Lens*. 1991;17(2):88–93.

39. Bhatoa NS, Hau S, Ehrlich DP. A comparison of a topography-based rigid gas permeable contact lens design with a conventionally fitted lens in patients with keratoconus. *Contact Lens and Anterior Eye.* 2010;33(3):128–35.

40. Bufidis T, Konstas AG, Mamtziou E. The role of computerized corneal topography in rigid gas permeable contact lens fitting. *Eye & Contact Lens.* 1998;24(4):206–9.

41. Romero-Jiménez M, Santodomingo-Rubido J, González-Méijome JM. An assessment of the optimal lens fit rate in keratoconus subjects using three-point-touch and apical touch fitting approaches with the Rose K2 lens. *Eye & Contact Lens.* 2013;39(4):269–72.

42. Romero-Jiménez M, Santodomingo-Rubido J, Flores-Rodríguez P, González-Méijome J-M. Short-term corneal changes with gas-permeable contact lens wear in keratoconus subjects: a comparison of two fitting approaches. *Journal of Optometry.* 2015;8(1):48–55.

43. Rajabi MT, Mohajernezhad-Fard Z, Naseri SK, Jafari F, Doostdar A, Zarrinbakhsh P, et al. Rigid contact lens fitting based on keratometry readings in keratoconus patients: predicting formula. *International Journal of Ophthalmology.* 2011;4(5):525.

44. Netto, A.L., Walline, J.J. (2004). *Contact Lens Fitting in Aphakia. In: Contact Lenses in Ophthalmic Practice.* Springer, New York. https://doi.org/10.1007/0-387-21758-4_13.

45. Sabesan R, Jeong TM, Carvalho L, Cox IG, Williams DR, Yoon G. Vision improvement by correcting higher-order aberrations with customized soft contact lenses in keratoconic eyes. *Optics Letters.* 2007;32(8):1000–2.

46. Smith KA, Carrell JD. High-Dk piggyback contact lenses over intacs for keratoconus: a case report. *Eye & Contact Lens.* 2008;34(4):238–41.

47. Sengor T, Kurna SA, Aki S, Özkurt Y. High Dk piggyback contact lens system for contact lens-intolerant keratoconus patients. *Clinical Ophthalmology.* 2011;331–5.

48. Barnett M, Mannis MJ. Contact lenses in the management of keratoconus. *Cornea.* 2011;30(12):1510–6.

49. Romero-Jiménez M, Santodomingo-Rubido J, González-Meijóme J-M, Flores-Rodriguez P, Villa-Collar C. Which soft lens power is better for piggyback in keratoconus? Part II. *Contact Lens and Anterior Eye.* 2015;38(1):48–53.

50. O'Donnell C, Maldonado-Codina C. A hyper-Dk piggyback contact lens system for keratoconus. *Eye & Contact Lens.* 2004;30(1):44–8.

51. Jalbert I, Sweeney DF, Holden BA. Epithelial split associated with wear of a silicone hydrogel contact lens. *The CLAO Journal: Official Publication of the Contact Lens Association of Ophthalmologists, Inc.* 2001;27(4):231–3.

52. Lin MC, Yeh TN. Mechanical complications induced by silicone hydrogel contact lenses. *Eye & Contact Lens.* 2013;39(1):115–24.

53. Baldone JA. Piggy-back fitting of contact lenses. *Eye & Contact Lens.* 1985;11(2):130–4.

54. Jinabhai A, Neil Charman W, O'Donnell C, Radhakrishnan H. Optical quality for keratoconic eyes with conventional RGP lens and simulated, customised contact lens corrections: a comparison. *Ophthalmic and Physiological Optics.* 2012;32(3):200–12.

55. González-Méijome JM, Jorge J, de Almeida JB, Parafita MA. Soft contact lenses for keratoconus: case report. *Eye & Contact Lens.* 2006;32(3):143–7.

56. Jinabhai A, O'Donnell C, Tromans C, Radhakrishnan H. Optical quality and visual performance with customised soft contact lenses for keratoconus. *Ophthalmic and Physiological Optics*. 2014;34(5):528–39.

57. Horst CR, Brodland B, Jones LW, Brodland GW. Measuring the modulus of silicone hydrogel contact lenses. *Optometry and Vision Science*. 2012;89(10):1468–76.

58. Marsack JD, Parker KE, Niu Y, Pesudovs K, Applegate RA. *On-eye performance of custom wavefront-guided soft contact lenses in a habitual soft lens-wearing keratoconic patient*. Slack Incorporated Thorofare, NJ; 2007. p. 960–4.

59. Katsoulos C, Karageorgiadis L, Vasileiou N, Mousafeiropoulos T, Asimellis G. Customized hydrogel contact lenses for keratoconus incorporating correction for vertical coma aberration. *Ophthalmic and Physiological Optics*. 2009;29(3):321–9.

60. Marsack JD, Parker KE, Applegate RA. Performance of wavefront-guided soft lenses in three keratoconus subjects. *Optometry and Vision Science: Official Publication of the American Academy of Optometry*. 2008;85(12):E1172.

61. Suzaki A, Maeda N, Fuchihata M, Koh S, Nishida K, Fujikado T. Visual performance and optical quality of standardized asymmetric soft contact lenses in patients with keratoconus. *Investigative Ophthalmology & Visual Science*. 2017;58(7):2899–905.

62. Schornack MM. Scleral lenses: a literature review. *Eye & Contact Lens*. 2015;41(1):3–11.

63. Bergmanson JP, Walker MK, Johnson LA. Assessing scleral contact lens satisfaction in a keratoconus population. *Optometry and Vision Science*. 2016;93(8):855–60.

64. Schornack MM, Patel SV. Relationship between corneal topographic indices and scleral lens base curve. *Eye & Contact Lens*. 2010;36(6):330–3.

65. Rathi VM, Mandathara PS, Taneja M, Dumpati S, Sangwan VS. Scleral lens for keratoconus: technology update. *Clinical Ophthalmology*. 2015:2013–8.

66. Fuller DG, Wang Y. Safety and efficacy of scleral lenses for keratoconus. *Optometry and Vision Science*. 2020;97(9):741.

67. Schornack MM, Fogt J, Harthan J, Nau CB, Nau A, Cao D, et al. Factors associated with patient-reported midday fogging in established scleral lens wearers. *Contact Lens and Anterior Eye*. 2020;43(6):602–8.

68. Walker MK, Bergmanson JP, Miller WL, Marsack JD, Johnson LA. Complications and fitting challenges associated with scleral contact lenses: a review. *Contact Lens and Anterior Eye*. 2016;39(2):88–96.

69. Fadel D, Kramer E. Potential contraindications to scleral lens wear. *Contact Lens and Anterior Eye*. 2019;42(1):92–103.

70. Van der Worp E. *A guide to scleral lens fitting: College of Optometry*. Pacific University, Forest Grove, OR; 2010.

71. Kloeck D, Koppen C, Kreps EO. Clinical outcome of hybrid contact lenses in keratoconus. *Eye & Contact Lens*. 2021;47(5):283–7.

72. Abdalla YF, Elsahn AF, Hammersmith KM, Cohen EJ. SynergEyes lenses for keratoconus. *Cornea*. 2010;29(1):5–8.

73. Leal F, Lipener C, Chalita MR, Uras R, Campos M, Höfling-Lima AL. Hybrid material contact lens in keratoconus and myopic astigmatism patients. *Arquivos Brasileiros de Oftalmologia*. 2007;70:247–54.

74. Hassani M, Jafarzadehpur E, Mirzajani A, Yekta A, Khabazkhoob M. A comparison of the visual acuity outcome between Clearkone and RGP lenses. *Journal of Current Ophthalmology*. 2018;30(1):85–6.

75. Harbiyeli II, Erdem E, Isik P, Yagmur M, Ersoz R. Use of new-generation hybrid contact lenses for managing challenging corneas. *European Journal of Ophthalmology*. 2021;31(4):1802–8.

76. Manczak H. Improving vision and comfort of patients with corneal deformations with implementation of ultraHealth and ultraHealth FC S-H hybrid lenses. *Acta Ophthalmologica*. 2015;93.

77. Fernandez-Velazquez FJ. Severe epithelial edema in Clearkone SynergEyes contact lens wear for keratoconus. *Eye & Contact Lens*. 2011;37(6):381–5.

78. Edmonds CR, Wung S-F, Husz MJ, Pemberton B. Corneal endothelial cell count in keratoconus patients after contact lens wear. *Eye & Contact Lens*. 2004;30(1):54–8.

79. Özkurt Y, Oral Y, Karaman A, Özgür Ö, Dogan ÖK. A retrospective case series: use of SoftPerm contact lenses in patients with keratoconus. *Eye & Contact Lens*. 2007;33(2):103–5.

80. Stapleton F. Contact lens-related corneal infection in Australia. *Clinical and Experimental Optometry*. 2020;103(4):408–17.

81. Schaumberg DA, Snow KK, Dana MR. The epidemic of Acanthamoeba keratitis: where do we stand? *Cornea*. 1998;17(1):3.

82. Hammersmith KM. Diagnosis and management of Acanthamoeba keratitis. *Current Opinion in Ophthalmology*. 2006;17(4):327–31.

83. Jackson AJ, Wolsley C, Briggs JL, Frazer DG. Acute rigid gas permeable contact lens intolerance. *Contact Lens and Anterior Eye*. 2001;24(4):161–7.

84. Luensmann D, Jones L. Protein deposition on contact lenses: the past, the present, and the future. *Contact Lens and Anterior Eye*. 2012;35(2):53–64.

85. Sharma N, Rao K, Maharana PK, Vajpayee RB. Ocular allergy and keratoconus. *Indian Journal of Ophthalmology*. 2013;61(8):407–9.

86. Ahuja P, Dadachanji Z, Shetty R, Nagarajan SA, Khamar P, Sethu S, et al. Relevance of IgE, allergy and eye rubbing in the pathogenesis and management of Keratoconus. *Indian Journal of Ophthalmology*. 2020;68(10):2067.

9 Corneal Cross-Linking

Epi-Off versus Epi-On versus Epi-Partially-Off Techniques

Mehrdad Mohammadpour and Masoud Khorrami-Nejad

INTRODUCTION

This chapter explores the different techniques of corneal cross-linking (CXL) for the treatment of keratoconus and corneal ectasia. It focuses on three main approaches: epithelium-off (epi-off), epithelium-on (epi-on), and partially epithelium-off techniques. The chapter begins by explaining keratoconus and the basic principles of CXL. It then delves into detailed descriptions of each technique, including their procedures, advantages, and limitations. The authors present a comprehensive comparison of epi-off and epi-on methods, discussing their relative efficacy, safety, and patient outcomes based on various clinical studies. Additionally, the chapter introduces newer variations such as the partial full-thickness epithelium removal and modified partial epithelial-off techniques. These emerging approaches aim to balance the benefits of traditional methods while minimizing their drawbacks. By examining the latest research and clinical outcomes, this chapter provides readers with a thorough understanding of current CXL techniques, their comparative effectiveness, and potential future directions in the treatment of keratoconus.

EPI-OFF TECHNIQUE

This technique is carried out under topical anesthesia. Firstly, 7 mm of the central corneal epithelium is removed (corneal thickness should be checked by pachymetry). Secondly, 0.1% riboflavin solution is applied prior to UV radiation every three minutes for 30 minutes. Riboflavin saturation is checked by slit lamp; this molecule produces oxygen-free radicals and protects the underlying structures. The UV is radiated from an optical instrument that comprises seven light-emitting diodes and a voltmeter to adjust the voltage. Before the procedure begins, the device should be set up, so the energy is 5.4 joules, the voltage is 3 mW/cm^2, and the working distance is 6 m.[1-2]

Another study was carried out by Kymionis et al. to explore the strong effect of pachymetric-guided CXL.[3] In this technique, after using pachymetry, two types of eyes were chosen: the KCN eyes and the ectatic eyes (after Lasik surgery), then the epithelium was debrided. Finally, CXL was performed using riboflavin hypo-osmolar and UV radiation. After nine months follow-up, the topographic data were stable and there was no damage to the endothelial cells.

A study by Hersh et al. in 2017 assessed the effectiveness and safety of CXL on 205 progressive KCN eyes. Patients were divided into two groups: the CXL treatment group (102 eyes) and the sham control group (103 eyes). In the CXL treatment group, after performing topical anesthesia and removing the central 9.0 mm of the epithelium, riboflavin (0.1%) in 20% dextran solution was administered topically every two minutes for thirty minutes. Then, 3.0 mW/cm^2 UV-A light was radiated to the aligned cornea for 30 minutes after ultrasound pachymetry was performed to ascertain that central corneal thickness (CCT) was more than 400 μm. During UV-A exposure, the riboflavin/dextran solution was administered again every two minutes. Finally, patients had antibiotic and corticosteroid drops applied (four times a day for two weeks) in addition to a therapeutic contact lens. In the sham control group, there was administration of riboflavin (0.1%) plus dextran solution (every two minutes for 30 minutes) without removal of the epithelium and an additional topical riboflavin administration (every two minutes for 30 minutes) was done on these patients during a turned-off UV-A light exposure to the cornea. Patients were followed up at one, three, six, and 12 months post-operatively in the first group, whereas patients in the second group were followed-up at the one and three months. After the three-month follow-up examination, these patients were allowed to cross over and receive the full treatment of CXL.

The outcomes demonstrated that the mean K_{max} value decreased and increased markedly by 1.6 ± 4.2 D and 1.0 ± 5.1 D from baseline to one year in the CXL treatment group and control group, respectively and the difference between K_{max} changed between groups was 2.6 D. Also, the maximum K_{max} decreased by 2.0 D or more in 28 eyes (31.4%) and increased by 2.0 D or more in five eyes (5.6%) in the treatment group. In addition, CDVA improved from 33.2 ± 13.4 D to 38.9 ± 11.8 D in the CXL treatment group and from 32.8 ± 13.6 D to 35.0 ± 13.8 D in the control group. Twenty-three eyes (27.7%) gained and five eyes lost (6.0%) 10 logMAR or more. Uncorrected distance visual acuity (UDVA) improved from 11.9 ± 12.2 D to 16.3 ± 14.5 D and from 8.2 ± 11.0 D to 10.8 ± 12.9 D in the first and second group, respectively. Corneal haze was the most reported CXL-related

DOI: 10.1201/9781003371601-9

adverse finding. There were no notable changes in endothelial cell count at the 12-month follow-up. They concluded that CXL was safe and efficacious in improving the K_{max} value, CDVA, and UCVA in progressive KCN eyes and was a new method to slow the KCN progression.[4]

EPI-ON CXL TECHNIQUE

Transepithelial or epi-on CXL is a technique accomplished without corneal epithelium debridement by using drugs like benzalkonium chloride, EDTA (ethylenediaminetetraacetic acid) and trometamol (Tris-hydroxymethyl aminomethane) as enhancers in order to loosen the corneal epithelial tight junctions and also increase riboflavin permeability through an intact epithelium. In this method, the complications of epithelial removal, such as post-operative pain and risk of infection (keratitis) and temporary worsening of vision, were fewer; so the tissue stress and treatment depth were dramatically reduced. Animal studies confirmed the fact that this method increases corneal rigidity.[2]

In recent years, several investigators carried out many studies regarding evaluation of this technique's safety and efficacy. For instance, Filippello et al. in 2012 used riboflavin 0.1%, dextrane T500 with trometamol and EDTA sodium salt for 30 minutes before 30 minutes of ultraviolet-A irradiation for 20 progressive KCN eyes. The corneal thickness was 412 ± 21 microns. After 18 months follow-up, it was revealed that the progression of KCN was halted, and the keratometric and visual results were also improved. In 2014, Lesniak et al.[5] performed transepithelial CXL in 30 keratoconic eyes by using proparacaine with benzalkonium chloride (BAK) 0.01% and riboflavin 0.10% without dextran. At the 6-month follow-up, a statistically significant improvement in maximum K values and CDVA was observed. In another study, Hersh et al. in 2018 treated 82 KCN eyes by applying riboflavin 0.1% and a topical anesthetic containing benzalkonium chloride every one or two minutes (two groups of randomized eyes) during ultraviolet-A irradiance at 3 mW/cm^2. Marked improvements in maximum K and UDVA were reported at the 1-year follow-up.[6] Spadea et al. in 2012[7] and Akbar et al., in 2017[8] used this protocol on thin corneas (less than 400 μm) of patients with progressive KCN, who were not treatable by standard CXL. Although different substances were added to enhance epithelial penetration, both studies came to the same conclusion that epi-on CXL is an effective method for ultra/thin corneas.[9]

COMPARISON OF EPI-OFF AND EPI-ON CXL TECHNIQUES

There have been several studies comparing epi-off and epi-on CXL. In the following section, some of the latest articles are represented. In 2017, Li et al. evaluated the safety and effectiveness of 244 KCN eyes. Although observing similar safety in both groups, the standard CXL group presented a more significant improvement of K_{max} while the transepithelial CXL group demonstrated greater improvement in CDVA.[10]

Some of the comparative studies demonstrated that the epi-off CXL technique was more effective and safer than the epi-on method. For example, in 2015, Al Fayez and colleagues conducted a study on 70 progressive KCN patients. When measuring K_{max} changes during the 3-year follow-up period, the epi-off group presented a more significant decrease (2.4 D) than the epi-on group (1.1 D). In addition, the authors concluded that the epi-off CXL technique was more efficacious with respect to halting KCN progression than the epi-on technique.[11]

Another comparative study was carried out by Kocak et al. on progressive KCN eyes in 2014. In their conclusion, epi-off CXL seemed to be effective in halting the progress of KCN and improving corneal parameters. In a study by Arance-Gil et al.[12] study (2020), 64 progressive KCN eyes were treated by epi-off CXL (31 eyes) or by epi-on CXL (33 eyes) procedures. Halting and stabilizing the KCN progression was observed in both groups; however, epi-off treatment appeared to be more efficacious. Furthermore, there was a greater improvement in CDVA with central than with paracentral KCN.[13]

Conversely, some studies demonstrated similar results from these two techniques. For instance, Çerman et al. in 2015 treated 60 progressive KCN eyes with epi-off and epi-on CXL methods. According to the results, epi-off CXL technique appeared to be more effective with respect to topographic indices, although, when the effects on visual acuity were compared, the two groups demonstrated similar consequences. Another study was conducted by Rossi and colleagues[14] in 2015 on 20 eyes with progressive KCN. There were remarkable improvements in UDVA, CDVA, topographic outcomes, and spherical equivalent (SE) in both groups at the 1-year follow-up post-operatively.[15]

Moreover, in some articles, better outcomes were observed from the epi-on CXL method than from the epi-off CXL technique. For instance, in 2018, a study was performed by Cifariello et al. on 40 progressive KCN patients with a 2-year follow-up. They reported that both procedures could slow KCN progression. Also, in both groups, the results and related complications were similar. In accordance with the outcomes, epi-on CXL technique was preferred to epi-off CXL as it maintained the corneal thickness and improved visual acuity (VA), while reducing the ocular complication post-operatively.[16]

In the Magli et al. study, two groups of pediatric patients with progressive KCN were treated by epi-off (23 eyes) or trans-epithelial CXL (TE-CXL) (14 eyes) techniques. In both the first (epi-off) and second (TE-CXL) groups, there were remarkable improvements in K_{max} (–1.11 and –1.14 D, respectively), Kmin (–3.2 and –2.4 D, respectively), mean-K (–1.47 and –1.63 D, respectively), surface asymmetry index (–0.64 and –0.86 D, respectively), I-S symmetry index (–0.54 and –0.55 D, respectively), index of height asymmetry (–2.97 and –2.95 D, respectively) and anterior elevation at the thinnest location (–2.82 and –2.96 D, respectively) and at the apex (–2.27 and –2.19 D, respectively). In addition, there was no corneal edema after TE-CXL post-operatively, whereas it lasted three months in 16 eyes and more than six months in two eyes after epi-off CXL treatment. At a 12-month follow-up, they reported that the TE-CXL technique was less painful and resulted in fewer postoperative complications than the epi-off method. However, there was no considerable difference between the two groups regarding the improvements of measured parameters.[17]

PARTIAL FULL-THICKNESS EPITHELIUM REMOVAL

In addition to compare epi-off and epi-on CXL techniques, several researchers introduced a new technique (partial corneal full-thickness de-epithelization) which is an improvement on the standard technique.

Razmjoo et al. published an article describing a study which was conducted on 44 keratoconic eyes in 2014. Their study aimed to report the corneal haze and visual outcome after collagen cross-linking to compare total epithelium removal and partial epithelium removal methods. In their study, two groups of patients were enrolled: in the first group of 22 eyes, the epithelium of the cornea was removed totally over the central 9 mm, whereas in the second group of 22 eyes, the central 3 mm was retained intact and the outer ring (3 mm width) of the epithelium was removed. In accordance with their method of surgery, first of all, pilocarpine 2% and then topical anesthesia were applied to all patients. Afterward, they performed epithelium removal by mechanical debridement and, after every one-minute administration of riboflavin (0.1% in 20% dextran solution) every 30 minutes, 3 mW/cm² UV-A was irradiated to the cornea for half an hour at a working distance of 5 cm. Finally, patients received therapeutic contact lenses, which were maintained for one week post-operatively. At the 6-month follow-up, the authors found that there was no significant difference between the two groups regarding corneal haze, intra ocular pressure (IOP), and improvement of sphere, cylinder, and visual acuity. However, by comparing parameters within each group pre- and post-operatively, Razmjoo et al. reported that patients in the first group manifested a marked decrease in K_{max}, Q-value, and index of height asymmetry (IHA), while eyes in the second group revealed greater improvements in BCVA and R-min. There was a considerable and similar increase in corneal density in both groups post-operatively. In their conclusion, the authors deduced that the partial de-epithelization technique improved corrected vision, whereas it was ineffective for decreasing corneal haziness. Conversely, patients treated with total removal CXL showed more significant improvement in K-max and Q-value. But, recently, however, this research team has announced that they had abandoned this technique due to the presence of haze, corneal thinning, and endothelial cell damage in the intact epithelial central region.[18]

In 2016, research was published, by Galvis et al., on 80 keratoconic eyes studied over a five-year period. In their study, pilocarpine 2% and proparacaine 0.5% were applied one hour and immediately before surgery. Then, the epithelium of the cornea in vertical full-thickness stripes and within 9 mm central of the cornea were removed. Subsequently, after riboflavin drops were placed into the cornea (every 5 minutes for 30 minutes), 3 mW/cm² UV-A light at a 5-cm work distance was used for 30 minutes by applying the UV-X Illumination System and every five minutes of topical riboflavin after the exposure. At the last follow-up, the authors reported that there were no marked improvements in the sphere, cylinder, SE, flatter, stepper, and average mean average K, CT, CH, and CRF. In contrast, there was a mild improvement in DCVA (from 20/39 to 20/36) and the endothelial cell count decreased by 4.7% ± 7.2%. According to the results, Galvis et al. concluded that this technique is safe and efficacious in halting KCN progression.[19]

Authors of both aforementioned studies[18,19] suggested that further studies with a more significant number of eyes and with longer follow-up times are needed to assess if this method (partial de-epithelization) could be considered a good alternative to the standard total corneal de-epithelization cross-linking procedure.

Two more studies on this topic were conducted by Hashemi et al. in 2013 and 2015.

The first study reported the results of a five-year study on corneal CXL with partial epithelium removal in 40 progressive KCN eyes. After local anesthesia by adding proparacaine hydrochloride 0.5% three times, 5 minutes apart, the 8 to 9 mm center of the epithelium was removed manually as three or four vertical strips (2 mm wide), with 1-mm strips of epithelium in between being kept intact. In addition, another strip was horizontally removed at the inferior third of the cornea. Then, riboflavin 0.1% in 20% dextran solution was added every three minutes onto the cornea for 30 minutes. At the final stage, to achieve UV irradiation (3 mW/cm^2) at a 5-cm perpendicular distance from the eye, the UV-X Illumination System was used for 30 minutes while riboflavin was instilled every three minutes. The results demonstrated that, in addition to UCVA and BCVA improvements, the mean MRSE and mean refractive cylinder error decreased from −3.18 ± 2.23 D to −2.77 ± 2.18 D and −3.14 ± 2.22 to −2.49 ± 1.71, respectively. Also, there was a slight decrease in mean max-K (0.24) and mean-K (0.11). In addition, the CCT changed from 483.87 ± 29.07 to 485.95 ± 28.43 μm. Based on these outcomes, the authors concluded that CXL treatment can halt KCN progression and can remove the keratoplasty requirement.[20]

Their second study compared total and partial epithelium removal in corneal cross-linking on 80 progressive KCN eyes for a one-year follow-up. Patients were divided into two groups: the total group (40 eyes) and the partial group (40 eyes). One year after CXL, the improvement of UDVA in the total and partial groups were 0.13 ± 0.42 and 0.12 ± 0.36 logMAR, respectively and CDVA improved by 0.00 ± 0.19 and 0.13 ± 0.20 logMAR in the first and second group, respectively. The decrease in SE in the total group and partial group was 0.44 ± 1.25 D and 0.56 ± 1.47 D. Also, max-K and mean-K decreased by 0.39 ± 0.93 D and 0.42 ± 0.93 D, respectively in the first group and 0.01 ± 0.95 D and 0.00 ± 0.65 D in the second one, respectively. In addition, CCT decreased by 18.39 ± 20.66 μm in the total group and 0.11 ± 13.29 μm in the partial group.

The authors concluded that both groups generated similar outcomes regarding UDVA, whereas there were small differences in CDVA and CCT (with better results in the partial group) and also corneal flattening (had better results in the total group). They also reported that long-term studies are required to compare both techniques regarding slowing the KCN progression and results stability.[21]

MODIFIED PARTIAL EPITHELIAL-OFF TECHNIQUE

Nattis et al. in 2018 evaluated a sequential treatment algorithm for visual and keratometric improvement after CXL followed by TG-PRK on 62 KCN eyes. There were two groups of patients: In the first group, 34 eyes had both topographic and refractive treatment, whereas, in the second group, 28 eyes had topographic irregularity treatment only. The time between CXL and Photorefractive keratectomy (PRK) was four to ten months.

The following procedures described the surgical technique of the CXL method. First, a topical proparacaine hydrochloride solution 0.5% was used for anesthetizing the ocular surface. To increase riboflavin penetration, they used a specific (cotton-tipped) applicator to make punctate ablations superficially on the corneal epithelium while performing a modified epi-on method. Then, after applying isotonic riboflavin 0.5% solution without dextran every two minutes for 1 hour, the eye was examined at the slit-lamp to evaluate stromal absorption of riboflavin. Afterward, the CCL-Vario 365 system (365 nm wavelength, 15 mW/cm^2 fluence) was applied for 5 minutes to achieve adequate riboflavin saturation of the cornea. In the last step, a therapeutic contact lens was inserted and medication with specific dosages were given to the patients, namely ofloxacin 0.3%, prednisolone acetate 1.0%, and bromfenac 0.07% (dosages were as follows: four times a day until epithelial closure, four times a day for one week, and twice a day for three days, respectively).

PRK was performed after CXL when there had been no changes in refraction or topographic parameters for at least three months. After analyzing topographic images, the surgeon carried out the appropriate PRK surgical plan. The aim of the plan was to treat as much refractive error as possible, in addition to corneal topographic irregularities. If the residual stromal bed (RSB) thickness was 300 mm or less, only topographic irregularities were treated, and a 6-mm optical zone was used for ablation. Otherwise, patients were treated with a 6.5 mm optical zone. PRK was performed in a standard manner and applied by an excimer laser. Similar to the CXL procedure, a topical proparacaine hydrochloride solution 0.5% was used for anesthesia. Then, epithelium removal was achieved using a blunt spatula. The eye was placed at the center, focused under the excimer laser, the image was registered, and then the eye was treated. Finally, after placing a bandage contact lens, ofloxacin 0.3%, prednisolone acetate 1.0%, and bromfenac 0.07% ophthalmic drops with specific dosages were applied (dosages were as follows: four times a day until epithelial closure, four times a day tapered over one month, and twice a day for three days, respectively).

After CXL, 3 months after PRK, and 6 months after PRK, the overall data across all groups demonstrated that, in terms of UDVA and CDVA, there was no change in UDVA and a 1-line gain in CDVA after CXL and three months after PRK, and there was a 1-line gain in UDVA and a 2-line gain in CDVA six months after PRK.

Regarding corneal astigmatism, there was a decrease by a mean of −0.41 D after CXL, a mean change of +0.26 D and +0.29 D at three and six months after PRK, respectively.

SE became more hyperopic by +1.37 D, +0.33 D, and +0.02 D in each of the groupings, respectively. With CCT, the mean decrease was 20.2 μm, −51.91 μm, and −58.07 μm in the three groupings, respectively. The mean K decreased by −0.05 D, and the mean maximum K decreased by −0.20 D after CXL. There was a mean change in steepest-K of +0.50 D and in the mean K of +1.50 D three months after PRK and there was a mean change in maximum K of −0.77 D and in mean K of +0.43 D six months after PRK. There was a considerable improvement in UDVA and CDVA in the refractive group (20/60 and 20/30, respectively) in comparison with the nonrefractive group (20/100 and 20/40, respectively) six months after PRK. The mean-K at baseline did not seem to have a statistically different effect on UDVA or CDVA six months after PRK. In addition, there was a statistically significant improvement in spherical equivalent toward emmetropia three and six months after PRK in the refractive group relative to the nonrefractive group. However, there was no significant difference between the two groups at baseline or after CXL. There was no statistically significant difference in corneal astigmatism, CCT, K_{max}, or mean-K between the two groups at baseline, after CXL, three months after PRK or six months after PRK. They suggested the use of refractive treatment in addition to topographic treatment for visual improvement in KCN patients who were treated with CXL and PRK.[22]

This chapter provides an in-depth comparative analysis of the epi-off and epi-on techniques based on various studies, assessing their safety, efficacy, and impact on patient outcomes. The authors include detailed descriptions of each procedure, focusing on their performance, outcome measurements, and potential complications. The chapter concludes with a discussion on the comparative studies between epi-off and epi-on CXL techniques, highlighting the strengths and weaknesses of both.

In this chapter, we focus on the comparative analysis of three different techniques of CXL, namely epi-off, epi-on, and epi-partially-off. The epi-off method involves the removal of corneal epithelium to allow penetration of riboflavin into the stroma, followed by UV radiation. Despite its effectiveness, it has limitations, such as post-operative pain, risk of infection, and delayed wound healing. On the other hand, the epi-on technique is performed without corneal epithelium debridement. It employs drugs to loosen the tight corneal epithelial junctions and increase riboflavin permeability through an intact epithelium. Although it has fewer complications compared to the epi-off technique, its efficacy in halting keratoconus progression is still under scrutiny. We also mention the partial full-thickness epithelium removal method and the modified partial epithelial-off technique. While epi-off CXL is reported to be more efficacious in halting keratoconus progression, epi-on CXL is found to have fewer complications.

REFERENCES

1. Nicula CA, Nicula D, Rednik AM, Bulboacă AE. Comparative results of "epi-off" conventional versus "epi-off" accelerated cross-linking procedure at 5-year follow-up. *Journal of Ophthalmology*. 2020;2020:4745101.

2. Beckman KA, Milner MS, Luchs JI, Majmudar PA. Corneal cross-linking: Epi-On vs. Epi-Off current protocols, pros, and cons. *Current Ophthalmology Reports*. 2020;8:99–103.

3. Kymionis GD, Diakonis VF, Coskunseven E, Jankov M, Yoo SH, Pallikaris IG. Customized pachymetric guided epithelial debridement for corneal collagen cross linking. *BMC Ophthalmology*. 2009;9(1):1–4.

4. Hersh PS, Stulting RD, Muller D, Durrie DS, Rajpal RK, Binder PS, et al. United States multicenter clinical trial of corneal collagen crosslinking for keratoconus treatment. *Ophthalmology*. 2017;124(9):1259–70.

5. Lesniak SP, Hersh PS. Transepithelial corneal collagen crosslinking for keratoconus: six-month results. *Journal of Cataract & Refractive Surgery*. 2014 Dec 1;40(12):1971–9.

6. Hersh PS, Lai MJ, Gelles JD, Lesniak SP. Transepithelial corneal crosslinking for keratoconus. *Journal of Cataract & Refractive Surgery*. 2018 Mar 1;44(3):313–22.

7. Spadea L, Mencucci R. Transepithelial corneal collagen cross-linking in ultrathin keratoconic corneas. *Clinical Ophthalmology*. 2012 Nov 2:1785–92.

8. Akbar B, Intisar-Ul-Haq R, Ishaq M, Arzoo S, Siddique K. Transepithelial corneal crosslinking in treatment of progressive keratoconus: 12 months' clinical results. *Pak J Med Sci*. 2017 May-Jun;33(3):570–75.

9. Filippello M, Stagni E, O'Brart D. Transepithelial corneal collagen crosslinking: bilateral study. *Journal of Cataract & Refractive Surgery*. 2012;38(2):283–91.

10. Li W, Wang B. Efficacy and safety of transepithelial corneal collagen crosslinking surgery versus standard corneal collagen crosslinking surgery for keratoconus: a meta-analysis of randomized controlled trials. *BMC Ophthalmology*. 2017;17(1):1–7.

11. Al Fayez MF, Alfayez S, Alfayez Y. Transepithelial versus epithelium-off corneal collagen cross-linking for progressive keratoconus: a prospective randomized controlled trial. *Cornea*. 2015;34:S53–S6.

12. Arance-Gil Á, Villa-Collar C, Pérez-Sanchez B, Carracedo G, Gutiérrez-Ortega R. Epithelium-Off vs. transepithelial corneal collagen crosslinking in progressive keratoconus: 3 years of follow-up. *J Optom*. 2021 Apr-Jun;14(2):189–98.

13. Kocak I, Aydin A, Kaya F, Koç H. Comparison of transepithelial corneal collagen crosslinking with epithelium-off crosslinking in progressive keratoconus. *Journal Français D'ophtalmologie*. 2014;37(5):371–6.

14. Rossi S, Orrico A, Santamaria C, Romano V, De Rosa L, Simonelli F, De Rosa G. Standard versus trans-epithelial collagen cross-linking in keratoconus patients suitable for standard collagen cross-linking. *Clinical Ophthalmology*. 2015 Mar 18:503–9.

15. Cerman E, Toker E, Ozcan DO. Transepithelial versus epithelium-off crosslinking in adults with progressive keratoconus. *Journal of Cataract & Refractive Surgery*. 2015;41(7):1416–25.

16. Cifariello F, Minicucci M, Di Renzo F, Di Taranto D, Coclite G, Zaccaria S, et al. Epi-off versus epi-on corneal collagen cross-linking in keratoconus patients: a comparative study through 2-year follow-up. *Journal of Ophthalmology*. 2018;2018.

17. Magli A, Forte R, Tortori A, Capasso L, Marsico G, Piozzi E. Epithelium-off corneal collagen cross-linking versus transepithelial cross-linking for pediatric keratoconus. *Cornea*. 2013;32(5):597–601.

18. Razmjoo H, Rahimi B, Kharraji M, Koosha N, Peyman A. Corneal haze and visual outcome after collagen crosslinking for keratoconus: A comparison between total epithelium off and partial epithelial removal methods. *Advanced Biomedical Research*. 2014;3(1):221.

19. Galvis V, Tello A, Carreño NI, Ortiz AI, Barrera R, Rodriguez CJ, et al. Corneal cross-linking (with a partial deepithelization) in keratoconus with five years of follow-up. *Ophthalmology and Eye Diseases*. 2016;8:S38364.

20. Hashemi H, Seyedian MA, Miraftab M, Fotouhi A, Asgari S. Corneal collagen cross-linking with riboflavin and ultraviolet a irradiation for keratoconus: long-term results. *Ophthalmology*. 2013;120(8):1515–20.

21. Hashemi H, Miraftab M, Hafezi F, Asgari S. Matched comparison study of total and partial epithelium removal in corneal cross-linking. *Journal of Refractive Surgery*. 2015;31(2):110–5.

22. Nattis A, Donnenfeld ED, Rosenberg E, Perry HD. Visual and keratometric outcomes of keratoconus patients after sequential corneal crosslinking and topography-guided surface ablation: early United States experience. *Journal of Cataract & Refractive Surgery*. 2018;44(8):1003–11.

10 Conventional versus Accelerated versus Customized Corneal Cross-Linking

Mehrdad Mohammadpour and Masoud Khorrami-Nejad

INTRODUCTION

In this chapter, we explore and compare different techniques used in corneal cross-linking procedures. Corneal cross-linking is a treatment method employed to strengthen the cornea in patients with keratoconus and corneal ectasia. The conventional approach involves the application of riboflavin drops followed by exposure to ultraviolet light. However, advancements in the field have led to the development of accelerated and customized techniques, which offer potential benefits in terms of treatment efficiency and personalized patient care. This chapter describes these three approaches, highlighting their similarities, differences, and potential clinical implications. By examining the various corneal cross-linking methods, readers will gain valuable insights into the evolving landscape of this important ophthalmological procedure.

CONVENTIONAL CXL

The conventional corneal cross-linking (CXL) method involves the application of riboflavin drops followed by exposure to ultraviolet (UV) light. When riboflavin is added, the corneal absorption of UV radiation increases significantly. In the conventional method, the UV region covers the wavelength range 360–375 nm, and its energy is 5.4 Joules. This amount of energy cannot damage the underlying tissue.[1] In this technique, the voltage is 3 mW/cm^2, and the time is 30 minutes. Usually, a change in the protocol is needed for thin corneas, such as adjusting the concentration of the light-sensitive material, voltage radiation, and duration of radiation exposure. The summary of the conventional CXL method highlights the role of riboflavin and UV radiation in strengthening the cornea and provides insights into potential protocol modifications based on individual patient needs.

ACCELERATED CXL

Accelerated CXL is classified into two main groups: pulse or continuous. In this technique, 34 thin corneas were treated by accelerated CXL, and after a one-year follow-up, it was revealed that the progression of KCN had been halted. Permanent UV radiation will de-oxygenize the cornea. Oxygen molecules play a prominent role in the cross-linking process. However, a challenging problem that arises in this domain is losing it. This problem is solved easily by using the pulse method.[2] CXL is carried out based on the photodynamic reaction type pulse or continuous.[3]

In 2017, an article was published by Toker et al. evaluating the effectiveness of various accelerated CXL protocols on 134 eyes with progressive KCN. The patients were divided into four groups: conventional CXL was done on 34 eyes, and 45, 28 and 27 eyes had accelerated CXL (9 mW/cm^2 for ten minutes), continuous-light accelerated CXL (30 mW/cm^2 for four minutes), and pulsed-light accelerated CXL (30 mW/cm^2 for eight minutes [one second on/one second off) CXL. The results demonstrated there was an increase in UDVA and CDVA in conventional and 9 mW accelerated CXL groups, whereas, in the continuous-light accelerated CXL group, only CDVA increased. In addition, there was no considerable improvement in UDVA and CDVA parameters in the pulsed-light accelerated CXL group. All K readings such as K1, K2, mean-K, and K_{max} decreased notably in conventional and 9 mW accelerated CXL groups; however, no significant decrease of K values was observed in the 30 mW accelerated CXL group. They concluded that 30 mW accelerated CXL protocols (continuous-light accelerated and pulsed-light accelerated CXL) were efficacious in stabilizing KCN progress; however, these two protocols resulted in lower improvement of topographic parameters.[4]

Another study was conducted by Kirgiz et al. in 2019 in which the consequences of two different protocols of accelerated CXL regarding visual, HOA, and topographic values were compared for 12 months. Sixty-six progressive KCN eyes were enrolled in this study and were divided into two groups: in the first group, 37 eyes were treated with 18 mW/cm^2 for five minutes and the 29 eyes in the second group were treated with 9 mW/cm2 for ten minutes. A marked increase in UCVA and BCVA and considerable improvement in corneal HOAs were observed in both groups. However, the corneal coma value and changes in K values (K1, K2, mean-K and K_{max}) were notably greater in the second group than the first one. They reported that the second accelerated CXL protocol (10

DOI: 10.1201/9781003371601-10

min of UV-A irradiance at 9 mW/cm²) demonstrated greater improvements regarding keratometry and coma values.[5]

Kinetic studies showed that UV radiation reduces corneal oxygen and, if it is stopped for three to four minutes, the oxygen level returns to its previous concentration again.[6] Oxygen-free radicals, especially singlet oxygen, are the main released molecule in this process. In aerobic conditions, photo-oxidation of proteoglycan and collagen with singlet oxygen occurs after 10–15 seconds of UV radiation and this is the second type of photochemical mechanism. After 10–15 seconds, the oxygen level decreases, and the first type of reaction occurs. Measured oxygen level has shown that it flows much better with on- and off-types and increases the CXL effect without high energy.[7] Another study was carried out on detached pigs' eyes; after de-epithelization and injection of riboflavin 0.1%, the eyes were kept in a beaker, filled with oxygen, and irradiated for three minutes continuously or six minutes with pulsed UV light. The results from continuous irradiation were much better than from the pulse type.[8]

A study was carried out by Kang et al. in 2019 to evaluate the effect of CXL for myopic correction on the alteration of epithelial thickness and refractive result after myopic TPRK for one year. Ninety-eight patients were enrolled in the study and were divided into two groups: 49 eyes in the first group underwent TPRK and the other 49 eyes had TPRK-CXL. In all patients, the SE refraction was in the range of −2.20 to −8.70 D, the refractive astigmatism was < 4.00 D, and the myopia was stable for at least one year. First, riboflavin 0.1% with hydroxypropyl methylcellulose was administered to the corneal surface for 90 seconds and after that it was rinsed entirely by 30 mL of a solution of chilled balanced salt. Then, by applying the KXL system, 30 mW/cm² UV-A light with a 9 mm diameter was irradiated onto the cornea in a similar circular pattern for 90 seconds. After UV-A irradiation cessation, mitomycin C 0.02% was used for 20 seconds and then a similar post-operative treatment was applied with TPRK. Finally, a therapeutic contact lens was placed on the cornea after the instillation of one drop of topical levofloxacin 0.5%. Topical levofloxacin 0.5% and fluorometholone 0.1% were used four times a day for one month post-operatively.

According to the results, CDVA was greater than 20/20 [with 44 (90%) eyes after TPRK and 45 (92%] eyes after TPRK-CXL). At the 12-month follow-up, the mean refractive errors were changed from 0.21 ± 0.31 to 0.07 ± 0.22 D after TPRK and from 0.01 ± 0.30 to 0.16 ± 0.24 D after TPRK-CXL. Regarding the keratometric power alterations, the outcomes demonstrated 0.47 D of steepening in the TPRK group and 0.19 D of flattening in the TPRK-CXL group. Despite the similar epithelial thickness in all the 17 segments of epithelial thickness map (using an automatic algorithm) in both groups pre-operatively, a marked thickening in all areas was observed in the epithelium, with the greatest thickening being in the temporal paracentral site in both groups. The mean epithelial thickness of the center (2 mm in diameter), paracenter (2 to 5 mm), and pericenter (5 to 6 mm) increased by 6.5 ± 3.1, 7.0 ± 2.9, and 4.9 ± 2.9 μm, respectively, after TPRK and 4.8 ± 3.0, 5.9 ± 2.8, and 4.8 ± 2.7 μm, respectively, after TPRK-CXL. The authors concluded that TPRK-CXL (because of the simultaneous CXL) caused less epithelial hyperplasia than TPRK. The thickening of corneal epithelium, presumably associated with myopic regression, and the combination with CXL decreased the regression risk.[9]

The accelerated technique decreases the patient's discomfort and reduces the surgery time, decreasing the corneal dehydration, thinning, and tonicity. A study was conducted by Sherif in 2014 on 25 eyes. They were randomly classified into two main groups. The first group was 14 eyes treated by the accelerated technique, and the second group was 11 eyes treated by the conventional technique, and the keratometric changes and visual improvements were found to be similar in the two groups.[10]

Alex Lapki carried out another study. The first group had 14 eyes treated by conventional technique and the second group had 12 eyes that had the protocol of 9 mW/cm² irradiance for ten minutes. In the first group, the CDVA improved significantly. By contrast, there was no dramatic change in the CDVA and K_{max} in the second group. After 12 months follow-up, the progression of KCN halted in both groups, but excessive corneal flattening was vividly seen in the conventional group.[11]

Another research study, by Elbaz, on 20 eyes (with the same protocol) produced similar results.[12]

Hashemi et al. did a study with the protocol of 18 mW/cm² irradiance for five minutes that had the same results as the Dresden protocol, with no difference being seen in any index. They also conducted another study with the protocol of 18 mW/cm² irradiance for three minutes. In this study, no difference in the keratometric data was seen, but there was a significant reduction in keratocytes density and basal nerves in the conventional group.[13]

CUSTOMIZED CXL

An article was published by Seiler et al. in 2016, describing the effectiveness of customized CXL in comparison with standard CXL for one year. Forty progressive primary KCN eyes were enrolled in the study and were divided into two groups: 20 eyes in the customized CXL group and 20 eyes in the control group.

In the control group, a 9.0 mm circular epithelium was first debrided and riboflavin 0.1% in 16% dextran was applied for thirty minutes. Then, UV-irradiation with 9 mW/cm^2 and a total energy of 5.4 J/cm^2 for ten minutes was performed on the cornea. The same procedure was done in the customized CXL group, although a smaller eccentric zone was debrided and there were three different customized UV-irradiation profiles. Customized irradiation patterns had an energy fluence of 9 mW/cm^2 and the energy levels were 5.4 J/cm^2 in the outer circle, 7.5 J/cm^2 in the middle circle, and 10 J/cm2 in the inner circle, and these three circular areas were centered on the maximum of the posterior float. (The diameter ranges of the inner and outer circles were from 1.9 mm to 2.9 mm and from 5.2 mm to 6.5 mm, respectively. Also, the diameter of the middle circle was the average of the inner and outer diameters.) Then, after the application of the antibiotic ointment and therapeutic contact lens, fluorometholone eye drops were the final topical treatment.

According to the results, K_{max} decreased by −1.7 ± 2.0 D in the first group and by −0.9 ± 1.3 D in the control group. In addition, the average regularization index (RI) demonstrated a marked difference between the groups: 5.2 ± 2.7 D in the first and 4.1 ± 3.1D in the control group. In total, the healing time of the epithelium, K_{max} alteration, and RI were considerably better in the customized CXL group. Two out of 19 eyes in the standard (control) group but 7 out of 19 eyes in the customized CXL group illustrated a flattening of 2 or more diopters.

The authors suggested that both the customized and standard CXL treatments were safe and effective, while customized CXL resulted in greater improvements in K_{max} flattening and RI and this procedure had faster epithelial healing time.[14]

THE SUB400 PROTOCOL: Individualized CXL With
Riboflavin and UV-A in Ultrathin Corneas

Individualized CXL with riboflavin and UV-A in ultrathin corneas (the Sub400 Protocol) was introduced by Hafezi et al. in 2020. Their study was performed on 39 eyes with progressive KCN and ultrathin corneas (214 to 398 μm). In this technique, UV irradiation was performed at 3 mW/cm^2 after epithelium removal, with irradiation times individually adapted to stromal thickness. They reported that this protocol individualized the fluence CXL protocol and standardized the treatment in patients with ultrathin corneas, and the success rate of halting KCN progression was 90% in one year.

This outcome extends the clinical range of patients that can be safely cross-linked to the stages of far-progressed KCN. In addition, a significant relationship was observed between irradiation and demarcation line (DL) depth. However, there was no significant correlation between K_{max} changes and DL depth; that is to say, treatment outcomes could not be predicted by DL depth. Hence, the depth of DL is most likely not related to the degree of corneal stiffening caused by CXL but to induced wound healing. The authors claimed that this protocol could apply not only to ultrathin corneas, but also to all patients with different corneal thicknesses.[15]

PACHYMETRY-BASED ACCELERATED CROSS-LINKING: The "M Nomogram"
for Standardized Treatment of All-thickness Progressive Ectatic Corneas

In 2018, Mazzotta et al. evaluated the effectiveness and safety of a novel customized epi-off accelerated CXL (ACXL) nomogram (M nomogram) based on the corneal optical thinnest point before surgery for progressive KCN and iatrogenic corneal ectasia. Patients were divided into four groups: the first 20 eyes were treated using conventional 3 mW/cm^2 CXL; the second 20 eyes were treated with 30 mW/cm^2 ACXL with continuous (10 eyes) or pulsed (10 eyes) UV-A irradiation (one second on and one second off); the third 20 eyes were treated applying 15 mW/cm2 pulsed light ACXL; and the last 20 eyes were treated with the 9 mW/cm^2 ACXL protocol. Comparing parameters, such as the demarcation lines' measured depths, was carried out using IVCM and corneal OCT. The mean demarcation depths were 350 ± 50 μm for the 3 mW/cm^2 conventional protocol, 200 ± 50 μm for the 30 mW/cm^2 continuous light ACXL, 250 ± 50 μm for the 30 mW/cm^2 pulsed light ACXL, and 280 ± 30 μm for the 15 mW/cm^2 pulsed light ACXL. The authors reorted that the accelerated CXL M nomogram was a standardized treatment for thin ectatic corneas and allowed efficacious and safe CXL parameter setting according to pre-operative thinnest cornea thickness

(250 to 400 μm) In addition, this nomogram, as a standardized management of thin ectatic corneas, can be performed for the treatment of all-thickness progressive KCN patients, as well as for all other iatrogenic ectasia cases, such as pellucid marginal degeneration, post-radial keratotomy hyperopic drift, post-LASIK, SMILE, and PRK ectasia.[16]

In another article, on research conducted by Mozzotta et al. in 2020, 27 progressive KCN eyes were treated with customized CXL applying a transepithelial approach and supplemental oxygen intra-operatively. In this study, 365 nm UV-A was used in a 30 mW/cm² pulsed-light UV light exposure in a two-zone elliptical pattern. After delivering a total dose of 10 J/cm² at the apex of the KCN and a 7.2 J/cm² broadbeam spot at the surroundings and then corneal soaking with 0.25% riboflavin, UV-A was irradiated while extra oxygen was present (using specific goggles linked to an oxygen delivery system (flow-rate 2.5 L/min) with ≥90% concentration). CDVA, AK, K1, K2, K-average, corneal HOAs and OCT, topographic, and manifest cylinder and endothelial cell count were measured and reported. Marked improvements in CDVA (from 0.19 ± 0.06 logMAR to 0.11 ± 0.04 logMAR), coma values (from 0.47 ± 0.28 μm to 0.28 ± 0.16 μm) and OCT (2 demarcation lines at mean depths of 218.23 ± 43.32 μm and 325.71 ± 39.70 μm) were observed in their results. Also, mean change in K2 was reported to be −1.9 D.[17]

In conclusion, this chapter has thoroughly examined and compared three techniques used in CXL procedures: conventional, accelerated, and customized CXL. Each approach has its unique characteristics and potential benefits, all with the ultimate goal of strengthening the corneal structure in patients suffering from conditions such as keratoconus and corneal ectasia. The conventional method, involving the use of riboflavin drops and UV radiation, is a tried and tested technique that has provided reliable results over the years. Modifications to the treatment protocol can be made to cater to individual patient needs, particularly in cases involving thin corneas. Accelerated CXL, on the other hand, offers the advantage of reducing procedure time and patient discomfort. Divided into two main groups, pulse and continuous, it has demonstrated promising results in arresting KCN progression and improving certain vision parameters. However, it has been observed that different accelerated CXL protocols may yield varying degrees of improvement in topographic parameters and visual outcomes, necessitating further research to optimize these procedures. It is clear that advancements in technology have opened up the possibility for even more personalized and efficient treatment strategies in CXL. Further research and clinical trials are essential to validate these methods, understand their long-term efficacy, and establish standardized protocols that can be universally adopted.

REFERENCES

1. Hafezi F, Kanellopoulos J, Wiltfang R, Seiler T. Corneal collagen crosslinking with riboflavin and ultraviolet A to treat induced keratectasia after laser in situ keratomileusis. *Journal of Cataract & Refractive Surgery*. 2007;33(12):2035–40.

2. Mazzotta C, Traversi C, Caragiuli S, Rechichi M. Pulsed vs continuous light accelerated corneal collagen crosslinking: in vivo qualitative investigation by confocal microscopy and corneal OCT. *Eye*. 2014;28(10):1179–83.

3. Kamaev P, Friedman MD, Sherr E, Muller D. Photochemical kinetics of corneal cross-linking with riboflavin. *Investigative Ophthalmology & Visual Science*. 2012;53(4):2360–7.

4. Toker E, Çerman E, Özcan DÖ, Seferoğlu ÖB. Efficacy of different accelerated corneal crosslinking protocols for progressive keratoconus. *Journal of Cataract & Refractive Surgery*. 2017;43(8):1089–99.

5. Kirgiz A, Eliacik M, Yildirim Y. Different accelerated corneal collagen cross-linking treatment modalities in progressive keratoconus. *Eye and Vision*. 2019;6(1):1–9.

6. Netto, E.A.T, Kling, S., Hafezi, F. (2019). The Role of Oxygen in Corneal Cross-Linking. In: Barbara, A. (eds) Controversies in the Management of Keratoconus . Springer, Cham. https://doi.org/10.1007/978-3-319-98032-4_7

7. Muller D, Kamaev P, Friedman M, Sherr E, Eddington W. Accelerated UVA-RF corneal cross-linking through pulsed UVA illumination and oxygen rich environments. *Investigative Ophthalmology & Visual Science*. 2013;54(15):5281.

8. Vetter JM, Brueckner S, Tubic-Grozdanis M, Voßmerbäumer U, Pfeiffer N, Kurz S. Modulation of central corneal thickness by various riboflavin eyedrop compositions in porcine corneas. *Journal of Cataract & Refractive Surgery*. 2012;38(3):525–32.

9. Kang DSY, Kim SW. Effect of corneal cross-linking on epithelial hyperplasia and myopia regression after Transepithelial photorefractive keratectomy. *Journal of Refractive Surgery*. 2019;35(6):354–61.

10. Sherif AM. Accelerated versus conventional corneal collagen cross-linking in the treatment of mild keratoconus: a comparative study. *Clinical Ophthalmology (Auckland, NZ)*. 2014;8:1435.

11. Ng ALK Chan TC, Cheng AC. Conventional versus accelerated corneal collagen cross-linking in the treatment of keratoconus. *Clinical & Experimental Ophthalmology*. 2016;44(1):8–14.

12. Elbaz U, Shen C, Lichtinger A, Zauberman NA, Goldich Y, Chan CC, et al. Accelerated (9-mW/cm2) corneal collagen crosslinking for keratoconus—a 1-year follow-up. *Cornea*. 2014;33(8):769–73.

13. Hashemi H, Fotouhi A, Miraftab M, Bahrmandy H, Seyedian MA, Amanzadeh K, et al. Short-term comparison of accelerated and standard methods of corneal collagen crosslinking. *Journal of Cataract & Refractive Surgery*. 2015;41(3):533–40.

14. Seiler TG, Fischinger I, Koller T, Zapp D, Frueh BE, Seiler T. Customized corneal cross-linking: one-year results. *American Journal of Ophthalmology*. 2016;166:14–21.

15. Hafezi F, Kling S, Gilardoni F, Hafezi N, Hillen M, Abrishamchi R, et al. Individualized corneal cross-linking with riboflavin and UV-A in ultrathin corneas: the Sub400 protocol. *American Journal of Ophthalmology*. 2021;224:133–42.

16. Mazzotta C, Romani A, Burroni A. Pachymetry-based accelerated crosslinking: the "M Nomogram" for standardized treatment of all-thickness progressive ectatic corneas. *International Journal of Keratoconus and Ectatic Corneal Diseases*. 2013;7(2):137–44.

17. Mazzotta C, Sgheri A, Bagaglia SA, Rechichi M, Di Maggio A. Customized corneal cross-linking for treatment of progressive keratoconus: Clinical and OCT outcomes using a transepithelial approach with supplemental oxygen. *Journal of Cataract & Refractive Surgery*. 2020;46(12):1582–7.

11 CXL under Special Conditions

Pediatrics, PACK CXL, PiXL, and Conductive Keratoplasty

Mehrdad Mohammadpour and Masoud Khorrami-Nejad

INTRODUCTION

Corneal crosslinking (CXL) has emerged as an effective treatment for halting the progression of keratoconus.[1-3] While the standard Dresden protocol is well-established for corneal crosslinking in adults, there has been increasing research into the use of CXL for pediatric keratoconus and other special situations.[4-10] This chapter reviews the evidence for accelerated CXL protocols in children, as well as novel applications of CXL technology for conductive keratoplasty, post-SMILE ectasia, and treatment of infectious keratitis (PACK-CXL). Key studies evaluating the safety and efficacy of these specialized CXL techniques are summarized. This chapter provides an overview of how collagen crosslinking is being adapted and utilized for a wider range of corneal conditions beyond traditional applications in adult keratoconus patients. Research continues to evolve in this exciting field

In 2017, Ulusoy et al. assessed the effectiveness and safety of accelerated CXL in 28 progressive keratoconic eyes of 19 pediatric patients for one year. Patients were divided into two groups in accordance with the magnitude of corneal thickness (CT). In the first group, 13 eyes were enrolled with CT ≥450 μm and 15 eyes with CT <450 μm were in the second group. All of the 28 eyes were treated by accelerated CXL, applying 9 mW/cm^2 UV-A irradiance for a total energy dose of 5.4 J/cm^2 for ten minutes. The first group demonstrated a marked improvement in UDVA of +0.12 logMAR at 3 months, whereas a considerable improvement of +0.3 logMAR was observed in the second group at one month post-operatively. However, 12 months after surgery, the increase in BCVA was +0.15 and +0.22 logMAR in the first and second groups, respectively. All mean-K values (such as K1 and K2) decreased by at least 1 D or stayed unchanged in both groups. The authors concluded that accelerated CXL was efficacious in halting or slowing down the keratoconus (KCN) progression, and no consistent complications were reported at six months post-operatively.[10]

Another study was carried out by Mazzotta et al. in 2018 in which the safety and effectiveness of CXL combined with riboflavin and UV-A light on patients under 18 years of age was evaluated for ten years. In their study, 62 progressive KCN eyes were treated by epi-off CXL [according to the Siena (modified Dresden) protocol]. The outcomes demonstrated an increase in UDVA (from 0.45 to 0.23 logarithm of the minimum angle resolution [logMAR]) and CDVA (from 0.14 to 0.1 logMAR), a marked decrease in K_{max} (six months after treatment up to the eight-year follow-up), notable improvement of the coma values (since the first month post-operatively), and a significant decrease in the minimum corneal thickness (at the first and third month after treatment, returning to baseline at the 6-month follow-up and remaining stable until the ten-year follow-up). The stability of KCN was reported in almost 80% of the patients at the ten-year follow-up and, at that time, the total progression rate was 24%, including 13 eyes of nine patients with the progression of K_{max} over 1 D and two eyes of two patients who had corneal grafting. In accordance with the results, the authors indicated that CXL decelerated the rate of KCN progression in pediatric patients.[6]

CONDUCTIVE KERATOPLASTY

Conductive keratoplasty (CK) is a non-invasive procedure that utilizes radiofrequency energy to correct presbyopia and astigmatism. In this method, the heat is transferred to the peripheral cornea, and the cornea is stretched against its astigmatism, so that vision is improved.

Regression and post-operative ectasia are among the most critical complications of refractive surgeries in high myopia with thin corneas. Relax SMILE is a flapless technique that removes a small corneal tissue by femtosecond laser. This technique has many advantages over the LASIK surgery; for instance, there are no flap-related complications, there is faster visual recovery, better long-term biomechanical stability, and less post-operative dry eye. In 2015, Sri Ganesh et al.[11] carried out research on 40 eyes that underwent SMILE surgery, then 0.25% riboflavin in saline was injected. The cornea was irradiated with the UV-A light of 45 mW/cm^2 for 75 seconds. After a one-year follow-up, the keratometric data and visual results improved dramatically.[11]

DOI: 10.1201/9781003371601-11

PHOTOREFRACTIVE INTRASTROMAL CORNEAL CROSSLINKING (PIXL)

PIXL, or photorefractive intrastromal CXL, is a non-invasive process without tissue removal. This mechanism flattens the cornea and changes its biomechanics without altering the whole structure. This study was conducted by Elling in 2017.[12] The research included 26 myopic or myopic astigmatism eyes. The riboflavin 0.1 % was injected, and the cornea was irradiated with the UV-A light (365 nm, 30 mW/cm²). The follow-up was at one, three, and six months. This method reduced corneal curvature significantly and dramatically improved the UCVA.[13] Another study was carried out by Wee Kiak Lim[13] on 14 eyes. The patients were non-ectatic and underwent PIXL procedure for their myopic treatment. After 12 months, the analysis led to the following conclusions: CDVA improved dramatically (20/20 or better), as a result of flattening the cornea and significantly reducing the SE.

PHOTOACTIVATED CHROMOPHORE FOR INFECTIOUS
KERATITIS - CORNEAL CROSSLINKING (PACK-CXL)

As mentioned earlier, CXL was originally a treatment to halt the progression of ectatic diseases such as KCN by applying the Dresden protocol. Then, scientists proved that it successfully treated iatrogenic ectasia developing after LASIK and PRK surgeries. Afterward, a novel and innovative technique was represented for infectious keratitis treatment: It had been presumed that ultraviolet light combined with riboflavin not only strengthened the cornea biomechanically but also appeared to have the ability to remove living cells and organisms such as keratocytes and pathogens. At first, only advanced infectious melting ulcers, which could not be treated with standard microbicidal methods, were treated with CXL, with standard therapy as the control. In later studies, CXL was also used to treat bacterial keratitis at the initial stage with no concomitant antibiotics, and it had positive outcomes in most patients. To distinguish the CXL usage for infectious keratitis therapy from its use for corneal ectatic disorders, a new term was adopted at the 9th CXL congress in Dublin for this new treatment as PACK-CXL (photoactivated chromophore for infectious keratitis – corneal collagen crosslinking). PACK-CXL is now the most used treatment for infectious corneal disorders from various infectious sources.[9]

Iseli et al. evaluated the efficiency of UV-A/riboflavin CXL for treating five patients who had advanced infectious melting keratitis in 2008 for nine months. Two patients had fungal keratitis, and the others were infected with the *Mycobacterium* spp. bacterial pathogen. Patients underwent CXL (3 mW/cm² CXL for 30 min) because the infection was unresponsive to full topical and systemic antibiotic treatment. The results demonstrated that the corneal melting was halted in all patients except one, who had a persistent corneal melt (due to an immune counteraction) without any active pathogens. In addition, there was no need for emergency keratoplasty in any case. The authors regarded CXL to be a satisfactory method for treating therapy-resistant infectious keratitis patients to avoid emergency keratoplasty.[14]

A study was carried out by Makdoumi et al. on seven eyes infected with severe keratitis and corneal melting, which were treated by CXL in 2010 for six months. The symptoms were observed a maximum of seven days before CXL surgery. Keratitis photodocumentation was achieved before the operation and at the follow-up. In addition to CXL, topical antibiotic treatment was performed on five patients. In the first 24 hours, the symptoms were improved in all eyes except one postoperatively and no symptoms were observed in two patients. In addition to halting the corneal melting, complete epithelialization was attained in all eyes, whereas, two days after CXL, this recurred in two cases with hypopyon. The authors concluded that CXL might be an efficacious treatment for eyes with infectious keratitis. However, despite its advantages, further studies would be required.[5]

Another study was carried out by Said et al. on 40 eyes to evaluate the PACK-CXL treatment for patients with advanced infectious keratitis and coexisting corneal melting in 2014. Two groups of patients were enrolled: the 21-eyes group had both PACK-CXL and antimicrobial treatments, whereas the 19-eyes control group underwent just antimicrobial treatment. The mean healing time for the first and second groups was 39.76 ± 18.22 days and 46.05 ± 27.44 days, respectively. According to the outcomes, CDVA was 1.64 ± 0.62 in the PACK-CXL group and 1.67 ± 0.48 in the control group, and the size of the corneal ulcer was markedly bigger in the first (treatment) group. Also, corneal puncture was observed in three patients of the second (control) group (with one regression of the infection). However, there were no significant complications in the first group. The authors deduced that PACK-CXL might effectively treat patients with infectious keratitis and corneal melting. However, it did not influence the time taken to achieve corneal healing.[8]

In another study, Price et al. in 2012 investigated the influence of adjunctive photoactivated riboflavin on infectious keratitis treated with CXL. In their study, 47 eyes were enrolled: seven eyes with prior PK, 24, seven, two, and one eye with bacterial, fungal, protozoan, and viral species, respectively, with no organism identified in six eyes. Eyes were treated with riboflavin 0.1% solution instillation for 30 minutes, after which they were irradiated with 365-nm UV-A light (3 mW/cm^2) at a range of 15 to 45 minutes while riboflavin was instilled. Then, the treatment of standard antibiotics was carried out on the eyes. The pre-operative maximum diameter of infiltration and epithelial defect increased from 1 to 12 mm and 0 to 8 mm, respectively.

The keratitis was not successfully treated in six eyes exposed to CXL (two bacterial, three fungal, and one with no improvement) and in one eye treated with PK. In addition, in one of the eyes with previous PK, the infectious keratitis was removed by the treatment, although to locate the puncture of the PK incision, a regraft was needed. In their conclusion, the authors reported that the riboflavin/UV-A treatment was not effective in eyes with previous herpes simplex infection; however, no risk to safety was observed and, if the degree of the infection was low, it seemed to have maximum effectiveness. In addition, the treatment was more successful against bacterial than fungal infections.[7]

A systematic review with a meta-analysis of reported cases on CXL and infectious keratitis was conducted by Alio et al. in 2013, summarizing 12 published articles, dealing with 104 eyes, regarding the effectiveness of this treatment. The eyes with infectious keratitis and bacteria were 58: 44 eyes with Gram-positive bacteria (four eyes had *Mycobacterium*) and 14 eyes with Gram-negative bacteria, 13 eyes with fungi and seven eyes with *Acanthamoeba*. The other 26 eyes had either negative microbiological culture results, or it was not performed. The mean re-epithelization after CXL was 20.7 ± 28.1 days. Also, there were 16 eyes with deep or lamellar keratoplasty. CXL had a desirable efficacy on halting corneal melting, and the pooled analysis supported this treatment for infectious keratitis.[4]

In summary, this chapter reviews specialized applications of CXL beyond its traditional use in adult keratoconus patients. Accelerated CXL protocols demonstrate early efficacy and safety in pediatric keratoconus. CXL also shows promise when combined with conductive keratoplasty for correction of presbyopia and astigmatism. CXL improves refractive and biomechanical outcomes as an adjunct to SMILE for myopia. Photorefractive intrastromal CXL (PiXL) is a non-invasive CXL technique to flatten the cornea and reduce myopia without tissue removal. Finally, photoactivated CXL (PACK-CXL) can effectively treat infectious keratitis, halting corneal melting and avoiding emergency keratoplasty. Key studies for each application are summarized. In conclusion, CXL continues to prove to be a treatment with widening possibilities for use in special situations like pediatric and infectious corneal diseases. Further research is warranted to refine protocols and indications.

REFERENCES

1. Mohammadpour M, Khoshtinat N, Khorrami-Nejad M. Comparison of visual, tomographic, and biomechanical outcomes of 360 degrees intracorneal ring implantation with and without corneal crosslinking for progressive keratoconus: a 5-year follow-up. *Cornea*. 2021;40(3):303–10.

2. Mohammadpour M, Heirani M, Khoshtinat N, Khorrami-Nejad M. Comparison of two different 360-degree intrastromal corneal rings combined with simultaneous accelerated-corneal crosslinking. *European Journal of Ophthalmology*. 2023:11206721231171420.

3. Mastropasqua L. Collagen crosslinking: when and how? A review of the state of the art of the technique and new perspectives. *Eye and Vision*. 2015;2(1):1–10.

4. Alio JL, Abbouda A, Valle DD, Del Castillo JMB, Fernandez JAG. Corneal cross linking and infectious keratitis: a systematic review with a meta-analysis of reported cases. *Journal of Ophthalmic Inflammation and Infection*. 2013;3(1):1–7.

5. Makdoumi K, Mortensen J, Crafoord S. Infectious keratitis treated with corneal crosslinking. *Cornea*. 2010;29(12):1353–8.

6. Mazzotta C, Traversi C, Baiocchi S, Bagaglia S, Caporossi O, Villano A, et al. Corneal collagen crosslinking with riboflavin and ultraviolet a light for pediatric keratoconus: ten-year results. *Cornea*. 2018;37(5):560–6.

7. Price MO, Tenkman LR, Schrier A, Fairchild KM, Trokel SL, Price FW. Photoactivated riboflavin treatment of infectious keratitis using collagen crosslinking technology. *Journal of Refractive Surgery*. 2012;28(10):706–13.

8. Said DG, Elalfy MS, Gatzioufas Z, El-Zakzouk ES, Hassan MA, Saif MY, et al. Collagen cross-linking with photoactivated riboflavin (PACK-CXL) for the treatment of advanced infectious keratitis with corneal melting. *Ophthalmology*. 2014;121(7):1377–82.

9. Tabibian D, Richoz O, Hafezi F. PACK-CXL: Corneal crosslinking for treatment of infectious keratitis. *Journal of Ophthalmic & Vision Research*. 2015;10(1):77.

10. Ulusoy DM, Göktaş E, Duru N, Özköse A, Ataş M, Yuvacı İ, et al. Accelerated corneal cross-linking for treatment of progressive keratoconus in pediatric patients. *European Journal of Ophthalmology*. 2017;27(3):319–25.

11. Ganesh S, Brar S. Clinical Outcomes of Small Incision Lenticule Extraction with Accelerated Cross-Linking (ReLEx SMILE Xtra) in Patients with Thin Corneas and Borderline Topography. *J Ophthalmol*. 2015;2015:263412. doi: 10.1155/2015/263412. Epub 2015 Jun 28. PMID: 26221538; PMCID: PMC4499409.

12. Elling M, Kersten-Gomez I, Dick HB. Photorefractive intrastromal corneal crosslinking for the treatment of myopic refractive errors: Six-month interim findings. *J Cataract Refract Surg*. 2017 Jun;43(6):789–95. doi: 10.1016/j.jcrs.2017.03.036. PMID: 28732613.

13. Lim WK, Soh ZD, Choi HK, Theng JT. Epithelium-on photorefractive intrastromal cross-linking (PiXL) for reduction of low myopia. *Clinical Ophthalmology*. 2017 Jun 27:1205–11.

14. Iseli HP, Thiel MA, Hafezi F, Kampmeier J, Seiler T. Ultraviolet A/riboflavin corneal cross-linking for infectious keratitis associated with corneal melts. *Cornea*. 2008;27(5):590–4.

12 Combined Corneal Cross-Linking Protocols

Masoud Khorrami-Nejad, Mehrdad Mohammadpor, and Kiana Raeesdana

INTRODUCTION

Corneal collagen cross-linking (CXL) has emerged as a pivotal treatment for halting the progression of this condition. Traditional CXL aims to fortify the corneal structure, thereby preventing further deterioration. However, recent advancements have seen the integration of CXL with additional refractive, topographic, or surface ablation procedures, creating combined protocols that offer a more comprehensive approach to managing keratoconus.[1-8]

This chapter delves into these combined CXL protocols, which have been designed not only to arrest the progression of ectasia but also to enhance visual outcomes. By merging CXL with other surgical techniques, these protocols seek to optimize refractive correction, minimize irregular astigmatism, and stabilize the anterior corneal surface topography. Some protocols also aim to address milder cases of keratoconus and reduce the risk of ectasia in high-risk refractive surgery patients.

We will explore several established combined CXL protocols, including the Prophylactic CXL protocol, Cretan protocol, Tehran protocol, Athens protocol, Modified Athens protocol, and Tel-Aviv protocol. Each protocol will be examined in detail, covering surgical techniques, reported outcomes, conclusions, and limitations. By providing an overview of these approaches, this chapter aims to highlight their roles in optimizing patient outcomes in refractive surgery and ectasia management.

PROPHYLACTIC CXL PROTOCOL

In 2014, Kanellopoulos et al. published an article assessing the topographic epithelial thickness remodeling after high myopic femtosecond LASIK with simultaneous prophylactic high-fluence CXL and standard femtosecond LASIK on 139 eyes. There were two groups of patients: in the first group, 67 eyes were treated with simultaneous prophylactic CXL (LASIK-Xtra) supplementally, whereas the other 72 eyes in the second group were treated with stand-alone femtosecond LASIK. The epithelial thickness was measured by optical coherence tomography over the 2-mm-diameter central disk, 5-mm mid-peripheral rim, and the total 6-mm-diameter disc zone.

The outcomes demonstrated that the epithelial thickness increase was markedly different between matched myopic correction subgroups (especially high myopia). According to the results, in LASIK-Xtra and stand-alone LASIK groups the increase in the mid-peripheral epithelial thickness were +3.79 μm and +3.95 μm and +9.75 μm and +7.14 μm for the "−8.00 to −9.00 D" and "−7.00 to −8.00 D" subgroups, respectively. The authors showed that prophylactic CXL combined simultaneously with high myopic LASIK surgery caused a marked reduction in the epithelial thickness increase compared with stand-alone LASIK (specifically between matched high myopic correction subgroups).[9]

A study was conducted by Taneri et al. in 2017 reporting a unilateral corneal ectasia after LASIK surgery combined with prophylactic CXL in a young patient for one year. Before the surgery, the minimum CT was 554 μm in the right eye and 546 μm in the left eye, the patient had a CDVA of 20/20 in both eyes and the refraction of the right and left eyes were +1.25 −2.75 × 10 and +0.50 −2.00 × 163, respectively. At the 12-month follow-up, the patient had a UDVA of 20/20 in both eyes and no significant changes were observed. At 2-year follow-up, a loss of vision (UDVA 0.25) and also an inferior steepening on topography were observed in the left eye. Therefore, the patient underwent standard CXL to prevent further progression. The authors indicated that prophylactic CXL combined with LASIK might not be effective at arresting corneal ectasia.[8]

CRETAN PROTOCOL

The Cretan protocol is a surgical treatment approach for keratoconus (KCN) patients developed at the University of Crete in Greece. In this method, after PTK, PRK, and CXL are carried out,[6] CXL alone strengthens the cornea but does not improve the vision, so the CXL PLUS is used, which involves PRK/LASIK/ICRS/IOL. PTK is a common surgical technique that treats some corneal pathologies, for instance, corneal dystrophies, degenerations, and nodule keratitis.[10] In this method, PTK is performed on eyes with KCN that allows excimer laser ablation to remove the corneal epithelium, thus regularizing the anterior corneal surface and improving the efficacy of the cross-linking. A study conducted by Kyminious on a KCN patient showed an improvement in the UCVA after the first month (of performing PTK). Reduced corneal tissue, especially at the corneal apex, imposed some limits on this technique.[6,10,11]

TEHRAN PROTOCOL

Mohammadpour et al., in 2020, investigated the simultaneous use of PRK and accelerated CXL in a high-risk refractive surgery called the Tehran protocol. To evaluate the efficiency and safety of this method, 17 eyes from 15 patients were examined.

The age of the patients was between 25 and 35 years and, within their topographic findings, there have been at least one of the following risk factors: the amount of K_{max} was between 48 and 50 D and the range of I-S value was from 1.4 to 1.9 D. In addition, the corneal center was in the 450–480 μm thickness range.

In their conclusion, except for a mild corneal haze at the first-month follow-up (which was later completely resolved), the authors reported that no other significant complications, particularly corneal ectasia, were observed. As a result, Mohammadpour et al., by the 3-year outcomes, assessed that a combination of PRK and accelerated CXL is an efficacious and secure procedure for patients with high-risk refractive surgery, which has no accrued risk of continuous corneal haze.[7]

ATHENS PROTOCOL

Kanellopoulos, in 2010, introduced the Athens protocol in which topography-guided partial PRK and CXL are performed in the same session by the surgeon to manage KCN and post-LASIK ectasia. The purpose of this protocol (done over the past ten years) is to normalize the corneal surface and improve the patient's functional vision by correcting the refractive error and irregular astigmatism and preventing the KCN progression. In this method, initially, 50 μm of epithelium is removed by a 6.5-mm phototherapeutic keratectomy. Then, topographic-guided ablation is performed (using mitomycin C [0.02% for 20 seconds]), and, using an excimer laser, micro-irregularities on the surface of the cornea are corrected. Finally, the CXL procedure is carried out (to increase the covalent bonds of collagen and stop the KCN progression) by applying riboflavin, which absorbs UV radiation.

In this study, the treatment outcomes from comparing two large groups of eyes were reported. In the first group, 127 eyes were treated by performing topography-guided surface ablation one year after the CXL procedure, whereas, in the second group, 198 eyes were treated pursuant to the Athens protocol. The increase in UCVA and CDVA and the decrease in MRSE and keratometry value in the simultaneous group (Athens protocol) was notably greater than those in the sequential group; furthermore, the mean haze scores in the first and second groups were 1.20 and 0.5, respectively. The reduction in CCT was 70 μm in either treatment and no marked change in endothelial cell count was observed in the two groups. Kanellopoulos concluded that this protocol is a therapeutic intervention in patients (thickness < 350 μm) with KCN and progressive post-LASIK ectasia and that it may reduce the requirement for ICRs and keratoplastic procedures in patients with highly irregular corneas.[4]

MODIFIED (ENHANCED) ATHENS PROTOCOL

In 2019, Kanellopoulos published a new article reporting a novel usage of partial TG-PRK combined with refractive, customized CXL for safe and efficacious KCN treatment in order to maximize the refractive normalization effect along with ectasia stabilization to eliminate some of the Athens protocol limitations, such as stromal tissue removal.

In his study, 25 progressive KCN eyes underwent the enhanced Athens protocol for 36 to 42 months. In this procedure, 50 μm of epithelium is removed by a 7-mm PTK treatment after applying a TG partial PRK treatment of a maximum 30 μm over the thinnest cone zone. Afterward, mitomycin 0.02% and then riboflavin solution 0.1% (for soaking the exposed stroma) were used for 20 seconds and 5 minutes, respectively. Then, to treat the cornea with a customized pattern, 20 mW/cm² UV light fluence was irradiated in three various and specific patterns continuously: the all inner-smaller curved trapezoid pattern, the intermediate, and the outer were centered at the thinnest zone of the cone and received 15 J, 10 J, and 5 J, respectively.

An increase in UDVA (from 20/80 to 20/25 at six months), an improvement in the severity of the KCN stage (from a mean of 3.2 to 1.8), 7.8 D decrease in the maximum astigmatism and a marked cornea surface normalization (at the first-month follow-up) were observed.

The author concluded that this technique might simplify the reduced use of tissue ablation versus application of a homogeneous UV light beam for CXL. In addition, this results in the increased number of cases with limitations in using this method (owing to the restrictions of tissue thickness).[5]

TEL AVIV PROTOCOL

Kaiserman et al., in 2019, presented the Tel Aviv protocol in which an epithelial PRK (ePRK), combined with CXL, is performed for keratoconic patients. This protocol aims to slow KCN progression, achieve reduction in astigmatism (including irregular), and achieve improvements in UDVA and CDVA without thinning or weakening the cornea unnecessarily.

In this retrospective study, 20 consecutive patients (13–40 years of age with CDVA of 20/40 or worse, SE of –10.00 D or less, K_{max} of 55.00 D or less, TCT of 430 μm or greater, and Amsler–Krumeich stages of 1 to 2) underwent CXL with the Tel Aviv protocol by the developer of the protocol, Igor Kaiserman. The authors followed-up over the 266- to 1749-day range.

This protocol contained ablation of the epithelial layer by using an excimer laser, with 50% of the manifest refractive astigmatism (on the same axis), then carrying out the spherical ablation (the ablation of the epithelial and anterior stroma did not exceed a total of 50 μm), and then performing CXL. A marked increase in UDVA (from 0.95 ± 0.73 to 0.22 ± 0.15 logMAR) and CDVA ((from 0.24 ± 0.13 to 0.13 ± 0.12 logMAR), a significant decrease in mean-K (from 46.86 ± 2.48 to 45.00 ± 2.27 D), K_{max} (from 48.18 ± 2.74 to 45.97 ± 2.55 D), Kmin (from 45.54 ± 2.35 to 44.03 ± 2.12 D), and TCT (from 450.90 ± 35.99 to 404.90 ± 43.96 μm) were observed at the end of the follow-up period. Moreover, no complications or KCN progression were reported. The authors concluded that the Tel Aviv protocol provides excellent improvements in VA and astigmatism and also stops KCN progression for patients with progressive KCN.[3]

The decision tree shown in Figure 12.1 outlines the management of patients with keratoconus. The first decision point is whether the patient has progressive keratoconus or not. Progressive keratoconus is defined as an increase in the K_{max} (steepest keratometric reading) of more than one diopter in one year.

In summary, this chapter discusses several combined CXL protocols that have been developed to arrest ectasia progression and improve visual outcomes. It begins by explaining that, while standard CXL aims to strengthen the cornea, combining it with additional refractive, topographic, or surface ablation procedures provides more comprehensive keratoconus management. Several notable protocols are then examined in detail, including the prophylactic CXL protocol, Cretan protocol, Tehran protocol, Athens protocol, modified Athens protocol, and Tel Aviv protocol. Each protocol outlines the surgical techniques used, reports on outcomes demonstrating improvements in areas like visual acuity and corneal stabilization, and concludes with discussions on efficacy and limitations. In summary, combining CXL with other vision-improving and -stabilizing

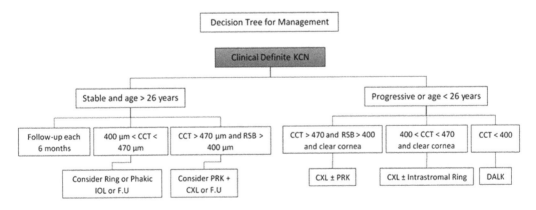

Figure 12.1 The decision tree of the management of patients with keratoconus. KCN: Keratoconus; CCT: Central corneal thickness; DALK: Deep anterior lamellar keratoplasty; RSB: Residual bed thickness.

treatments allows these protocols to offer better keratoconus and keratectasia management. However, outcomes can vary depending on patient factors and each protocol's specific constraints. Overall, this chapter provides an overview of established combined CXL approaches and their role in optimizing patient results for refractive surgery and ectasia handling.

REFERENCES

1. Mohammadpour M, Heirani M, Khoshtinat N, Khorrami-Nejad M. Comparison of two different 360-degree intrastromal corneal rings combined with simultaneous accelerated-corneal cross-linking. *European Journal of Ophthalmology*. 2023:11206721231171420.

2. Mohammadpour M, Khoshtinat N, Khorrami-Nejad M. Comparison of visual, tomographic, and biomechanical outcomes of 360 degrees intracorneal ring implantation with and without corneal crosslinking for progressive keratoconus: a 5-year follow-up. *Cornea*. 2021;40(3):303–10.

3. Kaiserman I, Mimouni M, Rabina G. Epithelial photorefractive keratectomy and corneal cross-linking for keratoconus: the TeL-Aviv protocol. *Journal of Refractive Surgery*. 2019;35(6):377–82.

4. Kanellopoulos AJ. Combining topography-guided PRK with CXL: the Athens protocol. *Cataract & Refractive Surgery Today Europe*. 2010:18–21.

5. Kanellopoulos AJ. Management of progressive keratoconus with partial topography-guided PRK combined with refractive, customized CXL–a novel technique: the enhanced Athens protocol. *Clinical Ophthalmology (Auckland, NZ)*. 2019;13:581.

6. Kymionis GD, Grentzelos MA, Kankariya VP, Liakopoulos DA, Karavitaki AE, Portaliou DM, et al. Long-term results of combined transepithelial phototherapeutic keratectomy and corneal collagen crosslinking for keratoconus: Cretan protocol. *Journal of Cataract & Refractive Surgery*. 2014;40(9):1439–45.

7. Mohammadpour M, Farhadi B, Mirshahi R, Masoumi A, Mirghorbani M. Simultaneous photorefractive keratectomy and accelerated collagen cross-linking in high-risk refractive surgery (Tehran protocol): 3-year outcomes. *International Ophthalmology*. 2020;40(10):2659–66.

8. Taneri S, Kiessler S, Rost A, Dick HB. Corneal ectasia after LASIK combined with prophylactic corneal cross-linking. *Journal of Refractive Surgery*. 2017;33(1):50–2.

9. Kanellopoulos AJ, Asimellis G. Epithelial remodeling after femtosecond laser-assisted high myopic LASIK: comparison of stand-alone with LASIK combined with prophylactic high-fluence cross-linking. *Cornea*. 2014;33(5):463–9.

10. Nagpal R, Maharana PK, Roop P, Murthy SI, Rapuano CJ, Titiyal JS, et al. Phototherapeutic keratectomy. *Survey of Ophthalmology*. 2020;65(1):79–108.

11. Wilson SE, Marino GK, Medeiros CS, Santhiago MR. Phototherapeutic keratectomy: science and art. *Journal of Refractive Surgery*. 2017;33(3):203–10.

13 Corneal Cross-Linking at the Slit Lamp

Farhad Hafezi, Emilio A Torres-Netto, and Mark Hillen

INTRODUCTION

The primary aim of corneal cross-linking (CXL) is to arrest the progression of corneal ectasias, such as keratoconus or post-operative ectasia.[1,2] The procedure has traditionally been performed in an operating room (OR) with the patient lying in a supine position, including the instillation of riboflavin, corneal pachymetry, and ultraviolet (UV-A) irradiation. The only instances where the patient is seated upright are during the pre- or post-operative slit-lamp examinations.

However, as our understanding of CXL, the UV-riboflavin photochemical reaction, and the underlying mechanisms continues to grow, it has become apparent that CXL can be safely and effectively performed outside of the OR at the slit lamp. This alternative approach brings several advantages, including reduced costs through eliminating the need to book and use an OR, plus it enables the technology to be more accessible in areas of low-to-middle-income countries (LMICs) where cost sensitivity is particularly high, and access to the technology is low.

This chapter examines the integration of CXL technology into the setting of a doctor's office (Figure 13.1), with consideration given to its various clinical applications, both in areas without access to an OR, and in large centers where efficiency and cost savings can be achieved.

TRANSITIONING FROM THE OR TO THE OFFICE

In medicine in general, there has been a trend to perform certain procedures, that were previously performed in an OR, in minor procedure rooms. If safety standards are maintained, then this approach should reduce costs and improve efficiency and patient convenience. This is not a new concept in ophthalmology. For several years now, retina specialists have been safely performing office-based intravitreal injections of anti-VEGF drugs for retinal disorders. In a retrospective consecutive case series review of over 11,700 intravitreal injections of anti-VEGF agents or triamcinolone acetonide for retinal disease treatment, Tabandeh et al. observed low rates of endophthalmitis in 2014, regardless of whether the procedure was performed in an OR or a doctor's office.[3]

Cataract surgery can also be safely performed in minor procedure rooms. In a study of over 21,000 eyes with an average patient age of 72 years, office-based cataract surgery was shown to be a safe and effective alternative to surgery performed in an OR. The study found no significant differences in visual outcomes, adverse events, or endophthalmitis rates between the two approaches.[4]

Although ORs offer a comfortable and familiar environment for surgeons, with equipment consistently available, they entail administrative and financial expenses. Booking an OR in advance and utilizing it result in additional expenses for both the physician and the patient. For a CXL procedure, a "clean, but not sterile" environment, similar to that in which retina specialists provide intravitreal anti-VEGF injections, is sufficient.

CXL EXERTS A PATHOGEN-KILLING EFFECT ON THE CORNEA

The CXL procedure reduces the presence of microorganisms on the cornea (Figure 13.2).[5,6] The application of UV light in CXL leads to the creation of photoactivated riboflavin molecules and reactive oxygen species (ROS),[1] which covalently bind together stromal molecules (mostly collagen and proteoglycans) that strengthen the cornea.[7] This cross-linking process also interferes with the ability of matrix metalloproteinases (MMPs) to degrade the cornea, as the binding of stromal molecules hides MMP-binding sites in a process called steric hindrance, making the stroma less easily digested. Additionally, photoactivated riboflavin and ROS can damage pathogen cell membranes and nucleic acids, resulting in high pathogen-killing rates, and leaving the post-CXL cornea effectively sterile.[8–11]

This pathogen-killing effect has led to the use of CXL in treating infectious keratitis in a procedure known as photoactivated chromophore for keratitis–corneal cross-linking (PACK-CXL),[12] reviewed below. In CXL for ectasia, given the sterilizing effect of CXL, it is not necessary to perform the procedure in an OR, particularly as antimicrobial prophylaxis is administered after the procedure. The post-operative handling of the exposed corneal surface is the primary infection concern after CXL, regardless of the clinical setting. Moreover, in terms of infectious keratitis,

DOI: 10.1201/9781003371601-13

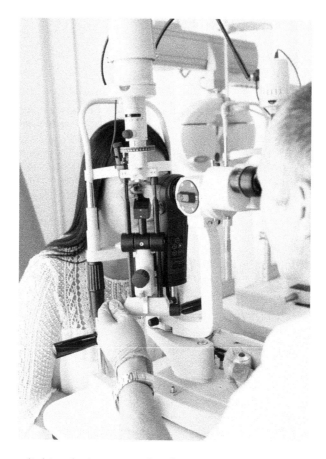

Figure 13.1 A cross-linking device mounted at the slit lamp.

rather than bringing an active infection to an OR, it is feasible to treat infectious keratitis with PACK-CXL at a slit lamp outside of one instead.

ADAPTING CXL TO THE SLIT-LAMP SETTING

After the completion of CXL, the microbial load on the corneal surface is potentially eliminated. However, almost all cases of infection following epi-off cross-linking procedures are attributed to mishandling of the cornea that occurs before complete regrowth of the corneal epithelium, during the healing phase. These factors apply equally whether the procedure is performed in an office-based, slit lamp setting or in an OR. The development of more effective epi-on CXL-for-ectasia protocols,[13] which so far demonstrate comparable short-term efficacy in biomechanical strengthening/ectasia halting to current epi-off protocols, and where the epithelium remains intact after the procedure is complete, should further enhance the safety of the post-operative handling period for CXL procedures in either setting.

Epithelium Abrasion for Epi-Off Protocols

For epithelium-off CXL procedures, various techniques can be employed to remove the epithelium, such as a hockey knife or an Amoils brush. However, these methods can prove challenging with the patient sitting upright, and extra care must be taken to avoid damaging Bowman's membrane during the epithelial removal process. In order to address these limitations, we developed a modified laser epithelial keratomileusis (LASEK) approach,[14] which involves using a sterile cotton swab soaked with 40% ethanol (Figure 13.3). This method is simple to perform, rapid, and safe, without risking harm to Bowman's membrane.[15]

A sterile cotton swab is dipped in a *freshly prepared* 40% ethanol solution to perform the epithelial removal procedure. The swab is then gently tapped on the center and periphery of the cornea in a circular pattern for 70 seconds. After approximately 45 seconds, the epithelium starts to loosen

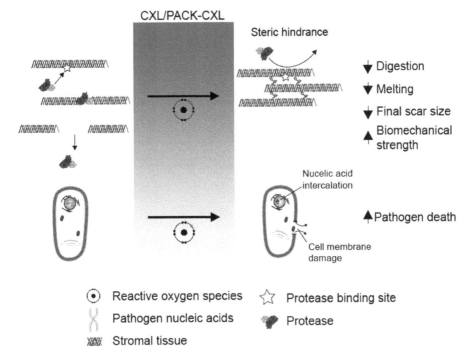

Figure 13.2 Mechanisms of action of CXL.

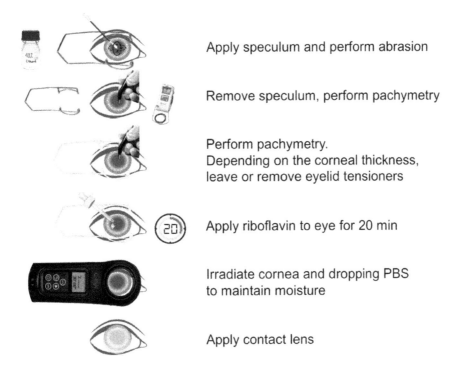

Figure 13.3 Key steps in performing CXL at the slit lamp.

and fold. The swab is applied with gentle pressure on the cornea in a circular motion to remove the loosened epithelium, resulting in an approximately 8 mm erosion. To maintain the effectiveness of the epithelium removal process, the 40% ethanol solution should not be exposed to the air for extended periods before use to prevent evaporation. After the removal, the cornea is rinsed with a balanced salt solution using a syringe with an irrigation cannula. For a PACK-CXL procedure, a dry, sterile triangular sponge is first used to remove the epithelial debris over or around the infiltrate.

Accelerated CXL Protocols

The use of CXL in the treatment of keratoconus has evolved over the past 20 years to include more efficient and faster protocols.[15–19] The traditional Dresden protocol, which involves a 30-minute period of UV irradiation, may not be ideal for all patients – particularly children – as prolonged periods of sitting upright can be uncomfortable.

With the advent of newer accelerated protocols, the duration of the required period of UV irradiation has been reduced by at least one-third.[19,20] As a result, in the majority of cases, the procedure can be performed in 10 minutes or less, which should be an acceptable length of time for most patients to comfortably sit at the slit lamp.

Riboflavin and Gravity

A hypothetical concern in CXL procedures is the potential redistribution of riboflavin in the cornea due to gravity during upright positioning. However, a 2017 laboratory study found no significant settling or shift in riboflavin concentration in the stroma even after one hour of upright positioning after saturation, indicating that performing CXL in seated patients is viable.[21]

CXL FOR INFECTIOUS KERATITIS

Infectious keratitis, referred to by the World Health Organization as a "silent epidemic,"[22] is a significant cause of visual impairment globally, particularly in developing countries where it affects agricultural workers in their most productive years, and the rapid progression of this condition highlights the importance of prompt diagnosis and treatment.[22,23] In temperate and developed countries, infections tend to be bacterial in nature, often resulting from micro-abrasions caused by contact lens wear. In warmer and more humid environments, prevalent in developing countries, fungal infections or mixed bacterial-fungal infections are more common.[24]

PACK-CXL has been shown to effectively treat early cases of bacterial, fungal, and mixed infectious keratitis without the use of antimicrobial drugs, thereby avoiding the issue of antimicrobial resistance.[8,25–36] Additionally, PACK-CXL increases the corneal resistance to digestion by pathogenic proteases,[37] which may reduce scarring. Results from a Phase III clinical trial have demonstrated the effectiveness of PACK-CXL in treating early bacterial, fungal, and mixed infections in a single accelerated treatment session without the use of antimicrobial drugs, effectively rivaling current standard-of-care antimicrobial therapy and avoiding the issue of antimicrobial resistance.[38]

This treatment is also characterized by a less stringent dependence on oxygen compared with traditional corneal cross-linking. As a result, higher intensities and shorter treatment times may be feasible.[31,32] The efficacy of PACK-CXL in killing pathogens is directly correlated with the total energy used, with higher fluences shown to be more effective.[25,26,33–36] While further research is required to determine the optimal role of PACK-CXL as a standalone therapy for infectious keratitis, multiple studies have already shown its positive impact as an adjuvant treatment.[32,39–41]

This one-time treatment outside of the OR may provide a more affordable option, especially for those in LMICs who would otherwise struggle to afford repeated doctor visits and intensive topical antimicrobial drug administration. Ultimately, PACK-CXL holds the potential to provide effective treatment for infectious keratitis to a wider population, and CXL at the slit lamp is an effective means to enable this delivery.

SUMMARY

The accessibility, cost, and convenience benefits of performing CXL at the slit lamp are numerous and compelling. This approach opens up access to CXL and PACK-CXL to a wider global demographic, particularly in LMICs where OR access is limited. The near-ubiquitous availability of the slit lamp in any eye care delivery setting – irrespective of whether it is in a rural region of a LMIC, or a hospital office in the capital city of a highly developed country – expands the reach of the procedure. This holds the potential for preserving and saving the vision of many who might otherwise ultimately have been blinded by a progressive ectasia or infectious keratitis.

REFERENCES

1. Randleman JB, Khandelwal SS, Hafezi F. Corneal cross-linking. *Surv Ophthalmol.* 2015;60(6):509–523. doi:10.1016/j.survophthal.2015.04.002

2. Wollensak G, Spoerl E, Seiler T. Riboflavin/ultraviolet-a-induced collagen crosslinking for the treatment of keratoconus. *Am J Ophthalmol.* 2003;135(5):620–627. doi:10.1016/s0002-9394(02)02220-1

3. Tabandeh H, Boscia F, Sborgia A, et al. Endophthalmitis associated with intravitreal injections: office-based setting and operating room setting. *Retina.* 2014;34(1):18–23. doi:10.1097/IAE.0000000000000008

4. Ianchulev T, Litoff D, Ellinger D, Stiverson K, Packer M. Office-based cataract surgery: population health outcomes study of more than 21 000 cases in the United States. *Ophthalmology.* 2016;123(4):723–728. doi:10.1016/j.ophtha.2015.12.020

5. Hafezi F, Randleman JB. PACK-CXL: defining CXL for infectious keratitis. *J Refract Surg.* 2014;30(7):438–439. doi:10.3928/1081597x-20140609-01

6. Kling S, Hufschmid FS, Torres-Netto EA, et al. High fluence increases the antibacterial efficacy of PACK cross-linking. *Cornea.* 2020;39(8):1020–1026. doi:10.1097/ico.0000000000002335

7. Hayes S, Boote C, Kamma-Lorger CS, et al. Riboflavin/UVA collagen cross-linking-induced changes in normal and keratoconus corneal stroma. *PLoS One.* 2011;6(8):e22405. doi:10.1371/journal.pone.0022405

8. Martins SA, Combs JC, Noguera G, et al. Antimicrobial efficacy of riboflavin/UVA combination (365 nm) in vitro for bacterial and fungal isolates: a potential new treatment for infectious keratitis. *Invest Ophthalmol Vis Sci.* 2008;49(8):3402–3408. doi:10.1167/iovs.07-1592

9. Naseem I, Ahmad M, Hadi SM. Effect of alkylated and intercalated DNA on the generation of superoxide anion by riboflavin. *Biosci Rep.* 1988;8(5):485–492. doi:10.1007/bf01121647

10. Pileggi G, Wataha JC, Girard M, et al. Blue light-mediated inactivation of enterococcus faecalis in vitro. *Photodiagnosis Photodyn Ther.* 2013;10(2):134–140. doi:10.1016/j.pdpdt.2012.11.002

11. Tsugita A, Okada Y, Uehara K. Photosensitized inactivation of ribonucleic acids in the presence of riboflavin. *Biochim Biophys Acta.* 1965;103(2):360–363. doi:10.1016/0005-2787(65)90182-6

12. Richoz O, Kling S, Hoogewoud F, et al. Antibacterial efficacy of accelerated photoactivated chromophore for keratitis-corneal collagen cross-linking (PACK-CXL). *J Refract Surg.* 2014;30(12):850–854. doi:10.3928/1081597x-20141118-01

13. Mazzotta C, Bagaglia SA, Sgheri A, et al. Iontophoresis corneal cross-linking with enhanced fluence and pulsed UV-A light: 3-year clinical results. *J Refract Surg.* 2020;36(5):286–292. doi:10.3928/1081597X-20200406-02

14. Browning AC, Shah S, Dua HS, Maharajan SV, Gray T, Bragheeth MA. Alcohol debridement of the corneal epithelium in PRK and LASEK: an electron microscopic study. *Invest Ophthalmol Vis Sci.* 2003;44(2):510–513. doi:10.1167/iovs.02-0488

15. Hafezi F, Richoz O, Torres-Netto EA, Hillen M, Hafezi NL. Corneal cross-linking at the slit lamp. *J Refract Surg.* 2021;37(2):78–82. doi:10.3928/1081597X-20201123-02

16. Lang PZ, Hafezi NL, Khandelwal SS, Torres-Netto EA, Hafezi F, Randleman JB. Comparative functional outcomes after corneal crosslinking using standard, accelerated, and accelerated with higher total fluence protocols. *Cornea*. 2019;38(4):433–441. doi:10.1097/ico.0000000000001878

17. Torres-Netto EA, Knyazer B, Chen S, Hosny M, Gilardoni F, Hafezi F. *Corneal cross-linking for treating infectious keratitis: final results of the prospective randomized controlled multicenter trial*. Paper presented at: ESCRS2020; Amsterdam (Virtual Meeting).

18. Torres-Netto EA, Kling S, Hafezi N, Vinciguerra P, Randleman JB, Hafezi F. Oxygen diffusion may limit the biomechanical effectiveness of iontophoresis-assisted transepithelial corneal cross-linking. *J Refract Surg*. 2018;34(11):768–774. doi:10.3928/1081597X-20180830-01

19. Mazzotta C, Raiskup F, Hafezi F, et al. Long term results of accelerated 9 mW corneal crosslinking for early progressive keratoconus: the Siena Eye-Cross Study 2. *Eye Vis (Lond)*. 2021;8(1):16. doi:10.1186/s40662-021-00240-8

20. Abrishamchi R, Abdshahzadeh H, Hillen M, et al. High-fluence accelerated epithelium-off corneal cross-linking protocol provides dresden protocol-like corneal strengthening. *Transl Vis Sci Technol*. 2021;10(5):10. doi:10.1167/tvst.10.5.10

21. Salmon B, Richoz O, Tabibian D, Kling S, Wuarin R, Hafezi F. CXL at the slit lamp: no clinically relevant changes in corneal riboflavin distribution during upright UV irradiation. *J Refract Surg*. 2017;33(4):281. doi:10.3928/1081597x-20161219-03

22. Whitcher JP, Srinivasan M. Corneal ulceration in the developing world--a silent epidemic. *Br J Ophthalmol*. 1997;81(8):622–623. doi:10.1136/bjo.81.8.622

23. Upadhyay MP, Karmacharya PC, Koirala S, et al. Epidemiologic characteristics, predisposing factors, and etiologic diagnosis of corneal ulceration in Nepal. *Am J Ophthalmol*. 1991;111(1):92–99. doi:10.1016/s0002-9394(14)76903-x

24. Flaxman SR, Bourne RRA, Resnikoff S, et al. Global causes of blindness and distance vision impairment 1990–2020: a systematic review and meta-analysis. *Lancet Glob Health*. 2017;5(12):e1221–e1234. doi:10.1016/S2214-109X(17)30393-5

25. Bamdad S, Malekhosseini H, Khosravi A. Ultraviolet A/riboflavin collagen cross-linking for treatment of moderate bacterial corneal ulcers. *Cornea*. 2015;34(4):402–406. doi:10.1097/ICO.0000000000000375

26. Price MO, Tenkman LR, Schrier A, Fairchild KM, Trokel SL, Price FW, Jr. Photoactivated riboflavin treatment of infectious keratitis using collagen cross-linking technology. *J Refract Surg*. 2012;28(10):706–713. doi:10.3928/1081597x-20120921-06

27. Iseli HP, Thiel MA, Hafezi F, Kampmeier J, Seiler T. Ultraviolet A/riboflavin corneal cross-linking for infectious keratitis associated with corneal melts. *Cornea*. 2008;27(5):590–594. doi:10.1097/ICO.0b013e318169d698

28. Makdoumi K, Mortensen J, Sorkhabi O, Malmvall BE, Crafoord S. UVA-riboflavin photochemical therapy of bacterial keratitis: a pilot study. *Graefes Arch Clin Exp Ophthalmol*. 2012;250(1):95–102. doi:10.1007/s00417-011-1754-1

29. Kasetsuwan N, Reinprayoon U, Satitpitakul V. Photoactivated chromophore for moderate to severe infectious keratitis as an adjunct therapy: a randomized controlled trial. *Am J Ophthalmol*. 2016;165:94–99. doi:10.1016/j.ajo.2016.02.030

30. Said DG, Gatzioufas Z, Hafezi F. Author reply: collagen cross-linking with photoactivated riboflavin (PACK-CXL) for the treatment of advanced infectious keratitis with corneal melting. *Ophthalmology.* 2014. doi:10.1016/j.ophtha.2014.06.044

31. Knyazer B, Krakauer Y, Baumfeld Y, Lifshitz T, Kling S, Hafezi F. Accelerated corneal cross-linking with photoactivated chromophore for moderate therapy-resistant infectious keratitis. *Cornea.* 2018;37(4):528–531. doi:10.1097/ICO.0000000000001498

32. Knyazer B, Krakauer Y, Tailakh MA, et al. Accelerated corneal cross-linking as an adjunct therapy in the management of presumed bacterial keratitis: a cohort study. *J Refract Surg.* 2020;36(4):258–264. doi:10.3928/1081597X-20200226-02

33. Seiler TG, Fischinger I, Koller T, Zapp D, Frueh BE, Seiler T. Customized corneal crosslinking - one year results. *Am J Ophthalmol.* 2016. doi:10.1016/j.ajo.2016.02.029

34. Kling S, Hufschmid FS, Torres-Netto EA, et al. High fluence increases the antibacterial efficacy of PACK cross-linking. *Cornea.* 2020. doi:10.1097/ICO.0000000000002335

35. Hafezi F, Munzinger A, Goldblum D, Hillen M, Tandogan T. Repeated high-fluence accelerated slitlamp-based photoactivated chromophore for keratitis corneal cross-linking for treatment-resistant fungal keratitis. *Cornea.* 2022;41(8):1058–1061. doi:10.1097/ico.0000000000002973

36. Lu NJ, Koliwer-Brandl H, Gilardoni F, et al. The antibacterial efficacy of high-fluence PACK cross-linking can be accelerated. *Transl Vis Sci Technol.* 2023;12(2):12. doi:10.1167/tvst.12.2.12

37. Spoerl E, Wollensak G, Seiler T. Increased resistance of crosslinked cornea against enzymatic digestion. *Curr Eye Res.* 2004;29(1):35–40. doi:10.1080/02713680490513182

38. Hafezi F, Hosny M, Shetty R, et al. PACK-CXL vs. antimicrobial therapy for bacterial, fungal, and mixed infectious keratitis: a prospective randomized phase 3 trial. *Eye Vis (Lond).* 2022;9(1):2. doi:10.1186/s40662-021-00272-0

39. Wei A, Wang K, Wang Y, Gong L, Xu J, Shao T. Evaluation of corneal cross-linking as adjuvant therapy for the management of fungal keratitis. *Graefes Arch Clin Exp Ophthalmol.* 2019;257(7):1443–1452. doi:10.1007/s00417-019-04314-1

40. Bonzano C, Di Zazzo A, Barabino S, Coco G, Traverso CE. Collagen cross-linking in the management of microbial keratitis. *Ocul Immunol Inflamm.* 2019;27(3):507–512. doi:10.1080/09273948.2017.1414856

41. Price MO, Price FW, Jr. Corneal cross-linking in the treatment of corneal ulcers. *Curr Opin Ophthalmol.* 2016;27(3):250–255. doi:10.1097/ICU.0000000000000248

14 Corneal Cross-Linking Combined With LASIK, LASEK, PRK, PTK, and SMILE Refractive Surgeries

Mehrdad Mohammadpour, Masoud Khorrami-Nejad, and Yasir Adil Shakor

INTRODUCTION

Corneal ectasia conditions like keratoconus (KCN) can lead to vision loss due to irregular astigmatism and corneal thinning.[1,2] Corneal cross-linking (CXL), using riboflavin and ultraviolet A irradiation, is an established treatment that halts the progression of ectasia by increasing corneal stiffness.[3,4] More recently, CXL has been combined with refractive surgeries like photorefractive keratectomy (PRK), laser-assisted *in-situ* keratomileusis (LASIK), and small incision lenticule extraction (SMILE) for treatment of keratoconus and post-refractive surgery ectasia.

Numerous studies have evaluated concurrent or sequential CXL with refractive surgeries and found visual, refractive, and keratometric improvements compared with refractive surgery alone. For a better explanation of the results of the studies, we have summarized them in the following table (Table 14.1). In Table 14.1, numerous studies have investigated the concurrent or sequential performance of refractive surgeries, such as PRK, LASIK, LASEK, and SMILE, in combination with CXL. As shown in Table 14.1, most of the articles have concluded that the patients who had CXL combined with PRK, in comparison with performing PRK alone, have attained better improvements of evaluated parameters.

Studies done by Kontadakis et al. and Lee et al. in 2016 and 2017, respectively, are examples for this assessment.[5,6] Others have evaluated the effectiveness and safety of PRK surgery in combination with CXL in both sequential and simultaneous groups. Furthermore, as mentioned in Table 14.1, a few studies have compared these combinations. To conclude from the outcomes of the studies, PRK surgery combined with CXL provides better improvement, especially in terms of refractive parameters and keratometric values.

In 2019, a ten-year study was carried out by Kanellopoulos on 144 progressive KCN eyes treated by topography-guided partial-refraction PRK combined with CXL (Athens protocol). Patients were followed up for 120 to 146 months. The outcomes showed remarkable improvement of mean UDVA at the first year follow-up (0.19 ± 0.17 D to 0.53 ± 0.21 D) and more improvement at the 10-year follow-up (0.55 ± 0.19 D). Also, CDVA improved from 0.59 ± 0.21 D to 0.80 ± 0.17 D at one year and to 0.81 ± 0.19 D at 10 years. Other parameters, such as corneal thickness, steep-K and K_{max}, decreased from 468.74 ± 35.05 to 391.14 ± 40.07 µm, 50.57 ± 2.80 to 45.87 ± 2.70 D, and 53.43 ± 2.97 to 46.17 ± 1.18 D, respectively, at one year and decreased by 395.42 ± 32.21 µm, 44.00 ± 3.22 D and 44.75 ± 2.14 D at 10 years, respectively. The majority of patients showed the stabilization of corneal ectasia, while progressive overcorrection or hyperopic alteration was observed in a few patients. In the conclusion, the author reported that the Athens protocol is safe and effective for corneal ectasia and visual function.[7]

In another study, Tsatsos et al. published an article in 2019, introducing a case in which a 29-year-old female was fully corrected by CXL with an excimer laser, with a BCVA of 20/20 (by soft contact lenses) and photophobia in both eyes pre-operatively. The refraction and CCT were −7.75/−0.75 × 10 and 465 µm, respectively, in the right eye and −7.50/−1.00 × 170 and 468 µm, respectively, in the left eye pre-operatively and there was no record of KCN in topography findings. The patient underwent PRK combined with mitomycin C 0.02% for 20 seconds and 18 mW/cm² accelerated CXL for 5 minutes 2 months earlier. At the one-month follow-up, she had a VA of 20/40 in the right and 20/50 in the left eye. First, bilateral epithelial defect was diagnosed and for the treatment, a therapeutic contact lens, autologous serum, topical dexamethasone, topical ofloxacin, and oral doxycycline 100 mg were applied. After continuous deterioration, she had bilateral amniotic membrane overlay in a specific place for two weeks and due to vision reduction and deterioration, another approach was required. During the examination, both her eyes had a VA of 20/100 and were acutely photophobic. There was a record of seborrhoeic blepharitis, a few staphylococcal collarettes were present, and there was dysfunction of the meibomian gland. Therefore, bilateral corneal melting was diagnosed due to the papillae reaction on the palpebral conjunctiva and corneal de-epithelialization with central corneal thinning. Her atopic conjunctivitis and ocular surface disease were treated by applying topical olopatadine (twice a day), copious ocular lubricants (every hour), punctal plugs, and mild topical steroid drops (six times a day), oral metalloproteinase inhibitor, and hygiene of the eyelid with hot compresses (twice a day). CCT decreased

DOI: 10.1201/9781003371601-14

from 466 μm to 188 μm in the right eye and from 339 μm to 256 μm at the thinnest point after this treatment and the epithelium was healed after five weeks. At the last follow-up, CCT and VA (with RGP) were 230 μm and 20/25 in the right eye and 310 μm and 20/23 in the left, respectively. However, despite good control of the lid disease, evidence of multiple stromal corneal opacities was observed.[8]

Several studies were done to compare CXL plus LASIK surgery (LASIK Xtra) with LASIK alone. Kanellopoulos et al. (2014) (two different studies), Tan et al. (2014), Kanellopoulos et al. (2015), Tomita et al. (2016) and Low et al. (2018) determined that there are better outcomes regarding refractive and keratometric parameters in the combined group than the other one.[9–13] However, Tomita et al. (2014) concluded that there were no significant differences between the two groups regarding UDVA, CDVA, MRSE, ECD, CH, CRF, and several other parameters.[14] In addition, Kymionis et al. (2009), Li et al. (2012), Richoz et al. (2013), Yildirim et al. (2014), Tong et al. (2017), and Sharif et al. (2019) studied performing CXL after LASIK surgery and there were successful results in all of these studies.[15–21]

On the other hand, Ng et al. (2016) and Osman et al. (2019) have compared SMILE surgery alone and in combination with CXL (SMILE Xtra).[22,23] They reported more significant improvements of refractive and keratometric values and other parameters in the SMILE Xtra group than the SMILE only group. Other researchers, such as Ganesh et al. (2015) and Zhou et al. (2018), have compared these surgeries simultaneously.[24,25] The outcomes have represented improvements in UDVA, CDVA, CCT, SE, and other values in response to SMILE Xtra.

Some studies were conducted by researchers comparing different types of surgeries. Hyun et al. (2016) compared the results of refractive errors, UDVA and corneal haze after SMILE, LASEK, and LASEK-CXL surgery.[26] For instance, no significant differences in UDVA were observed between the three groups. Studies conducted by Konstantopoulos et al. (2019) and Lim and Lim (2019) compared the outcomes between LASIK, LASIK Xtra, SMILE, and SMILE Xtra surgeries.[27,28] In Konstantinopoulos et al. study, K values and CT were reduced significantly following SMILE, SMILE Xtra, LASIK, and LASIK Xtra. In contrast, the Lim and Lim study showed better outcomes in SMILE Xtra and LASIK Xtra groups with regard to refractive and keratometric stabilities.

Cagil et al. (2019) conducted a study to assess the visual, refractive, topographic, and aberrometric results of CXL combined with transepithelial PTK treatment on 20 eyes with pellucid marginal degeneration over three years. As a result of the treatment, VA stabilized over the three-year follow-up. The cylindrical value, average-K readings, and the Baiocchi–Calossi–Versaci index decreased markedly from 4.97 ± 2.00 D, 47.12 ± 4.66 D and 3.21 ± 1.93 μm (at the baseline) to 3.28 ± 3.12 D, 46.27 ± 4.46 D and 2.86 ± 1.99 μm (at the 36-month follow-up), respectively. However, the K_{max}, HOA, trefoil, coma, and spherical aberration values remained unchanged during all follow-ups compared with the baseline. There was a notable decrease in SE at the one-year and three-year follow-ups. Also, a considerable decrease was observed regarding central and minimum corneal thicknesses during all follow-ups in comparison with the baseline. Therefore, they deduced that combining transepithelial PTK with accelerated CXL is an effective method to treat patients with pellucid marginal degeneration in the long term.[29]

Based on the summary of recently published results shown in Table 14.1, many studies evaluated combining CXL with refractive surgeries like PRK, LASIK, LASEK, and SMILE for the management of keratoconus and corneal ectasia. Follow-up periods ranged from one month to ten years. Most of these studies showed significant improvements in visual acuity (both uncorrected and corrected distance visual acuity), reduction in spherical equivalent refraction, cylinder, keratometry readings, and higher-order aberrations with combined CXL and refractive surgery compared with refractive surgery alone. Therefore, the combined procedures seem to offer better corneal stability and prevent progression of ectasia compared with refractive surgery alone.

Sequential CXL first followed by PRK or LASIK after 6–12 months offered better outcomes than simultaneous CXL with PRK/LASIK in some studies. Also, fewer complications like haze, regression, or hyperopic shift were noted with the combined approach compared with refractive surgery alone. No significant endothelial cell loss was seen.

Accelerated CXL protocols (high intensity, shorter duration) are preferred over standard Dresden protocol with combined surgeries to minimize damage. In addition, topography-guided or wavefront-guided ablation offers superior results compared with non-guided ablation when combined with CXL. SMILE Xtra (SMILE with CXL) shows comparable safety and efficacy as treatments for high myopes compared with LASIK Xtra and PRK Xtra.

In summary, combined corneal CXL with refractive surgery appears to be safe and effective approach for keratoconus and ectasia treatment with good long-term stability.

Table 14.1 Concurrent or Sequential Performance of Refractive Surgeries (PRK, LASIK, LASEK, SMILE) in Combination with CXL

Summary of Published Reports of CXL in Combination with PRK

Combining Sequence with CXL	Reference	Sample Size	Follow-Up Period	Additional Explanations	Outcome(s)
Simultaneous and sequential	Kanellopoulos (2009)[30]	325	24 to 68 months	Two groups: PRK 6 months after CXL, 127 eyes CXL and PRK simultaneously, 198 eyes	In both groups: Increase in UDVA, CDVA Decrease in spherical equivalent refraction, haze score, and K Unchanged endothelial cell count
Simultaneous	Kymionis et al. (2009)[31]	14	3–6 months	Progressive KCN TG-PRK with the Pulzar Z1 after CXL	Increase in UDVA and CDVA Decrease in SE refraction, defocus and steepest keratometry
Simultaneous and sequential	Kanellopoulos (2010)[32]	325	10 years	TG partial PRK and CXL for KCN and post-LASIK ectasia Two groups: TG surface ablation 1 year after CXL: 127 eyes The Athens protocol: 198 eyes	Increase in UDVA and CDVA and decrease in MRSE and K value (first group better than second group) Mean haze score: 1.20 in first and 0.5 in the second group 70 μm decrease in CCT and no marked change in endothelial cell count in either group
Simultaneous	Kymionis et al. (2011)[33]	31	12 to 25 months	CXL after TG-PRK Progressive KCN Epithelial removal by transepithelial PRK	Decrease in spherical equivalent, mean steep and flat K Increase in UDVA and CDVA
Simultaneous CXL after TG-PRK	Kymionis et al. (2011)[34]	A 39-year-old man	12 months	TG-PRK and CXL for post-LASIK ectasia (after 5 years)	Increase in UDVA and CDVA Decrease in astigmatism pattern and higher-order aberrations
Sequential	Lovieno et al. (2011)[35]	5	6 months	Same-day PRK and CXL after femtosecond laser-enabled placement of ICRSI (Intacs)	Increase in UDVA and CDVA Decrease in spherical equivalent refraction, keratometry, and total aberrations. No developed haze
Simultaneous	Tuwairqi et al. (2012)[36]	22	1 year	CXL combined with TG-PRK Low-grade KCN	Marked improvement in all study parameters
Simultaneous	Kremer et al. (2012)[37]	45	3, 6, and 12 months after PRK-CXL	Moderate KCN ICRSI 6 months before wavefront-guide PRK and ultraviolet-A CXL	Increase in UDVA and CDVA Decrease in the cylinder and apex K No marked changes in other corneal parameters Mild haze remained in 11.1% of eyes

Combining Sequence with CXL	Reference	Sample Size	Follow-Up Period	Additional Explanations	Outcome(s)
Sequential	Kymionis et al. (2012)[38]	A 36-year-old woman	4 months	tPRK 1 year after previous CXL for recrudescent of corneal erosions	Marked visual and topographic improvement No recurrence of corneal erosions after t-PRK
Simultaneous	Spadea et al. (2012)[39]	14	6–24 months	Outcomes of using PRK combined with CXL for residual RE after 27–52 months of performing ELLK in KCN patients	Improvement of at least one line of UDVA and three lines of CDVA (in four patients) Decrease in MRSE and topographic keratometric astigmatism Clear corneas in all patients
TG-PRK after ICRSI and CXL	Coskunseven et al. (2013)[40]	16	6 months after the last procedure	Topography-guided Transepithelial PRK Progressive KCN A 3-step procedure: 1. Keraring intracorneal ring segments implantation; 2. CXL; 3. TG-transepithelial PRK 6 months interval between stages	Increase in UDVA and CDVA Decrease in spherical equivalent refraction, steep, and flat keratometry
Simultaneous	Al-Tuwairqi et al. (2013)[41]	13	3 to 11 months	Same-day topography-guided PRK and CXL after ICRSI Low to moderate keratoconic eyes	Increase in UDVA (63% + two lines), CDVA (except 27%) Decrease in the sphere, astigmatism, mean-K, and coma
Simultaneous	Mukherjee et al. (2013)[42]	22	1, 3, 6, and 12 months	Combined tPRK with CXL Significant KCN	Increase in unaided vision, CDVA Decrease in cylinder Unchanged K_{max}
CXL after PRK	Alessio et al. (2013)[43]	34	2 year	Progressive KCN PRK-CXL: 17 worse eyes CXL alone: 17 better eyes	Considerable improvement of UDVA, CDVA, manifest SE refraction, cylindrical power, flattest, cylindrical simulated and apex keratometry, total, and coma-like aberrations in the first group, whereas significant improvement of spherical power, steepest and average simulated keratometry, and I-S value in both groups.
CXL immediately after TG-PRK	Zeraid et al. (2014)[44]	21	3 months (12 months generally)	Same-day TG-PRK and CXL 9 months after ICRSI Low-moderate KCN	Increase in UDVA Decrease in steep K, flat K, and mean-K value, sphere, cylinder Unchanged CDVA, CCT, and coma
Simultaneous	Fadlallah et al. (2014)[45]	140	6-month, 1-year, 2-year	Non-topography–guided PRK Early stage KCN Mild refractive errors	Increase in UDVA Unchanged CDVA Decrease in spherical equivalent, cylinder, steep and flat keratometry, and central corneal thickness.

(Continued)

Table 14.1 (Continued) Concurrent or Sequential Performance of Refractive Surgeries (PRK, LASIK, LASEK, SMILE) in Combination with CXL

Combining Sequence with CXL	Reference	Sample Size	Follow-Up Period	Additional Explanations	Outcome(s)
Simultaneous	Sakla et al. (2014)[46]	31	1, 3, 6, and 12 months	Partial TG-PRK combined with CXL	Increase in UDVA and CDVA Decrease in defocus, flat and steep K readings, refractive astigmatism
Combined PRK and CXL	Alessio et al. (2014)[47]	17	1, 3, 6, 12, and 48 months	Analyze corneal changes by confocal microscopy after combining PRK and CXL Progressive KCN	Unchanged superficial and basal epithelial cell density and endothelial cell density Decrease in anterior mid-stromal keratocyte density Increase in posterior stromal keratocyte density (1- and 3-month follow-up) Decrease in sub-basal and stromal nerve density parameters up to 6 months and then increase until 18 months follow-up
Simultaneous	Kymionis et al. (2014)[48]	8	1, 3, 6, and 12 months	Conventional PRK combined with CXL simultaneously for pellucid marginal corneal degeneration (Cretan Protocol Plus conventional photorefractive keratectomy) Removing corneal epithelium by t-PTK during treatment	No complications intra- and post-operatively Increase in UDVA Unchanged CDVA and endothelial cell density Decrease in mean spherical equivalent and mean corneal astigmatism
Simultaneous	Kymionis et al. (2014)[49]	23	1, 2, 3, and 4 years (24–56 months)	Progressive KCN tPRK combined with CXL (Cretan protocol)	No complications intra- and postoperatively Increase in UDVA and CDVA Decrease in mean steep and flat K readings, mean corneal astigmatism Unchanged endothelial cell density (ECD)
CXL after partial TG-PRK	Knezović et al. (2015)[50]	4	10 months	Same-day combined TG-PRK and CXL Progressive KCN	Increase in UDVA (except on eye), CDVA (1–5 lines) Decrease in MRSE and keratometry No corneal haze, prolonged epithelial healing, or endothelial cell
Accelerated CXL after TG-PRK	Shetty et al. (2015)[51]	29	1 year	KCN cone-location dependent results after combined TG-PRK and CXL Using riboflavin and enhanced intensity ultraviolet light in CXL procedure Mild to moderate KCN Two groups: cones located within and outside the central 2-mm zone (17 and 12 eyes, respectively)	Improvement of UDVA, CDVA (group 1 better than 2), sphere, cylinder, and simulated K in both Increase in CH and CRF in both (greater in group 2 than 1)

Combining Sequence with CXL	Reference	Sample Size	Follow-Up Period	Additional Explanations	Outcome(s)
CXL immediately after TG-PRK	Sherif et al. (2015)[52]	20	12 months	Mild and moderate KCN TG-PRK applying a Custom Ablation Transition Zone (CATz) and CXL Maximum of ablation: 58 μm	Remarkable increase in UDVA and CDVA Decrease in K_{max}, Kmin, and keratometric asymmetry Safety and efficacy index: 1.39 and 0.97, respectively
Two-step procedure for KCN: 1 KeraRing 2 TG-PRK & CXL (same-day)	Al-Tuwairqi et al. (2015)[53]	41	1 year	Femtosecond laser-enabled placement of ICRS: Intralase FS laser	Increase in UDVA (from 6 months to more than a year) Decrease in refraction SE, all keratometry readings, CCT, and corneal thickness at the thinnest point No marked improvement of CDVA and coma
Simultaneous	Sakla et al. (2016)[54]	85	1, 3, 6, and 12 months	TG-PRK and accelerated CXL Retrospective study	Increase in UDVA and 90.6% +1 line in CDVA Decrease in manifest SE refraction, flat, and steep keratometry
TG-PRK combined with CXL	Chen et al. (2016)[55]	53	1 to 3, 3 to 6, and more than 6 months	Corneal epithelial thickness change after combined TG-PRK and CXL for KCN Retrospective analysis	Increase in epithelial thickness at the thinnest area (no considerable change in other areas) Improvement of CDVA, refractive astigmatism, K_{max}, Kmin, and IRI
Simultaneous	Kontadakis et al. (2016)[5]	60	28—months	Progressive KCN Two groups: Group 1: CXL-alone (30 eyes) Group 2: tPRK-CXL (30 eyes and with a solid-state laser)	Increase in CDVA and UDVA in both groups (no case lost more than 2 lines of Snellen VA, while 8 and 19 eyes from first and second group, respectively, attained 2 or more lines of CDVA) Decrease in steep-K and flat-K at the last follow-up more significant in the second group than the first one (no marked difference between groups before surgery) Unchanged endothelial cell density
Simultaneous and sequential	Abou Sarma et al. (2016)[56]	62	1 year	Wavefront-guided (WFG) PRK and accelerated CXL Progressive KCN Two groups: First group: Simultaneous WFG PRK and accelerated CXL (30 eyes) Second group: WFG PRK 6 months after accelerated CXL (32 eyes)	Significant and stable improvement of all visual, refractive, and aberrometric parameters in both groups (no notable difference between groups) A marked improvement in keratometric and Q values

(Continued)

Table 14.1 (Continued)   Concurrent or Sequential Performance of Refractive Surgeries (PRK, LASIK, LASEK, SMILE) in Combination with CXL

Combining Sequence with CXL	Reference	Sample Size	Follow-Up Period	Additional Explanations	Outcome(s)
tPRK and CXL after ICRSI	Lee et al. (2017)[6]	23	1, 3, and 6 months after tPRK-CXL	Moderate KCN Combined corneal wavefront-guided transepithelial PRK and high-fluence accelerated CXL after ICRSI	Significant increase in UDVA and decrease in the sphere, MRSE, K_{max}, K at the apex, mean-K, and KCN index after ICRSI Remarkable improvement in UDVA and CDVA and decrease in cylinder and other corneal indices after tPRK and CXL Considerable decrease in HOAs, coma aberrations (with no changes after ICRSI), final radius, and deformation amplitude
TG-PRK combined with CXL	Müller et al. (2017)[57]	9	18 months	Use a different laser platform (AMARIS 500E) in KCN and PLE patients	Improvement of topography and VA (K_{max}, Kmean, RMS HOA, vertical coma, cylinder, CDVA, UDVA)
Simultaneous	Grentzelos et al. (2017)[58]	55	1,3,6, and 12 months	Combined transepithelial PTK and conventional PRK followed simultaneously by CXL (Cretan Protocol Plus) Progressive KCN	Increase in UDVA and CDVA Decrease in spherical equivalent, steep and flat keratometry readings No ECD alterations
Simultaneous	Cassagn et al. (2017)[59]	60	1 year	Progressive KCN Comparing customized TG-CXL with C-CXL Two groups: Group 1: 30 eyes treated with TG-CXL Group 2: 30 eyes treated with C-CXL (Dresden protocol)	Marked difference for both K_{max} and mean-K in the inferior part of the cornea (I index) between groups Increase in CDVA (significantly in TG-CXL group) Observation of a stromal marking line in both groups (equal depth at the top of the cone, but shallower depth at the circumambient area (less damage and quicker healing) in the first group)
TG-PRK and phakic IOL after ICRSI and CXL	Coşkunseven et al. (2017)[60]	11	Mean: 12 months after TG-PRK	Retrospective interventional patients Progressive KCN Four-stage combined treatment for KCN: 1 Keraring implantation 2 CXL 3 Phakic IOL implantation 4 TG-PRK At least 6-month interval between each stage	Increase in UDVA and CDVA Decrease in mean MRSE (from 16.78 ± 3.58 to 0.59 ± 0.89 D) and mean refractive astigmatism (from 5.16 ± 1.86 to 0.82 ± 0.28 D)
Simultaneous	Gore et al. (2018)[61]	47	24 months	Moderately keratoconic eyes Wavefront-guided transepithelial PRK and CXL	Increase in CDVA Decrease in maximum keratometry reading and coma Unchanged mean K values

Combining Sequence with CXL	Reference	Sample Size	Follow-Up Period	Additional Explanations	Outcome(s)
Simultaneous	Sachdev et al. (2018)[62]	227	1 year	PRK with concurrent half-fluence cross-linking (PRK Xtra) Two groups: Group A: PRK Xtra (109 eyes) Group B: PRK alone (118 eyes)	Increase in CDVA (96.3% A, 99.1% B) No iatrogenic ectasia or hyperopic shift secondary to progressive flattening in A No incidence of haze
Simultaneous	Al-Amri (2018)[63]	60	3 months 1, 2, 3, 4, and 5 years	Non-topography guided PRK combined with 15 min CXL Mild and non-progressive KCN	Increase in UDVA, CDVA Decrease in SE refraction, manifest sphere, manifest cylinder, steep and steepest keratometry.
Simultaneous PRK-CXL	Ohana et al. (2018)[64]	98	At least 1 year	Retrospective cohort study Patients without KCN only	Increase in UDVA Decrease in SE No corneal ectasia Corneal haze: a major complication
PTK combined with PRK and CXL sequentially on the same day	Zhou et al. (2019)[65]	16	6, 12, 24 months	Management of corneal ectasia after LASIK surgery	Increase in UDVA Decrease in cylinder equivalent refraction, flat K, and steep K values Unchanged endothelial count and morphology There is no obvious corneal haze and no significant reduction and change in spherical equivalent refraction and CCT, respectively.
Combined PRK-CXL	Kymionis et al. (2019)[66]	A 34-year-old man	12 months	Resolving the stromal interface epithelial ingrowth after combined PRK and CXL in a case with post-LASIK ectasia	Improvement of visual and topographic parameters without epithelial ingrowth relapse or progression of corneal ectasia
Combined PRK-AXL	Iqbal et al. (2019)[67]	125	3, 6, 12, 24 months	30 min Epi-off CXL versus PRK combined with accelerated epithelium-off cross-linking (AXL) Progressive KCN (CXL-Plus) Two groups: Standard CXL (58 eyes) PRK-AXL (67 eyes)	Increase in UDVA and CDVA Decrease in SE and cylinder Close results in both groups
Simultaneous	Kaiserman et al. (2019)[68]	20	266 – 1749 days	Performing an epithelial PRK (ePRK) combined with CXL for KCN (Tel Aviv protocol) Progressive KCN	Notable increase in UDVA and CDVA Marked decrease in mean keratometry, K_{max}, Kmin, and TCT No complications No KCN progression
Simultaneous	Makar et al. (2019)[69]	20	1 year	Evaluating corneal changes after TG-PRK combined with accelerated CXL (Athens protocol)	Increase in UDVA and CDVA Decrease in flat and steep K, mean post-operative index of surface variance, and index of high deceleration.

(Continued)

Table 14.1 (Continued) Concurrent or Sequential Performance of Refractive Surgeries (PRK, LASIK, LASEK, SMILE) in Combination with CXL

Combining Sequence with CXL	Reference	Sample Size	Follow-Up Period	Additional Explanations	Outcome(s)
TG partial-refraction PRK combined with CXL	Kanellopoulos (2019)[7]	144	10 years (120 to 146 months)	Progressive KCN Topography-guided partial-refraction PRK combined with CXL (the Athens protocol)	A notable increase in mean UDVA and CDVA (from 0.19 ± 0.17 to 0.53 ± 0.21 D and from 0.59 ± 0.21 to 0.80 ± 0.17 D respectively at first year and further to 0.55 ± 0.19 D and to 0.81 ± 0.19 D respectively at 10 years Decrease in corneal thickness from 468.74 ± 35.05 to 391.14 ± 40.07 μm at 1 first year and up to 395.42 ± 32.21 μm at 10 years. Decrease in steep-K and K_{max} from 50.57 ± 2.80 to 45.87 ± 2.70 D and from 53.43 ± 2.97 to 46.17 ± 1.18 D at first year, respectively and to 44.00 ± 3.22 D and to 44.75 ± 2.14 D respectively at 10 years Observation of ectasia stabilization and progressive "overcorrection" or "hyperopic" shift in 94.4% and 3.5%, respectively.
Partial TG-PRK combined with refractive, customized CXL	Kanellopoulos (2019)[70]	25	36 to 42 months	A novel usage (Modified (Enhanced) Athens protocol)	Increase in UDVA (from 20/80 to 20/25 at 6 months) Improvement in severity of KCN stage (from a mean of 3.2 to 1.8) Decrease in maximum astigmatism (7.8 D) A marked cornea surface normalization (at the first month)
Simultaneous	Mohammadpour et al. (2020)[71]	17	3 years (25 to 49 months)	Evaluating the combination of PRK and accelerated CXL in high- risk refractive surgeries (Tehran protocol)	Improvement of UDVA and CDVA (with no loss of lines) No late stromal haze, corneal ectasia, or other complications post-operatively

Summary of Recently Published Results for CXL Combined with LASIK

Combining Sequence with CXL	Reference	Sample Size	Follow-Up Period	Additional Explanations	Outcome(s)
CXL after LASIK	Kymionis et al. (2009)[15]	10	1 year	CXL in patients with post-LASIK keratectasia (5 eyes) and progressive KCN (5 eyes) Evaluating corneal remodeling by corneal *in vivo* confocal microscopy Control groups: three normal/healthy and three post-LASIK without ectasia eyes	Normal epithelial thickness pre- and postoperatively; Similar morphologic changes in both main groups; No subepithelial nerve plexus right away after surgery and appearance of nerve regeneration after 3 months; No keratocytes from the anterior 300 mum of the stroma at 3 months, while there was an increase in the keratocyte density in the posterior stroma (repopulation of full-thickness keratocytes in the anterior and mid-corneal stroma after 6 months); Uneven distribution of corneal collagen fibers in the anterior stroma in the form of a net; Unchanged corneal endothelium
CXL after LASIK	Li G, et al. (2012)[16]	20	1 year (1, 3, 6, and 12 months)	Preventing the progression of post-LASIK corneal ectasia by CXL without relevant complications	Increase in UDVA, CDVA, and thinnest cornea pachymetry; Decrease in flattest and steepest meridian keratometry; No deterioration in endothelial cell count
CXL after LASIK and PRK	Richoz et al. (2013)[17]	26	12–62 months (mean 25 months)	Post-operative progressive ectasia after LASIK (23 eyes) and PRK (3 eyes) Long-term follow-up	Increase in mean CDVA, minimum radius of curvature (R(min)); Decrease in K_{max} index of vertical asymmetry, KCN index, and the central KCN index
Same-day ICRS and CXL after LASIK	Yildirim et al. (2014)[19]	16	36–62 months	Post-operative ectasia after LASIK Long-term follow-up	Increase in UDVA and CDVA; Decrease in spherical and cylindrical refraction, maximum and minimum keratometry values; No serious complications
Simultaneous LASIK and CXL	Tomita et al. (2014)[14]	24	1 year	Evaluating morphologic changes by using *in-vivo* confocal laser microscopy Unilateral accelerated CXL (non-dominant eye) in bilateral myopic LASIK patients Two groups: First group: LASIK-CXL eyes Second group: LASIK-only eyes	No marked differences in UDVA, CDVA, MRSE, ECD, CH, CRF, KMI, and 37 additional parameters between groups; Increase hyper-reflectivity by observing a demarcation line (present in 23 eyes) in first group (well defined in 2 and faint in 21 eyes)
CXL after LASIK	Yildirim et al. (2014)[18]	20	36–60 months (mean 42 months)	Treatment of post-LASIK ectasia by CXL	Increase in UDVA and CDVA (no loss of lines); Decrease in spherical (non-significant) and cylindrical refraction and K_{max}; No notable complications

(Continued)

Table 14.1 (Continued) Concurrent or Sequential Performance of Refractive Surgeries (PRK, LASIK, LASEK, SMILE) in Combination with CXL

Combining Sequence with CXL	Reference	Sample Size	Follow-Up Period	Additional Explanations	Outcome(s)
Simultaneous	Kanellopoulos et al. (2014)[9]	139	6 months	Epithelial remodeling evaluation High myopia LASIK Xtra: LASIK + simultaneous prophylactic high-fluence CXL Group 1 : 67 (LASIK Xtra) Group 2:72 (femtosecond LASIK)	An increase in the epithelial thickness combined with notable differences, particularly between high-myopia subgroups. Significant reduction in epithelial increase in the first group in comparison with the second one
Simultaneous	Kanellopoulos et al. (2014)[10]	155	1 year	Femtosecond myopic LASIK with and without concurrent prophylactic high-fluence CXL (LASIK-CXL). Group A: LASIK combined with simultaneous prophylactic high-fluence CXL (73 eyes) Group B: stand-alone LASIK (82 eyes)	The outcomes of MRSE, flat and steep keratometry, are better in group A than B. The keratometric stability plots are constant for the first group and slightly retrogressing in the second group LASIK-CXL improves refractive and keratometric stability
Sequential	Tan et al. (2014)[72]	134	3 months	High myopia correction (−8.00 to −19.00 MRSE) Main group: consecutive LASIK and accelerated CXL (70) Control group: LASIK-alone (64 retrospective eyes)	Attainment of UDVA of 20/25: 98% of the first and 61% of the second group A greater proportion of eyes within ± 0.5 D of the intended: 88% in the first and 65% in the second group A tendency to greater refractive drift in LASIK Xtra (−0.04 D) and LASIK (−0.13 D) groups
Simultaneous	Kanellopoulos et al. (2015)[11]	140	2 year	High myopia Group 1: prophylactic high-fluence CXL combined with high-myopic LASIK (65 eyes) Group 2: myopic LASIK (75 eyes)	Mean MRSE, flat K, and steep K in group 1 are −0.18 ± 17.0, 37.67, and 38.38; whereas mean MRSE, flat K, and steep K in group 2 are 0.32 ± 0.24, 38.04, and 38.69, respectively A significant difference between the two groups at the 20/20 and 20/25 levels LASIK-CXL (probably by changing corneal biomechanical properties) improves refractive and keratometric stability
Simultaneous	Tomita (2016)[12]	673	3 months to 4.5 years	Comparison of combined LASIK and accelerated CXL with LASIK alone A review study Effective method for myopia and hyperopia correction and in patients with low predicted residual bed thickness	Less regression and better refractive and keratometric results by LASIK-accelerated CXL than LASIK alone No case of post-LASIK ectasia progression
Simultaneous	Taneri et al. (2017)[73]	1 patient (2 eyes)	12 months and 2 years	Combined CXL and LASIK Case report Post-LASIK unilateral corneal ectasia in combination with prophylactic CXL	Non-significant post-operative topography with UDVA of 1.0 in both eyes at first-year follow-up Loss of vision (UDVA 0.25) and steepening inferior on topography in left eye after 2 years

Combining Sequence with CXL	Reference	Sample Size	Follow-Up Period	Additional Explanations	Outcome(s)
CXL after LASIK	Tong et al. (2017)[20]	14	12–78 months	Epi-off CXL for post-LASIK ectasia A retrospective study	Increase in CDVA, index of height asymmetry No keratometric deterioration in 12 eyes No progression of corneal HOAs Unchanged CCT No significant complications post-operatively
Simultaneous	Low et al. (2018)[13]	50	1.5 to 13.3 months in first group and 1.7 to 4.2 months in second group	High myopia A retrospective study Two groups: First group: LASIK Xtra Second group: LASIK-only	Increase in UDVA to 20/40 or better in all eyes (20/20: 80.0% of first and 66.0% of second group) At 3 months, the proportion of eyes within ±0.5 D of attempted correction:was 72% in the first and 84% in the second group Achievement of good refractive stability at 6–12 months
CXL after LASIK	Sharif et al. (2019)[21]	17	57–102 months	Halting the progression of post-LASIK ectasia by CXL procedure Long-term follow-up	Increase in UDVA and CDVA Decrease in spherical and cylindrical refraction, K_{max}, Kmin, and corneal thickness (non-significant)

(Continued)

131

Table 14.1 (Continued) Concurrent or Sequential Performance of Refractive Surgeries (PRK, LASIK, LASEK, SMILE) in Combination with CXL

Summary of Recently Published Results for CXL Combined with SMILE

Combining Sequence with CXL	Reference	Sample Size	Follow-Up Period	Additional Explanations	Outcome(s)
Simultaneous	Ganesh et al. (2015)[24]	40	11–13 months	ReLEx SMILE Xtra Thinner corneas, borderline topography, and higher refractive errors	Decrease in SE, CCT, and keratometry Mean UCVA: 20/25 or better No lost lines of CDVA, haze, keratitis, ectasia, or regression
Simultaneous	Ng et al. (2016)[22]	53	1, 3, and 6 months	Group 1: SMILE Xtra (thinner preoperative CCT and residual stromal bed thickness) (21 eyes) Group 2: SMILE-only (32 eyes) Both groups: myopia with SEQ > 4.00 D	No eyes lost more than 1 line in CDVA The proportion of eyes within ±0.5 D of target refraction: 89% in the first and 94% in the second group The efficacy index: 0.88 ± 0.13 (group 1) and 0.97 ± 0.06 (group 2)
Simultaneous	Zhou et al. (2018)[25]	43	6 months	Assessment of microstructural modifications and security of SMILE Xtra in high myopia and thin corneas by IVCM and 3D-OCT	Slight damage in corneal epithelial cells up to 3 months Decrease in subepithelial nerve plexus Presence of strong reflective particles and cicatricial reaction in the anterior stroma within 6 months Increase in hyperreflectivity Unchanged corneal endothelium
Combined tPTK and CXL after SMILE	Ge et al. (2018)[74]	1	3 year	Uncommon corneal ectasia after SMILE	Improvement of K_{max}, mean corneal keratometry, SE, and UDVA
Simultaneous	Osman et al. (2019)[23]	60	24 months	Corneal safety and stability of SMILE Xtra procedure A retrospective study Two groups: SMILE Xtra and SMILE-alone Patients >18 years of age, myopic error >6D, thinner cornea <520 microns, and abnormal corneal topography	Considerable difference between the groups in terms of UDVA, CDVA, and MRSE at first-month follow-up At 24 months, UDVA in the first group 20/20 (90%) and 20/30 (97%), and the proportion of eyes within ±0.5 D of attempted correction in both groups were similar (87% vs 84%) MRSE improvement remained stable until at least 1-year follow-up CRF and corneal densitometry: higher in the first group
CXL after SMILE and PRK	Torres-Netto et al. (2020)[75]	26 paired corneas	Not mentioned	Evaluating the biomechanical efficacy of CXL surgery for post-operative ectasia after SMILE or PRK by an *ex-vivo* model in human corneas Two groups: Right corneas: PRK Left corneas: SMILE	The mean elastic modulus in corneas: 17.2 ± 5.3 MPa in the first and 14.1 ± 5.0 in the second group No marked biomechanical difference between the two groups

Summary of Recently Published Results for CXL Combined with PRK, LASIK, LASEK and SMILE Refractive Surgeries (Comparative Studies)

Combining Sequence with CXL	Reference	Sample Size	Follow-Up Period	Additional Explanations	Outcome(s)
SMILE, LASEK, and LASEK-CXL	Hyun et al. (2016)[26]	170	6 months	Comparing results of Group 1: SMILE (69) Group 2: LASEK (61) Group 3: LASEK-CXL (40) High-degree myopia (SE > −6.00 D)	No marked differences in UDVA between the various groups. The proportion of eyes with a residual refractive error within ±0.5 D: 84% in first, 65% in the second and 76% in the third group. Patients with UDVA better than 20/25 : 100%, 91% and 95% respectively. Post-operative corneal haze: 0, 18%, and 25% respectively
Simultaneous (LASIK Xtra and SMILE Xtra)	Konstantopoulos et al. (2019)[27]	21	2, 4, and 6 weeks	Corneal stability of LASIK and SMILE combined with CXL −5 D LASIK: 6 eyes −5 D SMILE: 6 eyes −5 D LASIK Xtra: 5 eyes −5 D SMILE Xtra: 5 eyes	Decrease in K values and CT in all surgical groups. Increase in MPE in all groups except LASIK Xtra. MPE after SMILE less than LASIK (not marked) and post-LASIK Xtra MPE less than that after LASIK
LASIK, PRK, and SMILE with simultaneous accelerated CXL	Lim et al. (2019)[28]	1189	≥ 1 year	Reducing complications of refractive surgical procedures by using LASIK Xtra, PRK Xtra, and SMILE Xtra. A review study. LASIK-only and Xtra: 300–347 PRK-only and Xtra: 204 –298 SMILE-only and Xtra: 0–40	Better outcomes regarding refractive and keratometric stability in refractive surgeries combined with simultaneous CXL than alone ones

PTK: Phototherapeutic keratectomy, PRK: Photorefractive keratectomy, LASIK: Laser Assisted *In-Situ* Keratomileusis, LASEK: Laser Assisted Sub-Epithelial Keratectomy. SMILE: Small Incision Lenticule Extraction, LASIK Xtra: LASIK surgery combined with CXL, PRK Xtra: PRK surgery combined with CXL, SMILE Xtra: SMILE surgery combined with CXL, CT: corneal thickness, MPE: maximum posterior elevation, SEQ: spherical equivalent refraction, KMI: keratoconus match index, MPa: megapascal, CCT: central corneal thickness, TG-PRK: Topography-Guided Photorefractive keratectomy, AXL: accelerated epithelium-off cross-linking, tPTK: Transepithelial Phototherapeutic keratectomy, PRK Xtra: PRK with concurrent half-fluence crosslinking, tPRK: Transepithelial Photorefractive keratectomy, MRSE: manifest refraction spherical equivalent, IRI: corneal irregularity index, RMS HOA: root mean square value for the higher order corneal aberrations, PLE: post-LASIK ectasia, TG-CXL: Topography-guided corneal collagen cross-linking, C-CXL: conventional corneal collagen cross-linking, WFG PRK: wavefront-guided photorefractive keratectomy, simulated K: simulated keratectomy, F/U: follow-up, CATz: Custom Ablation Transition Zone, ECD: endothelial cell density, K: keratometry, apex K: apex keratometry, ELLK: excimer laser-assisted lamellar keratoplasty, ICR: Intracorneal rings, ICRS: Intracorneal ring segment, ICRSI: Intracorneal ring segment implantation, K reading: Keratometry reading, MRSE: manifest refraction spherical equivalent, SE: spherical equivalent, RE: refractive error, flat-K: flat keratometry, steep-K: steep keratometry, mean-K: mean keratometry, average K: average keratometry, K values: keratometry values, steepest K values: steepest keratometry values, VA: visual acuity, Epi-off CXL: epithelium-off corneal crosslinking, CH: corneal hysteresis, CRF: corneal resistance factor, Km: mean keratometry, K_{max}: maximum keratometry, corneal HOAs: corneal higher-order aberrations, K1: flat keratometry, K2: steep keratometry, I-S difference: inferior-superior difference, toric pIOL: toric phakic intraocular lens, D: diopter, CH: corneal hysteresis, CRF: corneal resistance factor, TCT: thinnest corneal thickness

REFERENCES

1. Khorrami-Nejad M, Aghili O, Hashemian H, Aghazadeh-Amiri M, Karimi F. Changes in corneal asphericity after MyoRing implantation in moderate and severe keratoconus. *Journal of Ophthalmic & Vision Research*. 2019;14(4):428.

2. Naderi M, Karimi F, Jadidi K, Mosavi SA, Ghobadi M, Tireh H, et al. Long-term results of MyoRing implantation in patients with keratoconus. *Clinical and Experimental Optometry*. 2021;104(4):499–504.

3. Mohammadpour M, Khoshtinat N, Khorrami-Nejad M. Comparison of visual, tomographic, and biomechanical outcomes of 360 degrees intracorneal ring implantation with and without corneal crosslinking for progressive keratoconus: a 5-year follow-up. *Cornea*. 2021;40(3):303–10.

4. Mohammadpour M, Heirani M, Khoshtinat N, Khorrami-Nejad M. Comparison of two different 360-degree intrastromal corneal rings combined with simultaneous accelerated-corneal cross-linking. *European Journal of Ophthalmology*. 2024;34(1):126–39.

5. Kontadakis GA, Kankariya VP, Tsoulnaras K, Pallikaris AI, Plaka A, Kymionis GD. Long-term comparison of simultaneous topography-guided photorefractive keratectomy followed by corneal cross-linking versus corneal cross-linking alone. *Ophthalmology*. 2016;123(5):974–83.

6. Lee H, Kang DSY, Ha BJ, Choi JY, Kim EK, Seo KY. Visual rehabilitation in moderate keratoconus: combined corneal wavefront-guided transepithelial photorefractive keratectomy and high-fluence accelerated corneal collagen cross-linking after intracorneal ring segment implantation. *BMC Ophthalmology*. 2017;17(1):1–14.

7. Kanellopoulos AJ. Ten-year outcomes of progressive keratoconus management with the Athens Protocol (topography-guided partial-refraction PRK combined with CXL). *Journal of Refractive Surgery*. 2019;35(8):478–83.

8. Tsatsos M, Athanasiadis I, MacGregor C, Aristeidou A, Moschos MM, Ziakas N. Combined photorefractive keratectomy and cross-linking. Pushing the limits. *Taiwan Journal of Ophthalmology*. 2019;9(3):206.

9. Kanellopoulos AJ, Asimellis G. Epithelial remodeling after femtosecond laser-assisted high myopic LASIK: comparison of stand-alone with LASIK combined with prophylactic high-fluence cross-linking. *Cornea*. 2014;33(5):463–9.

10. Kanellopoulos AJ, Asimellis G, Karabatsas C. Comparison of prophylactic higher fluence corneal cross-linking to control, in myopic LASIK, one year results. *Clinical Ophthalmology (Auckland, NZ)*. 2014;8:2373.

11. Kanellopoulos AJ, Asimellis G. Combined laser in situ keratomileusis and prophylactic high-fluence corneal collagen crosslinking for high myopia: two-year safety and efficacy. *Journal of Cataract & Refractive Surgery*. 2015;41(7):1426–33.

12. Tomita M. Combined laser in-situ keratomileusis and accelerated corneal cross-linking: an update. *Current Opinion in Ophthalmology*. 2016;27(4):304–10.

13. Low JR, Lim L, Koh JCW, Chua DKP, Rosman M. Suppl-1, M3: Simultaneous accelerated corneal crosslinking and laser in situ keratomileusis for the treatment of high myopia in Asian Eyes. *The Open Ophthalmology Journal*. 2018;12:143.

14. Tomita M, Yoshida Y, Yamamoto Y, Mita M, Waring IV G. In vivo confocal laser microscopy of morphologic changes after simultaneous LASIK and accelerated collagen crosslinking for myopia: one-year results. *Journal of Cataract & Refractive Surgery*. 2014;40(6):981–90.

15. Kymionis GD, Diakonis VF, Kalyvianaki M, Portaliou D, Siganos C, Kozobolis VP, et al. One-year follow-up of corneal confocal microscopy after corneal cross-linking in patients with post laser in situ keratosmileusis ectasia and keratoconus. *American Journal of Ophthalmology.* 2009;147(5):774–8.e1.

16. Li G, Fan Z-J, Peng X-J. Corneal collagen crosslinking for corneal ectasia of post-LASIK: one-year results. *International Journal of Ophthalmology.* 2012;5(2):190.

17. Richoz O, Mavrakanas N, Pajic B, Hafezi F. Corneal collagen cross-linking for ectasia after LASIK and photorefractive keratectomy: long-term results. *Ophthalmology.* 2013;120(7):1354–9.

18. Yildirim A, Cakir H, Kara N, Uslu H, Gurler B, Ozgurhan EB, et al. Corneal collagen cross-linking for ectasia after laser in situ keratomileusis: long-term results. *Journal of Cataract & Refractive Surgery.* 2014;40(10):1591–6.

19. Yildirim A, Uslu H, Kara N, Cakir H, Gurler B, Colak HN, et al. Same-day intrastromal corneal ring segment and collagen cross-linking for ectasia after laser in situ keratomileusis: long-term results. *American Journal of Ophthalmology.* 2014;157(5):1070–6.e2.

20. Tong JY, Viswanathan D, Hodge C, Sutton G, Chan C, Males JJ. Corneal collagen crosslinking for post-LASIK ectasia: an Australian study. *The Asia-Pacific Journal of Ophthalmology.* 2017;6(3):228–32.

21. Sharif W, Ali ZR, Sharif K. Long term efficacy and stability of corneal collagen cross linking for post-LASIK ectasia: an average of 80mo follow-up. *International Journal of Ophthalmology.* 2019;12(2):333.

22. Ng AL, Chan TC, Cheng GP, Jhanji V, Ye C, Woo VC, et al. Comparison of the early clinical outcomes between combined small-incision lenticule extraction and collagen cross-linking versus SMILE for myopia. *Journal of Ophthalmology.* 2016;2016. https://doi.org/10.1155/2016/2672980

23. Osman IM, Helaly HA, Abou Shousha M, AbouSamra A, Ahmed I. Corneal safety and stability in cases of small incision lenticule extraction with collagen cross-linking (SMILE Xtra). *Journal of Ophthalmology.* 2019;2019. https://doi.org/10.1155/2019/6808062

24. Ganesh S, Brar S. Clinical outcomes of small incision lenticule extraction with accelerated cross-linking (ReLEx SMILE Xtra) in patients with thin corneas and borderline topography. *Journal of Ophthalmology.* 2015;2015. https://doi.org/10.1155/2015/263412

25. Zhou Y, Liu M, Zhang T, Zheng H, Sun Y, Yang X, et al. In vivo confocal laser microscopy of morphologic changes after small incision lenticule extraction with accelerated cross-linking (SMILE Xtra) in patients with thin corneas and high myopia. *Graefe's Archive for Clinical and Experimental Ophthalmology.* 2018;256(1):199–207.

26. Hyun S, Lee S, Kim J-h. Visual outcomes after SMILE, LASEK, and LASEK combined with corneal collagen cross-linking for high myopic correction. *Cornea.* 2016;36(4):399–405.

27. Konstantopoulos A, Liu Y-C, Teo EP, Nyein CL, Yam GH, Mehta JS. Corneal stability of LASIK and SMILE when combined with collagen cross-linking. *Translational Vision Science & Technology.* 2019;8(3):21.

28. Lim EWL, Lim L. Review of laser vision correction (LASIK, PRK and SMILE) with simultaneous accelerated corneal crosslinking–long-term results. *Current Eye Research.* 2019;44(11):1171–80.

29. Cagil N, Sarac O, Yesilirmak N, Caglayan M, Uysal BS, Tanriverdi B. Transepithelial photo-therapeutic keratectomy followed by corneal collagen crosslinking for the treatment of pellucid marginal degeneration: long-term results. *Cornea*. 2019;38(8):980–5.

30. Kanellopoulos AJ. Comparison of sequential vs same-day simultaneous collagen cross-linking and topography-guided PRK for treatment of keratoconus. *Journal of Refractive Surgery*. 2009;25(9):S812–S8.

31. Kymionis GD, Kontadakis GA, Kounis GA, Portaliou DM, Karavitaki AE, Magarakis M, et al. Simultaneous topography-guided PRK followed by corneal collagen cross-linking for keratoconus. *Journal of Refractive Surgery*. 2009;25(9):S807–S11.

32. Kanellopoulos AJ. Combining topography-guided PRK with CXL: the Athens protocol. *Cataract & Refractive Surgery Today Europe*. 2010:18–22.

33. Kymionis GD, Portaliou DM, Kounis GA, Limnopoulou AN, Kontadakis GA, Grentzelos MA. Simultaneous topography-guided photorefractive keratectomy followed by corneal collagen cross-linking for keratoconus. *American Journal of Ophthalmology*. 2011;152(5):748–55.

34. Kymionis GD, Portaliou DM, Diakonis VF, Karavitaki AE, Panagopoulou SI, Jankov II MR, et al. Management of post laser in situ keratomileusis ectasia with simultaneous topography guided photorefractive keratectomy and collagen cross-linking. *The Open Ophthalmology Journal*. 2011;5:11.

35. Iovieno A, Légaré ME, Rootman DB, Yeung SN, Kim P, Rootman DS. Intracorneal ring segments implantation followed by same-day photorefractive keratectomy and corneal collagen cross-linking in keratoconus. *Journal of Refractive Surgery*. 2011;27(12):915–8.

36. Tuwairqi WS, Sinjab MM. Safety and efficacy of simultaneous corneal collagen cross-linking with topography-guided PRK in managing low-grade keratoconus: 1-year follow-up. *Journal of Refractive Surgery*. 2012;28(5):341–5.

37. Kremer I, Aizenman I, Lichter H, Shayer S, Levinger S. Simultaneous wavefront-guided photorefractive keratectomy and corneal collagen crosslinking after intrastromal corneal ring segment implantation for keratoconus. *Journal of Cataract & Refractive Surgery*. 2012;38(10):1802–7.

38. Kymionis GD, Grentzelos MA, Mikropoulos DG, Rallis KI. Transepithelial phototherapeutic keratectomy for recurrent corneal erosions in a patient with previous corneal collagen cross-linking. *Journal of Refractive Surgery*. 2012;28(10):732–4.

39. Spadea L, Paroli M. Simultaneous topography-guided PRK followed by corneal collagen cross-linking after lamellar keratoplasty for keratoconus. *Clinical Ophthalmology (Auckland, NZ)*. 2012;6:1793.

40. Coskunseven E, Jankov MR, Grentzelos MA, Plaka AD, Limnopoulou AN, Kymionis GD. Topography-guided transepithelial PRK after intracorneal ring segments implantation and corneal collagen CXL in a three-step procedure for keratoconus. *Journal of Refractive Surgery*. 2013;29(1):54–8.

41. Al-Tuwairqi W, Sinjab MM. Intracorneal ring segments implantation followed by same-day topography-guided PRK and corneal collagen CXL in low to moderate keratoconus. *Journal of Refractive Surgery*. 2013;29(1):59–64.

42. Mukherjee AN, Selimis V, Aslanides I. Transepithelial photorefractive keratectomy with crosslinking for keratoconus. *The Open Ophthalmology Journal*. 2013;7:63.

43. Alessio G, L'abbate M, Sborgia C, La Tegola MG. Photorefractive keratectomy followed by cross-linking versus cross-linking alone for management of progressive keratoconus: two-year follow-up. *American Journal of Ophthalmology*. 2013;155(1):54–65.e1.

44. Zeraid FM, Jawkhab AA, Al-Tuwairqi WS, Osuagwu UL. Visual rehabilitation in low-moderate keratoconus: intracorneal ring segment implantation followed by same-day topography-guided photorefractive keratectomy and collagen cross linking. *International Journal of Ophthalmology*. 2014;7(5):800.

45. Fadlallah A, Dirani A, Chelala E, Antonios R, Cherfan G, Jarade E. Non-topography–guided PRK combined with CXL for the correction of refractive errors in patients with early stage keratoconus. *Journal of Refractive Surgery*. 2014;30(10):688–93.

46. Sakla H, Altroudi W, Muñoz G, Albarrán-Diego C. Simultaneous topography-guided partial photorefractive keratectomy and corneal collagen crosslinking for keratoconus. *Journal of Cataract & Refractive Surgery*. 2014;40(9):1430–8.

47. Alessio G, L'Abbate M, Furino C, Sborgia C, La Tegola MG. Confocal microscopy analysis of corneal changes after photorefractive keratectomy plus cross-linking for keratoconus: 4-year follow-up. *American Journal of Ophthalmology*. 2014;158(3):476–84.e1.

48. Kymionis GD, Grentzelos MA, Plaka AD, Tsoulnaras KI, Kankariya VP, Shehadeh MM, et al. Simultaneous conventional photorefractive keratectomy and corneal collagen cross-linking for pellucid marginal corneal degeneration. *Journal of Refractive Surgery*. 2014;30(4):272–6.

49. Kymionis GD, Grentzelos MA, Kankariya VP, Liakopoulos DA, Karavitaki AE, Portaliou DM, et al. Long-term results of combined transepithelial phototherapeutic keratectomy and corneal collagen crosslinking for keratoconus: cretan protocol. *Journal of Cataract & Refractive Surgery*. 2014;40(9):1439–45.

50. Knezović I, Belovari Višnjić M, Raguž H. Partial topography-guided photorefractive keratectomy followed by corneal cross linking in the management of progressive keratoconus: our initial ten-month results. *Acta Clinica Croatica*. 2015;54(2.):193–9.

51. Shetty R, Nuijts RM, Nicholson M, Sargod K, Jayadev C, Veluri H, et al. Cone location–dependent outcomes after combined topography-guided photorefractive keratectomy and collagen cross-linking. *American Journal of Ophthalmology*. 2015;159(3):419–25.e2.

52. Sherif A, Ammar M, Mostafa Y, Gamal Eldin S, Osman A. One-year results of simultaneous topography-guided photorefractive keratectomy and corneal collagen cross-linking in keratoconus utilizing a modern ablation software. *Journal of Ophthalmology*. 2015;2015. https://doi.org/10.1155/2015/321953

53. Al-Tuwairqi WS, Osuagwu UL, Razzouk H, Ogbuehi KC. One-year clinical outcomes of a two-step surgical management for keratoconus—topography-guided photorefractive keratectomy/cross-linking after intrastromal corneal ring implantation. *Eye & Contact Lens*. 2015;41(6):359–66.

54. Sakla H, Altroudi W, Munoz G, Sakla Y. Simultaneous topography-guided photorefractive keratectomy and accelerated corneal collagen cross-linking for keratoconus. *Cornea*. 2016;35(7):941–5.

55. Chen X, Stojanovic A, Wang X, Liang J, Hu D, Utheim TP. Epithelial thickness profile change after combined topography-guided transepithelial photorefractive keratectomy and corneal cross-linking in treatment of keratoconus. *Journal of Refractive Surgery*. 2016;32(9):626–34.

56. Abou Samra WA, El Emam DS, Farag RK, Abouelkheir HY. Simultaneous versus sequential accelerated corneal collagen cross-linking and wave front guided PRK for treatment of keratoconus: objective and subjective evaluation. *Journal of Ophthalmology.* 2016;2016. https://doi.org/10.1155/2016/2927546

57. Müller T, Lange A. Topography-guided PRK and crosslinking in eyes with keratoconus and post-LASIK ectasia. *Klinische Monatsblätter für Augenheilkunde.* 2017;234(04):451–4.

58. Grentzelos MA, Kounis GA, Diakonis VF, Siganos CS, Tsilimbaris MK, Pallikaris IG, et al. Combined transepithelial phototherapeutic keratectomy and conventional photorefractive keratectomy followed simultaneously by corneal crosslinking for keratoconus: cretan protocol plus. *Journal of Cataract & Refractive Surgery.* 2017;43(10):1257–62.

59. Cassagne M, Pierné K, Galiacy SD, Asfaux-Marfaing MP, Fournié P, Malecaze F. Customized topography-guided corneal collagen cross-linking for keratoconus. *Journal of Refractive Surgery.* 2017;33(5):290–7.

60. Coskunseven E, Sharma DP, Grentzelos MA, Sahin O, Kymionis GD, Pallikaris I. Four-stage procedure for keratoconus: ICRS implantation, corneal cross-linking, toric phakic intraocular lens implantation, and topography-guided photorefractive keratectomy. *Journal of Refractive Surgery.* 2017;33(10):683–9.

61. Gore DM, Leucci MT, Anand V, Cueto LF-V, Mosquera SA, Allan BD. Combined wavefront-guided transepithelial photorefractive keratectomy and corneal crosslinking for visual rehabilitation in moderate keratoconus. *Journal of Cataract & Refractive Surgery.* 2018;44(5):571–80.

62. Sachdev GS, Ramamurthy S, Dandapani R. Comparative analysis of safety and efficacy of photorefractive keratectomy versus photorefractive keratectomy combined with crosslinking. *Clinical Ophthalmology (Auckland, NZ).* 2018;12:783.

63. Al-Amri AM. 5-year follow-up of combined non-topography guided photorefractive keratectomy and corneal collagen cross linking for keratoconus. *International Journal of Ophthalmology.* 2018;11(1):48.

64. Ohana O, Kaiserman I, Domniz Y, Cohen E, Franco O, Sela T, et al. Outcomes of simultaneous photorefractive keratectomy and collagen crosslinking. *Canadian Journal of Ophthalmology.* 2018;53(5):523–8.

65. Zhou W, Wang H, Zhang X, Tian M, Cui C, Li X, et al. Management of corneal ectasia after LASIK with phototherapeutic keratectomy combined with photorefractive keratectomy and collagen cross-linking. *Journal of Ophthalmology.* 2019;2019. https://doi.org/10.1155/2019/2707826

66. Kymionis GD, Grentzelos MA, Voulgari N, Hashemi K, Mikropoulos D. Resolution of epithelial ingrowth after combined photorefractive keratectomy and corneal crosslinking in a patient with post-LASIK ectasia. *Journal of Cataract & Refractive Surgery.* 2019;45(7):1040–2.

67. Iqbal M, Elmassry A, Tawfik A, Elgharieb M, Nagy K, Soliman A, et al. Standard cross-linking versus photorefractive keratectomy combined with accelerated cross-linking for keratoconus management: a comparative study. *Acta ophthalmologica.* 2019;97(4):e623–e31.

68. Kaiserman I, Mimouni M, Rabina G. Epithelial photorefractive keratectomy and corneal cross-linking for keratoconus: the TeL-Aviv protocol. *Journal of Refractive Surgery.* 2019;35(6):377–82.

69. Makar WK, Marey HM, Khairy HA. Topography-guided photorefractive keratectomy combined with accelerated corneal collagen cross-linking (The Athens Protocol) for keratoconus. *Menoufia Medical Journal.* 2019;32(2):698.

70. Kanellopoulos AJ. Management of progressive keratoconus with partial topography-guided PRK combined with refractive, customized CXL–a novel technique: the enhanced Athens protocol. *Clinical Ophthalmology (Auckland, NZ)*. 2019;13:581.

71. Mohammadpour M, Farhadi B, Mirshahi R, Masoumi A, Mirghorbani M. Simultaneous photorefractive keratectomy and accelerated collagen cross-linking in high-risk refractive surgery (Tehran protocol): 3-year outcomes. *International Ophthalmology*. 2020;40(10):2659–66.

72. Tan J, Lytle GE, Marshall J. Consecutive laser in situ keratomileusis and accelerated corneal crosslinking in highly myopic patients: preliminary results. *European Journal of Ophthalmology*. 2015;25(2):101–7.

73. Taneri S, Kiessler S, Rost A, Dick HB. Corneal ectasia after LASIK combined with prophylactic corneal cross-linking. *Journal of Refractive Surgery*. 2017;33(1):50–2.

74. Ge Q, Cui C, Wang J, Mu G. Combined transepithelial phototherapeutic keratectomy and corneal collagen cross-linking for corneal ectasia after small-incision lenticule extraction—preoperative and 3-year postoperative results: a case report. *BMC Ophthalmology*. 2018;18(1):1–5.

75. Torres-Netto EA, Spiru B, Kling S, Gilardoni F, Lazaridis A, Sekundo W, et al. Similar biomechanical cross-linking effect after SMILE and PRK in human corneas in an ex vivo model for postoperative ectasia. *Journal of Refractive Surgery*. 2020;36(1):49–54.

15 Therapeutic Refractive Surgery for Regularly and Irregularly Irregular Astigmatism

Dan Z. Reinstein and Timothy J. Archer

INTRODUCTION

Visual symptoms such as reduced CDVA and contrast sensitivity, halos and starbursts, ghosting, and diplopia after corneal refractive surgery are usually found to be caused by irregular astigmatism. Irregular astigmatism can be classified in two categories: *regularly* irregular astigmatism and *irregularly* irregular astigmatism. The main examples of regularly irregular astigmatism are high spherical aberration (i.e., a small achieved optical zone) and decentration. In these situations, there is effectively one large "global" irregularity, but the topographic optical zone is otherwise symmetrical and round. On the other hand, in cases of irregularly irregular astigmatism, irregularities are localized to small regions resulting in an asymmetric or distorted topography, and often within the boundary of the optical zone.

The most important aspect of treating complications is first to make a confident diagnosis of the problem since some treatment options could actually be detrimental in certain circumstances. The introduction of custom ablation, based on either topography or wavefront, promised to be the answer to post-op complications. However, neither topography nor wavefront can measure the true source of the irregularity, the stromal surface. The natural compensatory mechanism of epithelial remodeling acts to mask a proportion of the stromal surface irregularity from front surface corneal topography (or from the wavefront).[1-5] If there is irregular astigmatism on the topography, then by definition there will be irregular epithelium; the epithelium overlying bumps in the stromal surface becomes progressively thinner, and the epithelium overlying troughs in the stromal surface becomes progressively thicker. Furthermore, the amount of epithelial remodeling has been shown to be correlated to the local curvature gradient of the stromal surface, with greater epithelial compensation for more localized irregularities.[1,6-8] In 1994, we summarized this phenomenon in the Law of Epithelial Compensation for irregular astigmatism: "Irregular astigmatism results in irregular epithelium."[9]

Therefore, in cases of local irregularities (irregularly irregular astigmatism), the majority of the stromal irregularity will be masked from topography by epithelial remodeling. In contrast, the stromal curvature gradient is more gradual for global irregularities, which reduces the amount of compensatory epithelial remodeling such that the majority of the stromal irregularity will be detectable on front surface corneal topography. Therefore, a topography-guided treatment can only be expected to be effective when used to treat global irregularities, and minimally effective in irregularly irregular astigmatism – which is exactly what has been reported for topography-guided custom ablation.[10] In some cases of irregularly irregular astigmatism, a topography-guided treatment can even make the irregularity worse.[1,2,4]

For this reason, an epithelial thickness profile is vital for an accurate diagnosis in cases of irregular astigmatism. In cases with localized irregularities where the epithelium has compensated for the majority of the irregularity, a different treatment option is required. Trans-epithelial PTK offers a solution by using the epithelium as a natural masking agent to focus the ablation onto the relative peaks in the stromal surface.

Thus, the decision process (Figure 15.1) for irregular astigmatism can be summarized as:

- "Global" regularly irregular astigmatism – dominant irregularity on topography – topography-guided custom ablation

- "Local" irregularly irregular astigmatism – dominant irregularity masked by epithelium – trans-epithelial PTK

TRANS-EPITHELIAL PHOTOTHERAPEUTIC KERATECTOMY
Understanding Epithelial Remodeling

As introduced above, epithelial remodeling is a well-known phenomenon and has been shown to occur in a wide range of situations. Somewhat surprisingly, we found that the epithelium was not uniform in thickness for a normal virgin eye as had previously been thought, but followed a very distinct pattern; on average, the epithelium was 5.7 μm thicker inferiorly than superiorly, and 1.2 μm thicker nasally than temporally, with a mean central thickness of 53.4 μm (Figure 15.2).[11]

DOI: 10.1201/9781003371601-15

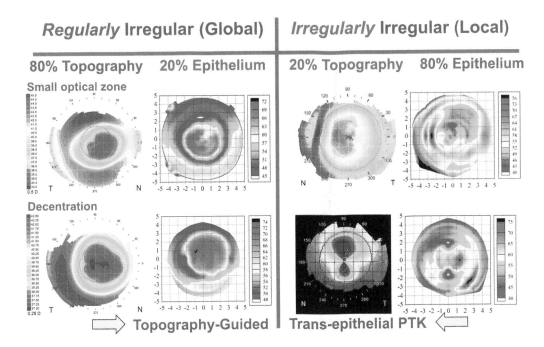

Figure 15.1 Diagram outlining the decision process for choosing the appropriate therapeutic treatment type for an eye that presents with irregular astigmatism after corneal laser refractive surgery. Topography-guided treatment is more effective for "global" irregularities such as small optical zones and decentration where the majority of the irregularity is on the topography. On the other hand, if there is irregularly irregular astigmatism, characterized by local irregularities, a significant proportion will have been compensated for by epithelial remodeling. Therefore, trans-epithelial PTK is a more effective treatment in these cases than topography-guided custom ablation.

This non-uniformity seemed to provide evidence that epithelial thickness is regulated by eyelid mechanics and blinking, as we suggested in 1994.[12]

Further evidence for this theory is provided by the epithelial thickness changes observed in orthokeratology.[13] In orthokeratology, a reversed geometry contact lens is placed on the cornea overnight that sits tightly on the cornea centrally, but leaves a gap in the mid-periphery. Therefore, the natural template provided by the posterior surface of the semi-rigid tarsus of the eyelid is replaced by an artificial contact lens template designed to fit tightly to the center of the cornea and loosely paracentrally. We found significant epithelial thickness changes with central thinning and mid-peripheral thickening (Figure 15.2), showing that the epithelium has remodeled according to the template provided by the contact lens – i.e., the epithelium is chafed and squashed by the lens centrally while the epithelium is free to thicken paracentrally where the lens is not so tightly fitted.

Epithelial thickness changes have been described after myopic excimer laser ablation,[14–17] hyperopic excimer laser ablation,[18] radial keratotomy,[19] intra-corneal ring segments,[20] irregularly irregular astigmatism after corneal refractive surgery,[1–4,21,22] and in keratoconus[23–27] and ectasia.[28] Figure 15.2 shows the epithelial thickness profile in a number of different situations.

In all of these cases, the epithelial thickness changes are clearly a compensatory response to the change to the stromal surface and can all be explained by the theory of eyelid template regulation of epithelial thickness. A further example is the epithelial thickness changes reported following the rotation of a LASIK free cap, in which dramatic changes were observed overnight once the asymmetric free cap was replaced in the correct anatomical position, demonstrating that the original stromal surface curvature had been restored.[29] Compensatory epithelial thickness changes can be summarized by the following rules:

1. The epithelium thickens in areas where tissue has been removed or the curvature has been flattened (e.g., central thickening after myopic ablation[14–16] or radial keratotomy,[19] and peripheral thickening after hyperopic ablation[18]).

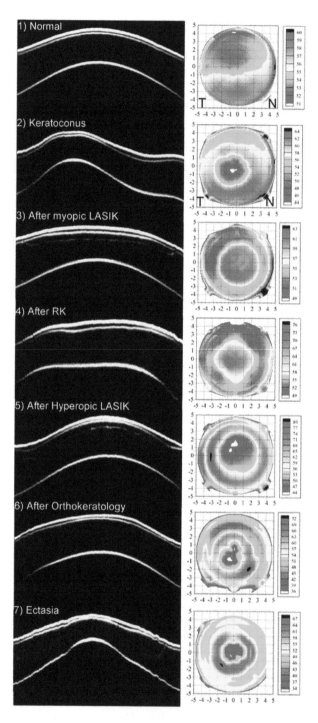

Figure 15.2 Artemis Insight 100 VHF digital ultrasound non-geometrically corrected B-scan (left) and epithelial thickness profile (right) for: (1) a population of 110 normal untreated eyes, (2) a population of 54 keratoconic eyes, (3) a population of 24 eyes after myopic LASIK, (4) a population of 14 eyes after radial keratotomy, (5) a population of 65 eyes after hyperopic LASIK, (6) a case example of one eye after two weeks wear of an orthokeratology lens, and (7) a case of post-LASIK ectasia.

2. The epithelium thins over regions that are relatively elevated or where the curvature has been steepened (e.g., central thinning in keratoconus,[23-27] ectasia,[28] and after hyperopic ablation[18]).

3. The magnitude of epithelial changes correlates to the magnitude of the change in curvature (e.g., more epithelial thickening for higher myopia,[14,15,17] higher hyperopia,[18] or more advanced keratoconus[23-27]).

4. The amount of epithelial remodeling is defined by the curvature gradient of an irregularity; there will be more epithelial remodeling for a more localized irregularity.[1-4,6-8] The epithelium effectively acts as a low-pass filter, smoothing small changes almost completely, but only partially smoothing large changes.

Trans-Epithelial PTK Treatment

As described earlier, despite all the advances in corneal topography and ocular wavefront measurement, it is not always possible to diagnose the cause of subjective visual complaints by these means alone because of the compensatory epithelial thickness changes that partially mask the true stromal surface irregularity. In applying the *Law of Epithelial Compensation*, if a patient presents with stable irregular astigmatism, by definition the epithelium has reached its maximum compensatory function. The epithelium can compensate almost completely for very localized irregularities. Therefore, topography or wavefront-guided treatments may lead to a sub-optimal treatment plan and potentially make things worse.[2-4] Instead, we need a method to target the irregularities masked by the epithelium, something that is achieved, by definition, by trans-epithelial PTK.[1-4]

We have described our treatment protocol for trans-epithelial PTK in detail in previous publications (Figure 15.3).[1-4] When planning these cases, we always obtain an epithelial thickness map in order to simulate the stromal ablation profile. We refer to this technique as digital subtraction pachymetry (DSP) as demonstrated in Figure 15.4, in which the breakthrough pattern and remaining epithelium at regular lamellar depths of trans-epithelial PTK ablation are simulated. This pattern can also be used to estimate the refractive effect; for example, a hyperopic shift would be expected if central stroma was being removed primarily. In our study, we found that trans-epithelial PTK resulted in a refractive shift of more than 0.50 D in 59% of eyes, equally split between myopic and hyperopic shifts.[1]

The PTK ablation is a uniform depth applied over a large diameter zone – the maximum zone is 8.0 mm for the MEL 80/90. Stromal tissue removal is defined by the epithelial thickness profile, so the optical zone diameter does not increase the ablation depth as for a refractive ablation. The ablation is centered in the same way as a refractive ablation, by centering the eye tracker on the coaxially sighted corneal light reflex. However, there is effectively no concern about centration as the PTK ablation is at a uniform depth across a wide 8-mm-diameter. In contrast, if a topography-guided ablation is slightly misaligned, then this may increase the irregularity, particularly in cases of very localized irregularities. This makes trans-epithelial PTK extremely easy to perform.

In our protocol, the first trans-epithelial PTK ablation is planned to expose a small area of stroma in the region of the thinnest epithelium. The initial transepithelial ablation depth data entry is calculated using a conversion factor of 1.14 times the intended depth based on our previous experience with the MEL 80 and MEL 90 excimer lasers. After the initial ablation, the epithelial DSP maps are compared to the observed epithelial breakthrough pattern to estimate the actual achieved ablation depth. This allows the conversion factor used for subsequent ablations to be calibrated individually for each case. Based on the remaining thickness of epithelium, trans-epithelial PTK ablations are applied in steps of 10–20 μm with the final goal of removing almost all of the epithelium up to the maximum thickness. In cases with very localized irregularities, we often choose not to remove the full thickness of epithelium in order to conserve stromal tissue.

On completion of the trans-epithelial PTK ablations, the stromal surface quality and smoothness is assessed. If there are fine irregularities visible, such as microfolds, a series of "wet" PTK ablations can be performed to smooth and polish the stromal surface.[2] The "wet" PTK ablations are done by first flooding the cornea with balanced salt solution (BSS), immediately followed by a PTK ablation of eight seconds duration in an 8-mm zone (equivalent to a readout of 20 μm on the MEL 80 PTK mode). The tendency for BSS surface tension to break up means that such PTK bursts must be kept short to avoid inadvertently ablating other areas of the stroma, which is why we limit each ablation to approximately 8 seconds. The BSS acts as a masking agent, in a similar way to the epithelium previously, and naturally spreads across the surface, leaving the ridges of any microfolds closer to the surface. The shockwaves of the excimer laser expose the peaks of the microfolds allowing them to be ablated in isolation from the rest of the stromal surface. This process is

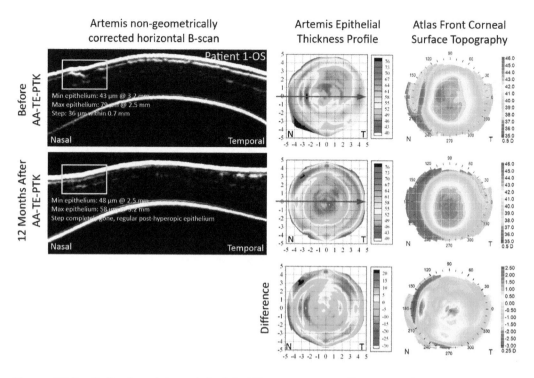

Figure 15.3 (Left column) Artemis Insight 100 non-geometrically corrected horizontal B-scans before and after an Artemis-assisted trans-epithelial PTK (AA-TE-PTK) procedure. The yellow box highlights the nasal region where the flap interface can be seen to stop abruptly. In this area, there is a crevice on the stromal surface over which the epithelium has thickened with thin epithelium overlying the adjacent ridge. (Middle column) Artemis Insight 100 epithelial thickness maps before and after the AA-TE-PTK procedure plotted on the same scale. These maps show that the nasal step in epithelial thickness has been completely smoothed after the procedure. The difference map is plotted underneath, which shows the significant epithelial remodeling in the nasal region after the procedure. (Right column) Atlas corneal front surface topography before and after the AA-TE-PTK procedure plotted on the same scale. The difference map is plotted underneath, which demonstrates the significant improvement in the topographic irregularity after the procedure. *Reproduced with permission from Reinstein DZ, Archer TJ, Gobbe M. Improved effectiveness of trans-epithelial phototherapeutic keratectomy versus topography-guided ablation degraded by epithelial compensation on irregular stromal surfaces [plus video]. J Refract Surg. 2013;29:526–533.*

usually repeated two to four times until the surface is visibly smoothed of microfolds on drying. In our population of eyes treated by trans-epithelial PTK, a "wet" PTK was performed in approximately half of the cases.[1]

In addition, a standard refractive, topography-guided or wavefront-guided ablation might be performed immediately following trans-epithelial PTK in selected cases. As described above, the DSP simulation can be used to estimate the refractive effect of the trans-epithelial PTK ablation, so a refractive ablation can be used in cases where the refractive shift is considered to be predictable. If the patient has a significant refractive error, then this might be treated simultaneously. Alternatively, if there is an obvious large-scale global irregularity in addition to the localized irregularities, then these might be treated by a topography-guided ablation. In theory, performing both a trans-epithelial PTK and a topography-guided treatment will correct the total stromal surface irregularity. However, if in doubt, it is preferable to do less and conserve tissue for future treatments.

Trans-Epithelial PTK without an Epithelial Thickness Measurement

While an epithelial thickness map and DSP can provide a confirmed diagnosis and expected treatment outcome, these are not compulsory for performing a trans-epithelial PTK treatment. As

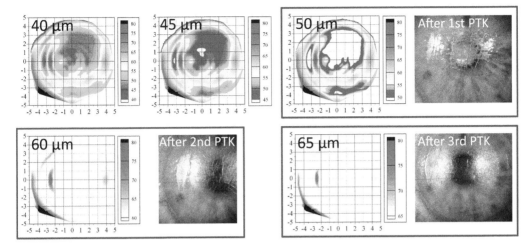

Figure 15.4   Digital subtraction pachymetry simulation of the pattern of remaining epithelium that would be expected after increasing trans-epithelial PTK ablations from 40 to 65 μm in 5 μm steps. The white areas on the colour map represents regions where all the epithelium would have been ablated after the labeled trans-epithelial PTK ablation, and hence the regions where ablation of stromal tissue would occur. Due to the epithelial masking, the stromal ablation was concentrated onto a nasal ridge immediately adjacent to a crevice on the stromal surface. During the procedure, the trans-epithelial PTK ablation was performed in three steps, with a planned 50 μm ablation as the first step. After the first ablation, the cornea was examined (as shown in the intraoperative photograph) and the areas of exposed stroma were compared with the Artemis simulated maps, which confirmed that the first ablation was close to 50 μm. The second and third trans-epithelial PTK ablations could then be planned to reach the intended end point of 65 μm accurately. The intraoperative photographs show that the pattern of remaining epithelium was similar to the predicted pattern with only a small line of epithelium remaining overlying the stromal crevice. *Reproduced with permission from Reinstein DZ, Archer TJ, Gobbe M. Improved effectiveness of trans-epithelial phototherapeutic keratectomy versus topography-guided ablation degraded by epithelial compensation on irregular stromal surfaces [plus video]. J Refract Surg. 2013;29:526–533.*

long as there is irregularly irregular topography, the epithelium must also be irregular, meaning that a trans-epithelial PTK treatment will afford some smoothing of the stromal surface. The mean central epithelial thickness in a normal eye is 53 μm,[11] so by definition the thinnest epithelium in an irregularly irregular cornea will most likely be less than this (as there must be compensatory thinning for an irregularity). This is confirmed by the distribution of minimum and maximum epithelial thicknesses in our trans-epithelial PTK population as shown in Figure 15.5.[1] The mean thinnest epithelial thickness was 43 μm (significantly thinner than normal) and the mean thickest epithelial thickness was 79 μm (significantly thicker than normal).

The goal of the initial trans-epithelial PTK ablation is to break through the epithelium in the region where it is thinnest to expose the peaks in the stromal surface to be ablated. The secondary goal of the initial trans-epithelial PTK ablation is to avoid removing the full thickness of epithelium as any ablation after complete removal of the epithelium will have no effect on stromal surface irregularities. This method therefore avoids wasting stromal tissue.

If no epithelial thickness measurement is available, the following standardized treatment method can be used based on the population minimum and maximum epithelial thicknesses. The highest minimum epithelial thickness was 54 μm, but, as this was a single outlier, the next lowest value of 51 μm is considered for this protocol. The lowest maximum epithelial thickness was 60 μm. Therefore, to achieve breakthrough but not complete removal of the epithelium, the first ablation should be targeted within the "therapeutic window" of 51–60 μm. We suggest an initial ablation depth of 55 μm, although this should be adjusted to take into account the epithelial ablation rate for the excimer laser being used (if this can be measured). Subsequent ablations can be performed in 102–0 μm steps, chosen intra-operatively after reviewing the coverage and pattern of epithelium remaining after each ablation. During this process, the pattern of remaining

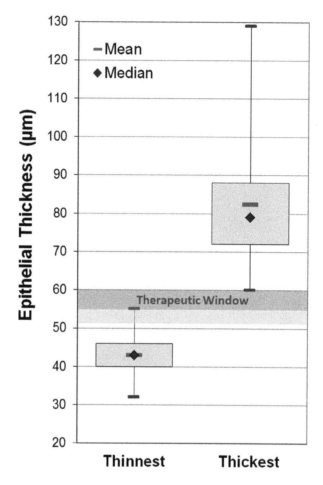

Figure 15.5 Boxplot displaying pre-operative Artemis Insight 100 VHF digital ultrasound epithelial thickness range for a population of 41 eyes with irregularly irregular astigmatism. The "therapeutic window" is defined as the region between the population's maximum thinnest epithelium and minimum thickest epithelium. The dark green color indicates the narrow "therapeutic window," including an anomalously high thinnest epithelium, and the light green color indicates a wider "therapeutic window" without this outlier. *Reproduced with permission from Reinstein DZ, Archer TJ, Dickeson ZI, Gobbe M. Trans-epithelial phototherapeutic keratectomy protocol for treating irregular astigmatism based on population epithelial thickness measurements by Artemis very high-frequency digital ultrasound. J Refract Surg. 2014;30:380–387.*

epithelium can be observed to identify the areas where the stroma is being ablated. The pattern of stromal ablation can then be correlated to corneal topography and wavefront to gain an understanding of the stromal surface irregularity being treated and evaluate potential postoperative changes. These stepwise ablations can be continued until the epithelium is completely removed or is restricted to an isolated area.

Alternatives and Weaknesses of Trans-Epithelial PTK

The effectiveness of trans-epithelial PTK is defined by the proportion of the irregularity that has been masked by the epithelial remodeling. A trans-epithelial PTK will therefore not treat the irregularity that is visible on front surface corneal topography, which in theory would become the post-operative stromal surface. After a trans-epithelial PTK treatment, the epithelium then remodels according to this new stromal surface, hence partially masking the remaining irregularity. In some cases, the remaining irregularity is small enough to be masked almost completely by the epithelium, resulting in an apparently normal front corneal surface topography, and no further therapeutic treatment is required. In other cases, the remaining irregularity is large enough that it cannot be completely compensated by the epithelium, in which case further treatment would be needed if the patient reports subjective symptoms. Depending on whether the remaining irregularity is global or local, further treatment can be performed as a topography-guided ablation or trans-epithelial PTK.

Another approach, described by Chen et al.,[30,31] is to combine a trans-epithelial PTK with a topography-guided ablation into a single treatment. The concept is that trans-epithelial PTK will treat the irregularity masked by the epithelium and the topography-guided treatment will treat the irregularity detectable on the front surface corneal topography, thereby treating the whole of the stromal surface irregularity. This treatment protocol has been used successfully in cases of flap and interface complications.[30,31] However, performing a trans-epithelial PTK alone can be a more conservative approach because the cornea can be regularized with less tissue removal by taking advantage of the epithelium masking the remaining irregularity that wasn't treated by the PTK. Furthermore, if the procedure is performed in one step, the predictability of the refractive outcome is likely to be less accurate given the power shifts that can be induced by epithelial compensation.[1-4]

Another method of treating irregular astigmatism has been described by Vinciguerra et al.[5] In their custom phototherapeutic keratectomy protocol, a topography-guided ablation is generated from a topography scan obtained after removing the epithelium, i.e., a topography of the stromal surface. After applying this ablation, another topography scan is obtained and a second topography-guided ablation is generated and applied. This process can be repeated numerous times, each time improving the regularity of the stromal surface.

The advantages of trans-epithelial PTK are that it is straightforward to perform, very low risk, and conservative. All excimer lasers include a PTK mode, so no extra repair software is required, and consequently no complicated ablation profile programming. By definition, the epithelium will be masking a proportion of the stromal surface irregularity, so it can be assumed that a trans-epithelial PTK will afford some smoothing of the stromal surface, but probably not as much as with other more complex techniques. Another advantage is that there is no concern about centration as the PTK ablation has a uniform depth across the whole diameter. In contrast, if a topography-guided ablation is slightly misaligned, then this may increase the irregularity, particularly in cases of very localized irregularities.

The weakness of trans-epithelial PTK is that the refractive shift is currently unpredictable, as demonstrated by our study reporting outcomes for a population of 41 eyes treated by trans-epithelial PTK.[1] A myopic shift was as likely as a hyperopic shift, and the change in spherical equivalent refraction was within ±0.50 D in only 41% of cases after a trans-epithelial PTK alone. In one case, a trans-epithelial PTK treatment induced a refractive change of +2.24 −3.97 × 120.[4]

CONCLUSION

In summary, there are now a number of different treatment options for therapeutic refractive surgery, meaning that virtually all refractive surgery complications can be resolved, or at least the visual quality can be improved. Topography-guided custom ablation provides a very effective solution for regularly irregular astigmatism, such as decentration and small optical zone, and trans-epithelial PTK provides a treatment option for even the most irregular corneas. Both procedures have now matured to the point where they can become part of mainstream refractive surgery; all surgeons should at least be aware of these and feel comfortable in referring patients to specialist therapeutic centers if they do not have the tools available. Epithelial thickness mapping plays a critical role for diagnostics in therapeutic cases due to the significant epithelial remodeling that occurs to compensate for stromal surface irregularities. Fortunately, this remodeling can be turned to our advantage as a natural masking agent to use trans-epithelial PTK to target the stromal irregularities.

Financial Disclosure: Dr Reinstein is a consultant for Carl Zeiss Meditec (Carl Zeiss Meditec AG, Jena, Germany). Dr Reinstein is also a consultant for CSO Italia (Florence, Italy) and has a proprietary interest in the Artemis Insight 100 technology (ArcScan Inc, Golden, Colorado) through patents administered by the Cornell Center for Technology Enterprise and Commercialization (CCTEC), Ithaca, New York. Timothy J Archer has no proprietary or financial interest in the materials presented herein.

REFERENCES

1. Reinstein DZ, Archer TJ, Dickeson ZI, Gobbe M. Trans-epithelial phototherapeutic keratectomy protocol for treating irregular astigmatism based on population epithelial thickness measurements by Artemis very high-frequency digital ultrasound. *J Refract Surg.* 2014;30:380–387.

2. Reinstein DZ, Archer TJ, Gobbe M. Improved effectiveness of trans-epithelial phototherapeutic keratectomy versus topography-guided ablation degraded by epithelial compensation on irregular stromal surfaces [plus video]. *J Refract Surg.* 2013;29:526–533.

3. Reinstein DZ, Archer T. Combined Artemis very high-frequency digital ultrasound-assisted transepithelial phototherapeutic keratectomy and wavefront-guided treatment following multiple corneal refractive procedures. *J Cataract Refract Surg.* 2006;32:1870–1876.

4. Reinstein DZ, Archer TJ, Gobbe M. Refractive and topographic errors in topography-guided ablation produced by epithelial compensation predicted by three-dimensional Artemis very high-frequency digital ultrasound stromal and epithelial thickness mapping. *J Refract Surg.* 2012;28:657–663.

5. Vinciguerra P, Camesasca FI. Custom phototherapeutic keratectomy with intraoperative topography. *J Refract Surg.* 2004;20:S555–563.

6. Reinstein DZ, Archer TJ, Gobbe M. Rate of change of curvature of the corneal stromal surface drives epithelial compensatory changes and remodeling. *J Refract Surg.* 2014;30:800–802.

7. Vinciguerra P, Azzolini C, Vinciguerra R. Corneal curvature gradient determines corneal healing process and epithelial behavior. *J Refract Surg.* 2015;31:281–282.

8. Vinciguerra P, Roberts CJ, Albe E, Romano MR, Mahmoud A, Trazza S, Vinciguerra R. Corneal curvature gradient map: a new corneal topography map to predict the corneal healing process. *J Refract Surg.* 2014;30:202–207.

9. Reinstein DZ, Aslanides IM, Silverman RH, Najafi DJ, Brownlow RL, Belmont S, Haight DM, Coleman DJ. Epithelial and Corneal 3D ultrasound pachymetric topography post excimer laser surgery. *Invest Ophthalmol Vis Sci.* 1994;35:1739.

10. Reinstein DZ, Archer TJ, Gobbe M. Combined corneal topography and corneal wavefront data in the treatment of corneal irregularity and refractive error in LASIK or PRK using the Carl Zeiss Meditec MEL80 and CRS master. *J Refract Surg.* 2009;25:503–515.

11. Reinstein DZ, Archer TJ, Gobbe M, Silverman RH, Coleman DJ. Epithelial thickness in the normal cornea: three-dimensional display with Artemis very high-frequency digital ultrasound. *J Refract Surg.* 2008;24:571–581.

12. Reinstein DZ, Silverman RH, Coleman DJ. High-frequency ultrasound measurement of the thickness of the corneal epithelium. *Refract Corneal Surg.* 1993;9:385–387.

13. Reinstein DZ, Gobbe M, Archer TJ, Couch D, Bloom B. Epithelial, stromal, and corneal pachymetry changes during orthokeratology. *Optom Vis Sci.* 2009;86:E1006–1014.

14. Gauthier CA, Holden BA, Epstein D, Tengroth B, Fagerholm P, Hamberg-Nystrom H. Role of epithelial hyperplasia in regression following photorefractive keratectomy. *Br J Ophthalmol.* 1996;80:545–548.

15. Reinstein DZ, Srivannaboon S, Gobbe M, Archer TJ, Silverman RH, Sutton H, Coleman DJ. Epithelial thickness profile changes induced by myopic LASIK as measured by Artemis very high-frequency digital ultrasound. *J Refract Surg.* 2009;25:444–450.

16. Reinstein DZ, Archer TJ, Gobbe M. Change in epithelial thickness profile 24 hours and longitudinally for 1 year after myopic LASIK: three-dimensional display with artemis very high-frequency digital ultrasound. *J Refract Surg.* 2012;28:195–201.

17. Kanellopoulos AJ, Asimellis G. Longitudinal postoperative lasik epithelial thickness profile changes in correlation with degree of myopia correction. *J Refract Surg.* 2014;30:166–171.

18. Reinstein DZ, Archer TJ, Gobbe M, Silverman RH, Coleman DJ. Epithelial thickness after hyperopic LASIK: three-dimensional display with artemis very high-frequency digital ultrasound. *J Refract Surg.* 2010;26:555–564.

19. Reinstein DZ, Archer TJ, Gobbe M. Epithelial thickness up to 26 years after radial keratotomy: three-dimensional display with artemis very high-frequency digital ultrasound. *J Refract Surg.* 2011;27:618–624.

20. Reinstein DZ, Srivannaboon S, Holland SP. Epithelial and stromal changes induced by intacs examined by three-dimensional very high-frequency digital ultrasound. *J Refract Surg.* 2001;17:310–318.

21. Reinstein DZ, Silverman RH, Sutton HF, Coleman DJ. Very high-frequency ultrasound corneal analysis identifies anatomic correlates of optical complications of lamellar refractive surgery: anatomic diagnosis in lamellar surgery. *Ophthalmology.* 1999;106:474–482.

22. Reinstein DZ, Gobbe M, Archer TJ, Youssefi G, Sutton HF. Stromal surface topography-guided custom ablation as a repair tool for corneal irregular astigmatism. *J Refract Surg.* 2015;31:54–59.

23. Reinstein DZ, Archer TJ, Gobbe M, Silverman RH, Coleman DJ. Epithelial, stromal and corneal thickness in the keratoconic cornea: three-dimensional display with artemis very high-frequency digital ultrasound. *J Refract Surg.* 2010;26:259–271.

24. Li Y, Tan O, Brass R, Weiss JL, Huang D. Corneal epithelial thickness mapping by Fourier-domain optical coherence tomography in normal and keratoconic eyes. *Ophthalmology.* 2012;119:2425–2433.

25. Rocha KM, Perez-Straziota CE, Stulting RD, Randleman JB. SD-OCT analysis of regional epithelial thickness profiles in keratoconus, postoperative corneal ectasia, and normal eyes. *J Refract Surg.* 2013;29:173–179.

26. Kanellopoulos AJ, Aslanides IM, Asimellis G. Correlation between epithelial thickness in normal corneas, untreated ectatic corneas, and ectatic corneas previously treated with CXL; is overall epithelial thickness a very early ectasia prognostic factor? *Clin Ophthalmol.* 2012;6:789–800.

27. Sandali O, El Sanharawi M, Temstet C, Hamiche T, Galan A, Ghouali W, Goemaere I, Basli E, Borderie V, Laroche L. Fourier-domain optical coherence tomography imaging in keratoconus: a corneal structural classification. *Ophthalmology.* 2013;120:2403–2412.

28. Reinstein DZ, Gobbe M, Archer TJ, Couch D. Epithelial thickness profile as a method to evaluate the effectiveness of collagen cross-linking treatment after corneal ectasia. *J Refract Surg.* 2011;27:356–363.

29. Reinstein DZ, Archer TJ, Gobbe M, Rothman RC. Epithelial thickness changes following the realignment of a malpositioned free cap. *J Cataract Refract Surg.* 2014;40:1237–1239.

30. Chen X, Stojanovic A, Zhou W, Utheim TP, Stojanovic F, Wang Q. Transepithelial, topography-guided ablation in the treatment of visual disturbances in LASIK flap or interface complications. *J Refract Surg.* 2012;28:120–126.

31. Chen X, Stojanovic A, Nitter TA. Topography-guided transepithelial surface ablation in treatment of recurrent epithelial ingrowths. *J Refract Surg.* 2010;26:529–532.

16 Intracorneal Ring Segments in Corneal Ectasia

Seyed Javad Hashemian and Yasaman Hadi

INTRODUCTION

Intracorneal ring segments (ICRS) are small circular arcs, made of poly(methyl methacrylate) (PMMA), which are placed in the posterior midperipheral corneal stroma in a lamellar channel, aiming to reshape the geometry of corneal tissue, alter its refractive properties, and improve corneal regularity and the patient's visual acuity. Because the ring segments are narrow, the overlying stroma can receive nutrients from surrounding tissue.

In 1987, Fleming et al. found that the insertion of an intracorneal device could diminish refractive errors in rabbit eyes and also reported that mechanically constricting or expanding the ring would increase or decrease the central corneal curvature, respectively.[1]

Reynolds (1978) was the first to use a 360-degree intracorneal ring for the management of myopia.[2] But Colin (2000) introduced the implantation of ICRSs for the management of keratoconus for the first time. Difficult implantation of the initial 360-degree implants and related complications lead to designing semicircular corneal implants which can be easily implantED into a corneal stromal tunnel.[3]

Nowadays ICRSs are known as a minimally invasive, potentially reversible, surgical alternative to avoid or postpone corneal transplantation in patients with ectatic corneal diseases, especially those with contact lens intolerance.

MECHANISM OF ACTION

The effects of ICRS implantation on the geometric and biomechanical corneal changes and the whole optical performance of the eye have been evaluated through algorithms, analytically solvable models, numerical studies, finite-element model (FEM), and clinically applied empirical nomograms. The consistent points in the results of these studies include that the insertion of an ICRS into the stroma changes the anterior and posterior corneal curvature as well as the corneal apex position. They also suggest a linear relation between refractive changes and ICRS thickness and diameter. The thicker the ICRS and the smaller the optical zone, the greater the corneal flattening effect.[4–8]

ICRS alter the corneal curvature through acting as a spacer element between the bundles of corneal lamellae, resulting in a shortening of central corneal arc length of these fibers proportional to the thickness of the device and inversely proportional to the corneal diameter of the implantation site.[2] Typically, the central cornea is steeper than the periphery, resulting in a positive shape factor or prolate shape, and there is a gradual increase in thickness from the central to the peripheral cornea.

The spherical 1–3-mm zone of the normal cornea is called the central zone, surrounded by the paracentral zone, a 3- to 4-mm-wide ring which gradually flattens from the center. The paracentral and central zones together are called the apical zone, which is the main target of refractive surgeries and contact lens fitting. Next is the peripheral zone, with the greatest flattening in the normal aspheric cornea and limbal zone.[9] ICRS insertion into the midperiphery of the cornea flattens the paracentral zone more than the central zone, maintaining the prolate shape of the cornea and improving contact lens tolerance.[10] In addition, ICRS implantation into the cornea redistributes stress and improves corneal biomechanics.[11]

A significant increase in corneal thickness up to several months after ICRS implantation has been observed which may be attributed to corneal edema caused by an alteration in endothelial cell function, especially in the area under the implants, or to collagen crowding and stromal infolding due to collagen remodeling, which means that the implant isolates and flattens a certain volume of the central cornea (i.e., the cone), thus compressing the corneal tissue and resulting in an increase in the thickness of the cornea.[11] ICRS implantation shifts the corneal apex of the keratoconic eyes more centrally and creates a second limbus of smaller diameter in the middle of the cornea which may add mechanical support to the ectatic cornea.[7,12]

DOI: 10.1201/9781003371601-16

Table 16.1 Types of Intracorneal Ring Segments

	Intacs	Intacs SK	Keraring SI5	Keraring SI6	Ferrara	Myoring
Arc length (degrees)	150	90–210	90–355	90-210	90–320	360
Cross-section	Oval/ hexagonal	Oval	Triangular	Triangular	Triangular	Triangular
Thickness (mm)	250–450	210–500	150–350	150–350	150–350	150–350
Optical zone (mm)	7	6	5	5.5–6.0	AFR: 5 AFR6: 6	
FDA	Yes	Yes				
Inner diameter	6.77	6	6		4.8	5–8
Outer diameter	8.10	7	7		5.4	5–8

TYPES OF INTRACORNEAL RING SEGMENTS

Currently, there are various types of ICRSs, all of which are made of PMMA, but what distinguishes them from one another includes arc length, cross section, thickness, optical zone size, inner, and outer diameter which are presented for each type in Table 16.1.

Intacs Ring Segment (AdditionTechnology Inc, Sunnyvale, CA, USA) is one of the most widely used corneal ring segment and the only commercially available ICRS in the USA, and consists of a single 210° implant or two semicircular implants of fixed 150° arc length designed for low refractive error corrections.

Intacs SK (Figure 16.1) has two modifications relative to the standard Intacs: a smaller inner diameter of 6.0 mm instead of 6.8 mm and an elliptical, instead of a hexagonal, cross-section. Intacs SK has a greater corneal flattening effect and may be implanted in keratoconic corneas with higher refractive errors and higher stages of ectasia.

Keraring Intrastromal Corneal Ring Segment (Mediphacos, Belo Horizonte, Brazil) comes in two types: standard ring segment with constant thickness (SI5 and SI6) (Figure 16.2) and Keraring AS (Figure 16.3) with progressive thickness (from 150 to 250 μm or from 200 to 300 μm) within the same implant. The AJL pro + ring, was introduced with an asymmetric design both in base width (600–800 μm) and in thickness, with the designs being available in both clockwise and counterclockwise forms, so that the thinnest part of the ring is located near the corneal incision. This type of ICRS can be useful for keratoconic patients with irregular non-orthogonal corneal topography.

Ferrara Ring Segment (Ferrara Ophthalmics Ltd., Belo Horizonte, Brazil) (Figure 16.4) consists of a semicircular segment and a fixed triangular section, AFR (0.60 mm base) or AFR6 (0.80 mm

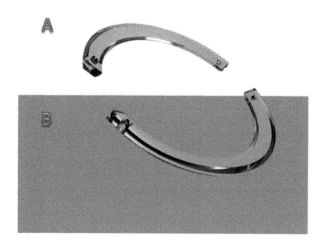

Figure 16.1 Intacs SK intracorneal implants

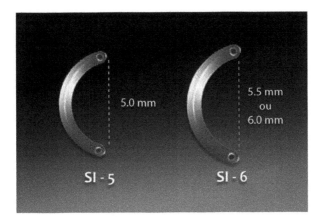

Figure 16.2 Standard ring segment with constant thickness (SI5 and SI6)

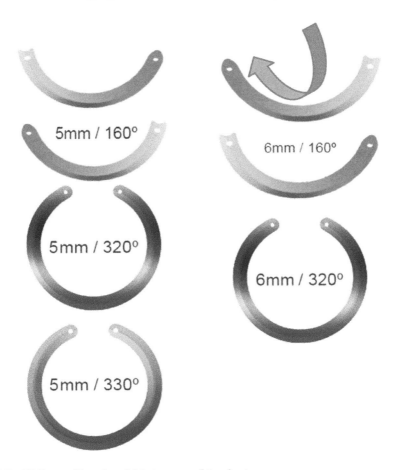

Figure 16.3 Different Keraring AS intracorneal implants

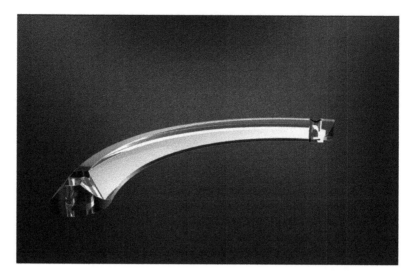

Figure 16.4 Ferrara Intrastromal Corneal Ring

base), and different arc lengths. Each segment has a 0.20-mm orifice at each end to facilitate the implantation.

MyoRing intracorneal continuous ring (Dioptex GmbH, Linz, Austria), suggested by Albert Daxer (2007), is the only ICRS with a 360° arc length that should be inserted into the corneal pocket, using a high-precision microkeratome (PocketMaker Microkeratome).[13]

INDICATIONS

It has been suggested that those who have mild to moderate corneal ectasis, without central corneal scars and with contact lenses intolerance, benefit most from intrastromal corneal implantation.[16]

In order to obtain the best results and the least amount of complications, it is necessary to consider most of the following criteria:[15,17]

- Age > 18-21 years

- A clear optical zone

- Corneal thickness greater than 400 μ in the thinnest location and greater than 450 μ in the area of implantation

- Corrected distance visual acuity worse than 0.6 on the decimal scale

- Mean keratometry less than 58.0 D (excluding stage 4 Amsler–Krumeich classification)

- Alignment (between 0 and 15°) of refractive, corneal, and internal (comatic) astigmatism.

MyoRing 360° and Keraring 355° (with 0.20 and 0.30 mm thickness, respectively) are proposed for treatment of moderate to advanced central nipple-shaped keratoconus.[16,17]

CONTRAINDICATIONS

Most studies on intrastromal corneal ring segment implantation exclude patients with mean keratometry greater than 58 due to the lower chance of success, and Krachmer et al. believe that intra corneal implants are contraindicated in patients with keratometry readings steeper than 70.0 D. Other contraindications for intracorneal ring segments include:[16]

- Central corneal opacities

- Corneal hydrops

- Uncontrolled allergic disease with chronic eye rubbing

- Active infection

- Localized or systemic collagen vascular, autoimmune, or immunodeficiency disease

- Ocular comorbidities that may predispose the patient to future complications, including recurrent corneal erosion, herpetic eye disease, and corneal dystrophy

- Pregnant or nursing women

NOMOGRAMS

Implantation of a suitable intracorneal ring requires the determination of several parameters, like arc length, thickness, and location of incision; thus, the surgeon must consider manifest refraction, topography and tomography, coma map/axis, the extent of ectatic area, cone location, mesopic pupil diameter, and corneal thickness before making the final decision. There are several nomograms, published in the literature, as well as nomograms suggested by each implant manufacturer as guidelines to help the clinician achieve the best post-operative results. Most authors recommend drawing a line along the steepest axis of the cornea and to make the incision on this axis to reduce astigmatism. Temporal incisions are suggested for inferior cones to implant the segments superiorly and/or inferiorly and superior incisions are recommended for central cones so that the segments could be implanted nasally and/or temporally. Two symmetric implants may be used when the steepest axis line divides the conical area into two equal parts, or when the conical area is on the central 3- to 5-mm corneal zone of the posterior float map. A single segment or two asymmetric segments can be utilized in asymmetrical cases.[16]

Table 16.2 shows some of the preferred nomograms for different types of ICRSs.

SURGICAL TECHNIQUES

Intracorneal ring segments are implanted deep into the stromal channels (created manually or with femtosecond (FS) lasers) at a depth of 70% to 80% of pachymetry on the desired location.[15]

Mechanical Technique

After instillation of anesthetic eye drop, the geographical center of the cornea and the steep axis and incision sites are marked. A radial incision of 1.2–1.8 mm width is created using a diamond knife which is set for a depth of between 70 and 80% of the pachymetry. Then, using a pocketing hook and two semicircular dissectors (one clockwise and the other counter-clockwise), two semicircular tunnels are dissected deep into the stroma by rotational movements. Ring segments should be inserted into the tunnels at least 1 mm away from the incision site.[15]

Femtosecond Laser Technique

The procedure is initiated by topical anesthesia and marking a reference point for centration (the pupil center or the Purkinje reflex). The single-use suction ring is centered and the disposable glass lens is applanated to the cornea for a safe fixation. Continuous circular stromal tunnel is created at 75–80% depth of the thinnest pachymetry and an entry cut is created. After dilating the tunnel using a blunt dilator, ring segments are introduced into the tunnels created.

Compared with the exclusively manual surgical technique, the femtosecond laser reduces intraoperative and post-operative complications, makes tunnel creation more comfortable and easier for both the patient and the surgeon, and also allows precise personalization of tunnel depth, width, and diameter. Using mechanical dissection, the tunnel depth may become shallower than intended throughout the tunnel dimension.[14,15] Different procedures, including crosslinking and refractive surgery, can be combined with femtosecond laser-assisted corneal ring implantation.[14]

EFFICACY

Different studies suggested that the following parameters maybe beneficial for predicting visual rehabilitation after ICRS implantation.[18–21]

- Mean simulated keratometry (SimKavg)

- Index of surface variance (ISV) value

- Difference between the pre-operative UDVA and CDVA (the greater the better)

- Coincidence of the most elevated points of the anterior and posterior corneal surfaces on the elevation maps

Table 16.2 Preferred Nomograms for Different Types of Intracorneal Ring Segments (ICRSs)

Symmetric SK; CC   Myopia>Astigmatism; or
Myopia=Astigmatism:

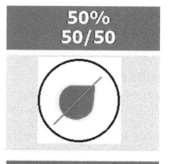

1 Seg SK 6.0 mm; DC   Astigmatism>Myopia/ Astigmatis +
Hyperopia:
the apex of the cone from 3 mm to 5 mm
topographical zone

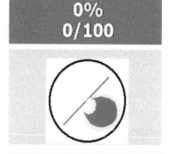

Asymmetric 2 Seg   Myopia=Astigmatism: In a de-centered
SK; DC   cone

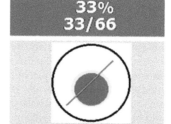

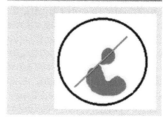

Intacs SK 90°/130° 2   Astigmatism>Myopia/Astigmatism +
Seg 7.0 mm   Hyperopia

1 Seg SK 6.0 mm   Astigmatism>Myopia/ Astigmatis +
Hyperopia: DC
DC with the apex of the cone from 3 mm
to 5 mm topographical zone

1 Seg 7.0 mm   Astigmatism>Myopia/ Astigmatism +
Hyperopia: DC
DC with the apex of the cone from 5 mm
to 7 mm topographical zone

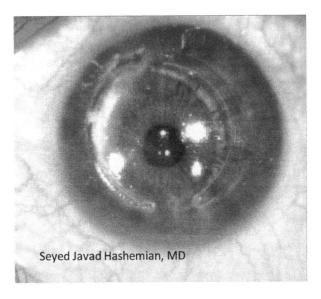

Seyed Javad Hashemian, MD

Figure 16.5   Extrusion of intrastromal corneal ring segments

The mean spherical equivalent and mean keratometry has been shown to decrease, from 1 to 7.6 D and 6.43 D to 2.16 D, respectively, while 34% to 100% of eyes showed visual improvement in different studies.[17]

COMPLICATIONS OF INTRACORNEAL RING SEGMENT IMPLANTATION

With the development of femtosecond laser-assisted implantation technique and advancements in the design of implants, complications of ICRS implantation in keratoconic patients have become minimal.

Intra-operative complications, such as incomplete stromal tunnel creation, perforation of anterior corneal surface, and perforation through the corneal endothelium into the anterior chamber are uncommon and more associated with the mechanical dissection technique.

Moreover, the post-operative complications described in most studies accounting for most cases of implant removal include functional failure (refractive or visual), implant migration, extrusion (Figure 16.5), corneal thinning, corneal melting, and infectious keratitis. Other complications are glare, halos, photophobia, visual fluctuation, neovascularization, milky infiltrates around segments, foreign body sensation, or pain.[22,23]

In general, ICRSs are an effective and safe surgical treatment in the management of corneal ectasia and is well tolerated in most patients over several years. Appropriate patient selection and surgical planning based on the available nomograms help to minimize adverse events.

Intrastromal Corneal Ring Segment in the Pediatric Population

Pediatric keratoconus is more progressive, especially when associated with allergic diseases and eye rubbing. Since corneal transplantation at a young age brings important complications, the viability of intracorneal ring segment implantation as an option in pediatric patients has been investigated. Although acceptable visual and topographic results has been shown for pediatric ICRS, the concern about the factors which may predispose the patient to future complications, such as eye rubbing, trauma, and rapid progression of disease, still remains.[17]

REFERENCES

1. Fleming JF, ReynoldsAlvin E, Kilmer LG, Burris TE, Abbott RL, Schanzlin DJ. The intrastromal corneal ring: two cases in rabbits. *Journal of Refractive Surgery.* 1987;3:227–32.

2. Burris TE. Intrastromal corneal ring technology: results and indications. *Current Opinion in Ophthalmology.* 1998;9(4):9–14.

3. Colin J, Cochener B, Savary G, Malet F. Correcting keratoconus with intracorneal rings. *Journal of Cataract & Refractive Surgery.* 2000;26(8):1117–22.

4. Sakellaris D, Balidis M, Gorou O, Szentmary N, Alexoudis A, Grieshaber MC, et al. Intracorneal ring segment implantation in the management of keratoconus: an evidence-based approach. *Ophthalmology and Therapy.* 2019;8(Suppl 1):5–14.

5. Patel S, Marshall J, Fitzke FW, 3rd. Model for deriving the optical performance of the myopic eye corrected with an intracorneal ring. *Journal of Refractive Surgery (Thorofare, NJ: 1995).* 1995;11(4):248–52.

6. Djotyan GP, Kurtz RM, Fernández DC, Juhasz T. An analytically solvable model for biomechanical response of the cornea to refractive surgery. *Journal of Biomechanical Engineering.* 2001;123(5):440–5.

7. Kling S, Marcos S. Finite-element modeling of intrastromal ring segment implantation into a hyperelastic cornea. *Investigative Ophthalmology & Visual Science.* 2013;54(1):881–9.

8. García de Oteyza G, Álvarez de Toledo J, Barraquer RI, Kling S. Refractive changes of a new asymmetric intracorneal ring segment with variable thickness and base width: A 2D finite-element model. *PLoS One.* 2021;16(9):e0257222.

9. Krachmer JH, Mannis MJ, Holland EJ. *Cornea Fundamentals, Diagnosis and Management.* 3rd ed. New York: Elsevier Inc.; 2011.

10. Piñero DP, Alio JL, Barraquer RI, Michael R. Corneal biomechanical changes after intracorneal ring segment implantation in keratoconus. *Cornea.* 2012;31(5):491–9.

11. Zare MA, Mehrjardi HZ, Afarideh M, Bahrmandy H, Mohammadi SF. Visual, keratometric and corneal biomechanical changes after intacs SK implantation for moderate to severe keratoconus. *Journal of Ophthalmic & Vision Research.* 2016;11(1):17–25.

12. Mounir A, Radwan G, Farouk MM, Mostafa EM. Femtosecond-assisted intracorneal ring segment complications in keratoconus: from novelty to expertise. *Clinical Ophthalmology.* 2018;12:957–64.

13. Ertan A, Colin J. Intracorneal rings for keratoconus and keratectasia. *Journal of Cataract & Refractive Surgery.* 2007;33(7):1303–14.

14. Tognon T, Campos M, Wengrzynovski JP, Barella KA, Pasqualotti A, de Brito Martins LA, et al. Indications and visual outcomes of intrastromal corneal ring segment implantation in a large patient series. *Clinics (Sao Paulo, Brazil).* 2017;72(6):370–7.

15. Kymionis GD. Actual indications for intracorneal ring segment implantation in keratoconus. *ESASO Course Series,* 66–73. https://doi.org/10.1159/000381493

16. Krachmer JH, Mannis MJ, Holland EJ. *Cornea e-book.* Elsevier Health Sciences; 2016.

17. Peña-García P, Alió JL, Vega-Estrada A, Barraquer RI. Internal, corneal, and refractive astigmatism as prognostic factors for intrastromal corneal ring segment implantation in mild to moderate keratoconus. *Journal of Cataract & Refractive Surgery.* 2014;40(10):1633–44.

18. Sedaghat M-R, Momeni-Moghaddam H, Piñero DP, Akbarzadeh R, Moshirfar M, Bamdad S, et al. Predictors of successful outcome following intrastromal corneal ring segments implantation. *Current Eye Research.* 2019;44(7):707–15.

19. Utine C, Durmaz Engin C, Ayhan Z. Effects of preoperative topometric indices on visual gain after intracorneal ring segment implantation for keratoconus. *Eye & Contact Lens: Science & Clinical Practice*. 2018;44 Suppl 2:1.

20. Hashemian SJ, Farshchian N, Foroutam-Jazi A, Jafari ME, Hashemian MS, Hashemian SM. Visual and refractive outcomes and tomographic changes after femtosecond laser-assisted intrastromal corneal ring segment implantation in patients with keratoconus. *Journal of Ophthalmic and Vision Research*. 2018;13:376–82.

21. Hashemian SJ, Abdolalizadeh P, Ghiasian L, Aghaei H, Hadavandkhani A, Semnani FN, Jafari ME, Hashemian SM, Hashemian MS. Outcomes of a single-segment intrastromal corneal ring in early keratoconus and early pellucid marginal degeneration. *International Ophthalmology*. 2022 Oct;42(10):2987–2996. https://doi.org/10.1007/s10792-022-02284-8

22. Bautista-Llamas MJ, Sánchez-González MC, López-Izquierdo I, López-Muñoz A, Gargallo-Martínez B, De-Hita-Cantalejo C, et al. Complications and explantation reasons in intracorneal ring segments (ICRS) implantation: a systematic review. *Journal of Refractive Surgery (Thorofare, NJ: 1995)*. 2019;35(11):740–7.

23. D'Oria F, Abdelghany AA, Ledo N, Barraquer RI, Alio JL. Incidence and reasons for intrastromal corneal ring segment explantation. *American Journal of Ophthalmology*. 2021;222:351–8.

17 Corneal Cross-Linking Combined with Intracorneal Ring Segments

Mehrdad Mohammadpour and Masoud Khorrami-Nejad

INTRODUCTION

Corneal collagen cross-linking (CXL) is known as an established treatment for halting the progression of keratoconus and corneal ectasia. Intracorneal ring segments (ICRS) are semicircular inserts implanted in the corneal stroma to regularize the abnormal corneal shape and improve vision in keratoconus patients. Both CXL and ICRS aim to improve vision and stabilize keratoconus progression through different mechanisms.[1-4] Based on recent studies, this chapter evaluates the visual, refractive, and keratometric outcomes of various approaches that combine CXL with ICRS implantation. These include ICRS followed by CXL; simultaneous ICRS and CXL; CXL first followed by ICRS; and comparative studies evaluating different sequences.

Some researchers such as Ertan et al., Awady et al., Saelens et al., and Mounir et al. have reported improvements of visual, refractive and keratometric values.[5-8] Also, two studies conducted done by Abozaid and by Abdelmassih et al. on pediatric patients have represented these improved parameters, whereas others, like Chan et al., Cakir et al., and Elsaftawy et al. have evaluated the clinical outcomes by dividing the patients into two groups: patients receiving ICRS alone and patients receiving ICRS before CXL surgery.[9-13] The results demonstrated greater improvements in the combined group in some studies (Chan et al. study). At the same time, there were no significant differences between groups regarding visual, refractive, and topographic results in the Elsaftawy et al. study.

Some other studies did another type of combination (performing ICRS and CXL simultaneously). The outcomes of this type of combination showed improvements in all parameters studied.

The final type of combination (performing ICRS after CXL) had similar consequences to previous studies, although El-Raggal et al., in their study, evaluated the influence of CXL surgery on femtosecond laser channel creation for ICRS implantation by using different power settings of the femtosecond machine, with patients having ICRS implantation six months later.[14] In their conclusion, they have reported that it is better to perform ICRS implantation before or concurrent with CXL.

In comparative studies, some researchers have assessed sequential ICRS and CXL combinations. For instance, Liu et al. (2015) reported that there were no marked differences in improvement of each of the parameters between the groups of ICRS implantation only, ICRS after CXL, and CXL after ICRS.[15] In other studies, Hersh et al. (2019) and Greenstein et al. (2020) compared simultaneous combination and the sequential CXL after ICRS implantation combination; the results showed no marked differences between the two groups.[16,17] However, the studies conducted by Coskunseven et al. (2009) and Nicula et al. (2017) showed better improvements of refractive and keratometric results in the "CXL after ICRS implantation" group than in the "ICRS implantation after CXL" group.[18,19] Hashemi et al. (2018) compared patients in three ICRS/CXL combinations groups: simultaneous, ICRS first, and CXL first,[20] and reported visual, refractive, and keratometric improvements in all groups. There were no notable differences in UCVA, BCVA, and cylindrical refractive error between the three groups, although the outcomes of same-day surgery were better than the ICRS-first group with respect to steep-K, and CXL-first group was superior in terms of spherical refractive errors and flat-K.

A study was conducted by Koh et al. (2019), evaluating the outcomes for one year of a modified version of a two-stage multimodal surgical protocol (PRK and accelerated CXL after Intacs SK ICRS implantation) on 30 eyes with moderate KCN. The interval between ICRS implantation and PRK-CXL was three months approximately. In addition, the optical zone was from 6.0 to 6.6 mm and the average maximum ablation profundity was 67.62 ± 26.52 μm for PRK-CXL.

First, the authors implanted an Intacs SK ICRS in the corneas. The inner and outer diameters of the channel were designed to be 5.8–5.95 mm and 7.05–7.2 mm, respectively (contingent on keratometry reading and the thickness of the ring). In addition, the ring tunnel profundity was set to 75 to 80% of the thinnest corneal thickness of the selected channel, and a 1.35-mm cut was made for the radial entrance. Then, after one drop of moxifloxacin 0.5% instillation, a therapeutic contact lens was located on the cornea. After contact lens removal, topical medications were used in particular dosages for two weeks. In the second step, CWG-transPRK was administered by applying the trans-epithelial mode of the Schwind Amaris 1050 RS excimer laser. Then, mitomycin C 0.02% was used immediately for 20 seconds to prohibit the regression of corneal haze. Afterward, they performed accelerated CXL a short time after completion of ablation. They instilled VibeX Rapid

DOI: 10.1201/9781003371601-17

Table 17.1 Summary of recently published results for CXL combined with ICRS implantation.

Reference	Sample Size	Follow-Up Period	Additional Explanation(s)	Outcome(s)
			Sequence: Intrastromal Corneal Ring Segments Implantation before CXL	
Chan et al. (2007)[11]	25	Group 1: 59 to 135 days Group 2: 63 to 141 days	A retrospective study Two groups: Group 1: Intacs and C3-R (13 eyes) Group 2: Intacs implantation alone (12 eyes)	A marked decrease in cylinder, steep, and mean-K and L–U ratios in both groups (greater improvement in group 1 than 2) No significant difference between the two groups regarding CDVA and UDVA improvement
Ertan et al. (2009)[5]	25	3 months	Bilateral KCN Trans-epithelial cross-linking Mean interval between procedures: 3.98 months	Improvement of UDVA (1.9 lines) and CDVA (1.7 lines) after Intacs and additional increase in UDVA (1.2 lines) and CDVA (0.36 lines) after CXL Decrease in SE (2.8 D), cylinder (0.47 D), mean-K (2.22 D), and steepest K (1.27 D) values after Intacs with further decreases of 0.5 D, 0.15 D, 0.35 D, and 0.76 D after CXL, respectively.
Saelens et al. (2011)[7]	7	3, 6, and 12 months	CXL immediately after Ferrara ICRS Progressive mild to severe KCN and contact lens intolerance	Increase in mean UDVA (from 0.10 ± 0.07 to 0.60 ± 0.24 D) and CDVA (from 0.56 ± 0.08 to 0.82 ± 0.25 D) Decrease in mean spherical equivalent (3.5 D) and mean K values (from 46.81 ± 2.13 D to 43.97 ± 2.22 D) No notable change in the average post-operative thinnest pachymetry
El Awady et al. (2012)[6]	21	Mean 5.67 ± 1.89 months after CXL	CXL after at least 3 months (mean 4.56 ± 3.2 months) of KeraRing implantation Mild to moderate KCN No corneal scarring and corneal thickness > 400 µm and endothelial cell count > 3000 per mm²	Increase in mean UDVA (from 0.05 ± 0.02 to 0.23 ± 0.17 D) and CDVA (from 0.18 ± 0.1 to 0.41 ± 0.18 D) after CXL Decrease in the SE (2.91 D), cylinder (2.11 D), and mean keratometric value (2.59 D) after CXL
Coşkunseven et al. (2013)[21]	14	At least 1 year after pIOL implantation	Progressive KCN 3-stage procedure for KCN: 1. ICRS implantation 2. CXL 3. Collagen copolymer toric pIOL implantation For residual myopic astigmatism Minimum 6 months between procedures (7 months between first and second stage and 8.4 months between second and third stage)	Increase in UDVA (from 0.01 to 0.44 D) and CDVA (from 0.14 to 0.57 D) Decrease in mean MRSE (from −16.40 ± 3.56 to −0.80 ± 1.02 D), mean refractive astigmatism (from −4.73 ± 1.32 to −0.96 ± 0.35 D), mean steep-K (from 60.57 to 54.48 D) and flat-K (from 56.16 to 53.57 D) No complications intra- and post-operatively.
Çakir et al. (2013)[12]	166	3, 6, and 12 months	Progressive KCN Two groups: First group: ICRSI-only Second group: CXL combined with ICRSI	Increase in UDVA and CDVA Decrease in spherical and cylindrical error and mean K-values No statistical difference in any parameters between groups Ring removal (in 3 eyes) owing to the melting of the cornea

(Continued)

Table 17.1 (Continued) Summary of recently published results for CXL combined with ICRS implantation

Reference	Sample Size	Follow-Up Period	Additional Explanation(s)	Outcome(s)
Elsaftawy et al. (2015)[13]	40	1, 3, and 6 months	Progressive mild to moderate KCN Two groups: Group 1: KeraRing implantation (20 eyes) Group 2: Transepithelial CXL 1 month after KeraRing insertion (20 eyes)	Increase in UDVA and CDVA Decrease in the refractive error and K values No marked difference between both groups regarding visual, refractive and topographic results, but a more significant decrease in spherical refraction after 3 and a highly significant reduction after 6 months
Ferenczy et al. (2015)[23]	32	2 years	Femtosecond-assisted ICRSI with and without CXL Two groups: Group 1: ICRSI alone (22 eyes) Group 2: ICRSI-CXL (10 eyes)	Increase in CDVA in both groups Decrease in spherical and cylindrical errors, mean-K values, and SE in both groups VA ≥ 20/60 in 78% of cases (72% of group 1 and 90% of group 2) with spectacles
Abozaid (2017)[9]	18	1 year	Trans-epithelial accelerated CXL two weeks after femtosecond laser-assisted Keraring implantation in children with KCN and VKC	Increase in UDVA and CDVA Significant decrease in all keratometry values: flat-K (from 47.9 ± 2.6 D to 44.7 ± 2.2 D), steep-K (from 52.8 ± 3.1 D to 47.7 ± 3.5 D) and mean-K (from 50.3 ± 2.7 D to 45.8 ± 3.1 D) Decrease in manifest sphere, manifest cylinder, and mean spherical equivalent.
Abdelmassih et al. (2017)[10]	17	6 months, 1, 2, and 4 years	A retrospective study Pediatric patients (aged ≤ 14 years) with KCN and poor CDVA CXL 1 month after ICRS implantation A 9-year-old patient: CXL 7 years after ICRSI, in 8-year follow-up: visual improvements and a stable cornea (the patient was not included in the statistical analysis)	At the 6-month follow-up: A significant increase in UDVA and CDVA A marked decrease in both K readings and SE after ICRS implantation At the 1, 2, and 4-year follow up: Unchanged refractive values compared with the 6-month follow-up (except for a considerable but non-significant decrease in cylinder and at 4 years in UDVA) No complications intra- and post-operatively (except for removing 1 ring segment after 2 years due to corneal thinning and vascularization)
Abdelmassih et al. (2017)[24]	16	6 months and 2 years	3-step procedure: 1. ICRSI 2. CXL 3. Toric ICL 4 weeks interval between ICRSI and CXL and at least 6 months between toric ICL and CXL Moderate to severe KCN	At 6 months: Marked decrease in steep-K, flat-K, K_{max} sphere, and SE Considerable increase in UDVA and CDVA Unchanged UDVA and K readings at 2 years, but improvements in CDVA, sphere, and cylinder
Sachdev et al. (2020)[25]	3	1, 3, 12, and 36 months	The combination of ICRS implantation and CXL, applying a SMILE lenticule for intra-operative reinforcement of stroma in thin corneas (< 400 μm) Progressive KCN or post-operative corneal ectasia and contact lens intolerance	Decrease in mean K_{max} (from 63.17 ± 9.31 D to 54.77 ± 9.47 D) Increase in CDVA No marked loss of endothelial cells Using a SMILE lenticule for augmentation of the thickness of stroma in ultrathin corneas allows efficacious CXL combined with ICRS.

Reference	Sample Size	Follow-Up Period	Additional Explanation(s)	Outcome(s)
			Sequence: Simultaneous Intrastromal Corneal Ring Segments Implantation and CXL	
Kılıç et al. (2012)[26]	131	2–11 months	Intra-corneal riboflavin injection for CXL combined with ICRS implantation	Increase in UDVA Decrease in mean manifest spherical refraction (from -3.87 ± 4.55 D to -1.25 ± 2.31 D), and cylinder (from -3.89 ± 1.97 D to -2.27 ± 2.18 D) and mean-K reading (from 50.50 ± 5.26 D to 46.03 ± 4.51 D) No complications intra- and post-operatively.
Yeung et al. (2013)[27]	3	3 years	ICRS implantation in KCN patients after ICRS (Intacs) combined with same-day CXL A retrospective study	No loss of lines in CDVA Topographic changes may be preserved in some cases after one or both segments implantation despite refractive results reversal.
Yeung et al (2013)[28]	85	1 year	Femtosecond laser-assisted ICRSI combined with same-day CXL Two groups: Group 1: paired ICRS combined with UV–A and riboflavin CXL (47 eyes) Group 2: single ICRS combined with UV–A and riboflavin CXL (38 eyes)	Increase in UDVA (2.7 lines in group 1 vs 3.4 lines in group 2) Unchanged CDVA (no lines lost) Remarkable decrease in mean cylinder (single ICRS: -3.84 ± 1.72 to -2.19 ± 1.54 D; and paired ICRS: -3.91 ± 1.45 to -2.96 ± 1.92 D) No considerable difference in total HOAs Equivalence of all refractive parameters in both groups
Hosny et al. (2018)[29]	20	6 months	Moderate-to-severe KCN Two groups: Group A: ICRSI with simultaneous intra-tunnel CXL (10 eyes) Group B: ICRSI with epi-off CXL (10 eyes)	Marked increase in UDVA and CDVA and non-significant increase in CRF (no significant difference between groups) Considerable decrease in manifest cylinder (in both groups) and manifest sphere (notably in group A and non-significantly in group B with no notable difference between groups), Kmin and K_{max} and CH (with no significant difference between groups) No complications intra- and post-operatively
Mounir et al. (2020)[8]	A 27-year-old male	12 months	Advanced superior KCN Accelerated CXL combined with KeraRing implantation by femtosecond laser Left eye: grade 3 KCN with superior cone Right eye: previous penetrating keratoplasty	Increase in UDVA and CDVA Decrease in keratometry reading at the superior cone, both anterior and posterior elevations

(Continued)

Table 17.1 (Continued) **Summary of recently published results for CXL combined with ICRS implantation**

Reference	Sample Size	Follow-Up Period	Additional Explanation(s)	Outcome(s)
			Sequence: Intrastromal Corneal Ring Segments Implantation after CXL	
El-Raggal et al. (2011)[14]	15	1 day, 1 week, 1, 3, and 6 months	ICRS implantation 6 months after CXL Grade II or III of KCN Influence of CXL on IntraLase FS-60 femtosecond laser channel creation for ICRS implantation The femtosecond machine power setting: First group: 1.5 mJ Second group: 1.6 mJ Third group: 1.7 mJ A control group: 1.5 mJ without CXL	Incomplete channel creation by power setting of 1.5 and completed one by 1.6 mJ and 1.7 mJ (increase in power setting led to increase in corneal haze) No corneal haze and other complications after 6 weeks Increase in UDVA and CDVA Decrease in spherical and cylindrical error, steep, and flat K No significant difference between the three groups except steep and flat K between groups 1 and 2 ICRS implantation should be before or simultaneous with CXL
Renesto Ada et al. (2012)[30]	39	1, 3, 6, 12, and 24 months	Two groups: 1: CXL group with riboflavin and UV-A light 2: riboflavin eyedrops group with riboflavin 0.1% in 20% dextran solution	Increase in UDVA and CDVA Decrease in flattest-K1, steepest-K2 and average keratometry in both groups with no significant difference between groups.
Henriquez et al. (2012)[31]	9	6 months after CXL and 6 months after FR implantation	CXL before Ferrara intrastromal corneal ring segment (FR) implantation Progressive KCN Cylinder value ≥ 5 D	Increase in UDVA and CDVA Marked decrease in mean spherical equivalent, minimum, and maximum K values
Comparative Studies				
Coskunseven et al. (2009)[18]	48	12–14 months	Progressive KCN Two groups: Group 1: ICRS after CXL Group 2: CXL after ICRS Mean interval between treatments: 7 ± 2 months	Increase in UDVA (from 0.07 ± 0.09 to 0.25 ± 0.12 D in first group and from 0.11 ± 0.09 to 0.32 ± 0.21 D in second group) and CDVA (from 0.24 ± 0.11 to 0.41 ± 0.20 D in first and from 0.22 ± 0.16 to 0.55 ± 0.2 D in second group) Decrease in the mean SE, cylinder, and mean K values (both groups) More improvement in mean-K, SE, and CDVA in group 2 than 1
Liu et al. (2015)[15]	86	1 year	A retrospective study 41 eyes with complete follow-ups Three groups: Group normal: ICRS implantation only (25) Group CXL-S: CXL immediately after ICRS (8) Group CXL-B: ICRS long after CXL (8)	Increase in UDVA and CDVA (improvement of both parameters for all the patients in group CXL-B) Improvements of refractive and topographic results No significant differences between groups (all the P values above 0.05)

Reference	Sample Size	Follow-Up Period	Additional Explanation(s)	Outcome(s)
Nicula et al. (2017)[19]	71	1, 3, 6, and 12 months	A retrospective study Two groups: Group 1: CXL after ICRS (41 eyes) Group 2: ICRS after CXL (30 eyes)	Decrease in Km values (1.5 D in group 1 and 1 D in group 2), SE, and cylinder Better improvement of VA in group 1 than in group 2
Hashemi et al. (2018)[20]	120 articles	12 months	Comparing the proper sequence of CXL and ICRS combination (sequential and simultaneous) A systematic review and meta-analysis Three groups (simultaneous, ICRS first, and CXL first)	Visual, refractive, and keratometric improvement in all groups No significant difference in UDVA, CDVA, and cylindrical refractive error between the three groups (albeit, the outcomes of same-day surgery were better than the ICRS-first group regarding steep-K and the CXL-first group regarding spherical refractive errors and flat-K)
Hersh et al. (2019)[16]	198	6 months	Two groups: Group 1: CXL immediately after ICRS in the same session (104 eyes) Group 2: CXL 3 months after ICRS (94 eyes)	Decrease in K_{max} (by 2.5 D) and I-S difference (improved by 3.9 D) and average maximum fattening (−7.5 D) Increase in UDVA and CDVA (1.1 lines) Equivalent results in both groups
Greenstein et al. (2020)[17]	158	6 months	Evaluating HOAs after CXL and Intacs Two groups: Group 1: Intacs and CXL simultaneously (81 eyes) Group 2: CXL 3 months after Intacs (77 eyes)	Improvement in UDVA (−0.22 ± 0.34 D), CDVA (−0.13 ± 0.24 D), I-S value (−4.2 ± 5.0 D) and significant improvement in total anterior corneal HOA (−1.05 ± 0.93 μm - no significant difference between groups), vertical coma (−1.53 ± 1.18 μm), and horizontal coma anterior corneal HOAs (−0.35 ± 0.57 μm) Decrease in K_{max} (−3.1 ± 3.0 D) and K_{max} flat (−7.9 ± 4.0 D) Increase in spherical anterior corneal HOAs (0.24 ± 0.70 μm) No significant change in trefoil

ICR: Intracorneal rings, ICRS: Intracorneal ring segment, CXL: Corneal cross-linking, CDVA: Best-corrected distance visual acuity in the LogMar system, UDVA: Uncorrected distance visual acuity in the LogMar system SMILE: Small Incision Lenticule Extraction, KCN: Keratoconus, ICRSI: Intracorneal ring segment implantation, K reading: Keratometry reading, SE: spherical equivalent, VKC: vernal keratoconjunctivitis, flat-K: flat keratometry, steep-K: steep keratometry, mean-K: mean keratometry, K values: keratometry values, steepest K values: steepest K values, VA: visual acuity, C3-R: Corneal collagen cross-linking with riboflavin, L–U ratio: lower-upper ratio, Epi-off CXL: epithelium-off corneal cross-linking, CH: corneal hysteresis, CRF: corneal resistance factor, Km: mean keratometry, K_{max}: maximum keratometry, corneal HOAs: corneal higher-order aberrations, UV-A light: Ultraviolet A light, K1: flat keratometry, K2: steep keratometry, I-S difference: inferior-superior difference, toric pIOL: toric phakic intraocular lens, ICL: implantable collamer lens, D: diopter

in the examined eye every two minutes for ten minutes. Then, the surface of the cornea was rinsed thoroughly using a sterile, balanced saline solution. Next, the cornea was irradiated with 30 mW/cm² UV-A at a wavelength of 365 nm for three minutes. After accelerated CXL was completed, the surface of the cornea was irrigated with a cold balanced salt solution and then a therapeutic contact lens was placed on the cornea. Levofloxacin 0.5% and fluorometholone 0.1% were applied four times daily for one week and twice daily for eight weeks, respectively.

According to the results, the mean UDVA and CDVA were improved from 6/38 to 6/12 and from 6/19 to 6/7.5, respectively, over a one-year follow-up period after CWG-transPRK and accelerated CXL.In addition, all eyes attained one or more lines of CDVA, which was better than 6/12 (no single line was lost). The amount of myopia, the mean-K, steep K, and maximum K were decreased after both ICRS implantation and PRK-CXL. The cylindrical value decreased from 4.8–7.8 D to 2.5–4.0 D. After ICRS implantation, coma was not changed, whereas spherical aberration was increased. However, after PRK-CXL, both coma and spherical aberration decreased in the first month and subsequently remained unchanged at one year. The thinnest corneal thickness increased slightly after ICRS but decreased after PRK-CXL, and was stabilized for three months. No serious complications were observed, such as a continuous corneal epithelial deficiency, ICRS protrusion, ICRS dislocation, profound corneal vascularization, or corneal infection.

The authors reported that this technique could improve the vision of patients with moderate KCN without contact lens requirements. Also, this method was safe and efficacious throughout the one-year follow-up period.[22] A summary of recently published results for CXL, combined with ICRS implantation, is shown in Table 17.1.

In conclusion, most studies show visual and topographic improvements with combination approaches compared with ICRS or CXL alone. However, the optimal sequence and timing of ICRS and CXL need further elucidation. While long-term data are limited, the combination therapies appear to be safe and effective in managing keratoconus progression and irregular astigmatism. Further research is required to establish standardized protocols for combining ICRS and CXL in keratoconus treatment.

The summary of recently published results for CXL combined with ICRS implantation is reported in Table 17.1. This table demonstrates that combining CXL with ICRS implantation is an effective approach for managing keratoconus. Most studies found improvements in uncorrected distance visual acuity, corrected distance visual acuity, and keratometric values when CXL was performed sequentially or simultaneously with ICRS placement. While some studies showed slightly better outcomes with one sequence over the other, many found no significant differences between doing CXL first versus ICRS. Both sequential and same-day procedures were found to be safe with minimal risks or complications. Overall, the combination of CXL and ICRS provides better visual, refractive, and topographic results than either treatment alone in keratoconus patients. Performing CXL strengthens the cornea and halts disease progression, while ICRS implantation flattens the cone and provides visual rehabilitation. Most studies noted long-term stability up to 2–4 years after the combination treatment.

In conclusion, the current body of evidence supports using combined CXL and ICRS implantation as an effective option for keratoconus management. Both sequential and same-day procedures have high safety and efficacy. More randomized controlled trials are still needed to compare techniques and optimize protocols. However, the combination approach appears to be a promising long-term solution for stabilizing and improving vision in keratoconus.

REFERENCES

1. Khorrami-Nejad M, Aghili O, Hashemian H, Aghazadeh-Amiri M, Karimi F. Changes in corneal asphericity after MyoRing implantation in moderate and severe keratoconus. *Journal of Ophthalmic & Vision Research*. 2019;14(4):428.

2. Kymionis GD, Grentzelos MA, Kankariya VP, Liakopoulos DA, Karavitaki AE, Portaliou DM, et al. Long-term results of combined transepithelial phototherapeutic keratectomy and corneal collagen cross-linking for keratoconus: Cretan protocol. *Journal of Cataract & Refractive Surgery*. 2014;40(9):1439–45.

3. Mohammadpour M, Heirani M, Khoshtinat N, Khorrami-Nejad M. Comparison of two different 360-degree intrastromal corneal rings combined with simultaneous accelerated-corneal cross-linking. *European Journal of Ophthalmology*. 2023:11206721231171420.

4. Mohammadpour M, Khoshtinat N, Khorrami-Nejad M. Comparison of visual, tomographic, and biomechanical outcomes of 360 degrees intracorneal ring implantation with and without corneal cross-linking for progressive keratoconus: a 5-year follow-up. *Cornea.* 2021;40(3):303–10.

5. Ertan A, Karacal H, Kamburoglu G. Refractive and topographic results of transepithelial cross-linking treatment in eyes with intacs. *Cornea.* 2009;28(7):719–23.

6. El Awady H, Shawky M, Ghanem AA. Evaluation of collagen cross-linking in keratoconus eyes with Kera intracorneal ring implantation. *European Journal of Ophthalmology.* 2012;22(7_suppl):62–8.

7. Saelens IE, Bartels MC, Bleyen I, Van Rij G. Refractive, topographic, and visual outcomes of same-day corneal cross-linking with Ferrara intracorneal ring segments in patients with progressive keratoconus. *Cornea.* 2011;30(12):1406–8.

8. Mounir A, Mostafa EM. Combined accelerated corneal collagen cross-linking and intrastromal Kerarings implantation for treatment of advanced superior keratoconus. *GMS Ophthalmology Cases.* 2020;10.

9. Abozaid MA. Sequential Keraring implantation and corneal cross-linking for the treatment of keratoconus in children with vernal keratoconjunctivitis. *Clinical Ophthalmology (Auckland, NZ).* 2017;11:1891.

10. Abdelmassih Y, El-Khoury S, Dirani A, Antonios R, Fadlallah A, Cherfan CG, et al. Safety and efficacy of sequential intracorneal ring segment implantation and cross-linking in pediatric keratoconus. *American Journal of Ophthalmology.* 2017;178:51–7.

11. Chan CC, Sharma M, Wachler BSB. Effect of inferior-segment Intacs with and without C3-R on keratoconus. *Journal of Cataract & Refractive Surgery.* 2007;33(1):75–80.

12. Çakir H, Pekel G, Perente I, Genç S. Comparison of intrastromal corneal ring segment implantation only and in combination with collagen cross-linking for keratoconus. *European Journal of Ophthalmology.* 2013;23(5):629–34.

13. Elsaftawy HS, Ahmed MH, Saif MYS, Mousa R. Sequential intracorneal ring segment implantation and corneal transepithelial collagen cross-linking in keratoconus. *Cornea.* 2015;34(11):1420–6.

14. El-Raggal TM. Effect of corneal collagen cross-linking on femtosecond laser channel creation for intrastromal corneal ring segment implantation in keratoconus. *Journal of Cataract & Refractive Surgery.* 2011;37(4):701–5.

15. Liu X-L, Li P-H, Fournie P, Malecaze F. Investigation of the efficiency of intrastromal ring segments with cross-linking using different sequence and timing for keratoconus. *International Journal of Ophthalmology.* 2015;8(4):703.

16. Hersh PS, Issa R, Greenstein SA. Corneal cross-linking and intracorneal ring segments for keratoconus: a randomized study of concurrent versus sequential surgery. *Journal of Cataract & Refractive Surgery.* 2019;45(6):830–9.

17. Greenstein SA, Chung D, Rosato L, Gelles JD, Hersh PS. Corneal higher-order aberrations after cross-linking and intrastromal corneal ring segments for keratoconus. *Journal of Cataract & Refractive Surgery.* 2020;46(7):979–85.

18. Coskunseven E, Jankov II MR, Hafezi F, Atun S, Arslan E, Kymionis GD. Effect of treatment sequence in combined intrastromal corneal rings and corneal collagen cross-linking for keratoconus. *Journal of Cataract & Refractive Surgery.* 2009;35(12):2084–91.

19. Nicula C, Pop RN, Nicula DV. Comparative results in a combined procedure of intrastromal corneal rings implantation and cross-linking in patients with keratoconus: a retrospective study. *Ophthalmology and Therapy*. 2017;6(2):313–21.

20. Hashemi H, Alvani A, Seyedian MA, Yaseri M, Khabazkhoob M, Esfandiari H. Appropriate sequence of combined intracorneal ring implantation and corneal collagen cross-linking in keratoconus: a systematic review and meta-analysis. *Cornea*. 2018;37(12):1601–7.

21. Koh IH, Seo KY, Park SB, Yang H, Kim I, Kim JS, et al. One-year efficacy and safety of combined photorefractive keratectomy and accelerated corneal collagen cross-linking after Intacs SK intracorneal ring segment implantation in moderate keratoconus. *BioMed Research International*. 2019;2019.

22. Coşkunseven E, Sharma DP, Jankov II MR, Kymionis GD, Richoz O, Hafezi F. Collagen copolymer toric phakic intraocular lens for residual myopic astigmatism after intrastromal corneal ring segment implantation and corneal collagen cross-linking in a 3-stage procedure for keratoconus. *Journal of Cataract & Refractive Surgery*. 2013;39(5):722–9.

23. Ferenczy PAvH, Dalcegio M, Koehler M, Pereira TS, Moreira H, Luciane Bugmann M. Femtosecond-assisted intrastromal corneal ring implantation for keratoconus treatment: a comparison with cross-linking combination. *Arquivos Brasileiros de Oftalmologia*. 2015;78(2):76–81.

24. Abdelmassih Y, El-Khoury S, Chelala E, Slim E, Cherfan CG, Jarade E. Toric ICL implantation after sequential intracorneal ring segments implantation and corneal cross-linking in keratoconus: 2-year follow-up. *Journal of Refractive Surgery*. 2017;33(9):610–6.

25. Sachdev GS, Sachdev R, Sachdev MS. Intra corneal ring segment implantation with lenticule assisted stromal augmentation for cross-linking in thin corneas. *American Journal of Ophthalmology Case Reports*. 2020;19:100726.

26. Kılıç A, Kamburoglu G, Akıncı A. Riboflavin injection into the corneal channel for combined collagen cross-linking and intrastromal corneal ring segment implantation. *Journal of Cataract & Refractive Surgery*. 2012;38(5):878–83.

27. Yeung SN, Lichtinger A, Ku JY, Kim P, Low SA, Rootman DS. Intracorneal ring segment explantation after intracorneal ring segment implantation combined with same-day corneal collagen cross-linking in keratoconus. *Cornea*. 2013;32(12):1617–20.

28. Yeung SN, Ku JY, Lichtinger A, Low SA, Kim P, Rootman DS. Efficacy of single or paired intrastromal corneal ring segment implantation combined with collagen cross-linking in keratoconus. *Journal of Cataract & Refractive Surgery*. 2013;39(8):1146–51.

29. Hosny M, Nour M, Azzam S, Salem M, El-Mayah E. Simultaneous intratunnel cross-linking with intrastromal corneal ring segment implantation versus simultaneous epithelium-off cross-linking with intrastromal corneal ring segment implantation for keratoconus management. *Clinical Ophthalmology (Auckland, NZ)*. 2018;12:147.

30. da Candelaria Renesto A, Melo Jr LAS, de Filippi Sartori M, Campos M. Sequential topical riboflavin with or without ultraviolet a radiation with delayed intracorneal ring segment insertion for keratoconus. *American Journal of Ophthalmology*. 2012;153(5):982–93.e3.

31. Henriquez MA, Izquierdo Jr L, Bernilla C, McCarthy M. Corneal collagen cross-linking before Ferrara intrastromal corneal ring implantation for the treatment of progressive keratoconus. *Cornea*. 2012;31(7):740–5.

18 Complete 360-Degree Intrastromal Corneal Rings with and without Corneal Cross-Linking in the Management of Keratoconus

Masoud Khorrami-Nejad, Mehrdad Mohammadpour, and Rua Abulhosein

INTRODUCTION

An effective therapeutic option for individuals with keratoconus (KCN) is the intrastromal corneal ring (ICR), a type of implant that is either segmental arc-shaped or 360-degree annular-shaped.[1,2] ICRs were initially designed by Barraquer (1949) to correct myopia. The surgical principle was based on placing a complete biocompatible rigid ring, centered on the pupil, between the corneal lamellae through the opening of a superficial flap previously cut with a microkeratome.[3,4] This approach allowed flattening of the center of the cornea.[5] However, the early results were not conclusive because of the cutting of the flap. It was the work of Fleming and Reynolds (1987) that produced the first promising results.[6] They were the first to envisage the introduction of a segmental ring into a preformed tunnel with the help of metal guides, allowing the stabilization of the device while completely sparing the optical axis. Thus, they benefited from a so-called "additive" approach, sparing the corneal tissue, limiting the risks of reduced vision, and making it reversible. This technique was applied by different commercial companies, such as Keravision™ and then Addition Technologie™ for Intacs® type ICR and Mediphacos™ for Ferraring® or Keraring® type of ICR. However, the advent of the excimer laser and LASIK procedure in the 1990s greatly inhibited the growth of ICRs in the refractive surgery market. The problem was the poor predictability of the correction obtained with ICR, which depended on numerous parameters that were difficult to control for a refractive outcome as accurate as half a diopter. However, laser photo-ablation offered considerably greater refractive precision. It was not until 1997 that Fleming and Colin were the first to propose using ICR for managing corneal ectasia in patients with KCN.[7] Secondly, the first case of ICR implantation for treating one of the first post-LASIK ectasias was described by Lovisolo et al. (1999).[8]

ICRs are now utilized to correct refractive errors of patients with mild-to-moderate KCN.[9] They work as spacers between corneal layers, and the main purpose of their use is to provide central and peripheral flattening of the cornea.[7] These corneal implants have the main advantages of safety, stability, and reversibility.[10] Various corneal implants, in particular intracorneal segments (Ferrara, Intacs, Keraring) and 360-degree rings (MyoRing and AICI), are used in the treatment of corneal ectatic disorders to correct ametropia. The FDA-approved segments were first used in 1999 for the surgical treatment of mild myopia (–1.0 to 3.0 D). Since 2004, they have been used for treating KCN in the USA.[7] In 2007, Daxer suggested a method of correcting high myopia (6 to 18 D), combined with astigmatism (1 to 4 D), by implanting an intrastromal ring (MyoRing) into the corneal stroma. Since 2008, this has been used for the treatment of corneal ectasia.[11] The essence of the method is to place an annular ICR made of polymethylmethacrylate (PMMA) into a stromal pocket, which is formed using the PocketMaker microkeratome. In recent years, an advanced version of continuous annular ICR (labeled as AICI and produced by Ophthalight cor. in Tehran, Iran) has also become available.[12,13] Similar to MyoRing, the AICI is a one-piece annular-shaped ICR that comes in different thicknesses with a rectangular cross-section to manage various stages of KCN.[14]

COMPLETE 360-DEGREE INTRASTROMAL CORNEAL RINGS

MyoRing

In 2007, at the European Society of Cataract and Refractive Surgeons Congress in Stockholm, Professor A. Daxer presented the concept of CISIS (Corneal Intrastromal Implantation Surgery). This concept aimed to correct high myopia with a thin cornea and secondary keratectasia after refractive laser surgery by implanting the MyoRing. The MyoRing is implanted into a corneal pocket which is 9 mm in diameter, and formed by a PocketMaker microkeratome or a Femtosecond laser at a depth of 300 µm.[15] This method can be used to treat myopia by compensation of the spherical component up to –20.0 D and the cylindrical component up to –4.5 D at different stages of KCN, provided that the corneal thickness is more than 350 µm.

MyoRing is made of a PMMA-based polymer; it is both rigid and elastic, which allows it to be implanted through a small incision.[16,17] The ring has a trapezoidal profile and is available in a 5- to 8-mm diameter in 1-mm increments, the base curve of 8.0 mm, and the 200- to 400-µm thickness in 20 µm increments (Figure 18.1).[11] The front surface of the ring is convex, and the back is concave.

DOI: 10.1201/9781003371601-18

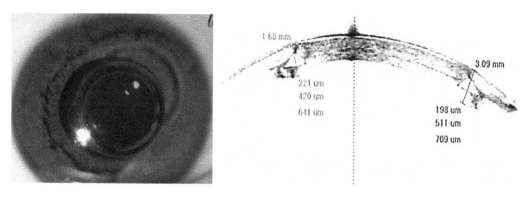

Figure 18.1 The appearance of the eye after MyoRing implantation (left), and anterior-segment OCT after surgery (right).

MyoRing parameters are calculated according to a nomogram, which considers the cornea's minimum thickness and the average keratometry value.[2,18]

Annular-Shaped Intracorneal Implant (AICI)

Annular-shaped intracorneal implant (AICI) is another complete 360-degree intrastromal ring with a rectangular-shaped profile (Figures 18.2 and 18.3).[12,19] This ICR comprises Hexafocon A, which has excellent oxygen permeability, with an estimated Dk value of around 100. The manufacturer of AICI has specified the external diameter, internal diameter, and base curve radius parameters to be 6 mm, 4 mm, and 7.4 mm, respectively. AICI is offered in four thicknesses: 140, 160, 180, and 200 microns. To ensure optimal results based on corneal topography features and refractive status, the manufacturer has established selection criteria for AICI (Table 18.1).

Mechanism of Action

Volumetric or Tomographic Action A concept for the action of the ICR is that the implantation of the ICR into the posterior lamellae results in localized thickening and bulging.[20] The ring protrudes more on the posterior surface than on the anterior surface due to its posterior implantation and the less compact nature of the deep lamellae than the superficial lamellae.[21]

Topographical Action The ICRs exert a pulling force on the cornea, which spaces the collagen fibers[22] and flattens the cornea.[23] This event is accompanied by an increase in peripheral corneal thickness, which is due to the addition of an external component on the periphery, and by an increased synthesis of collagen around the ring tunnel, allowing maximum curvature flattening.[20] The area around the ring forms a second zone of inflection of the ocular surface after that of the corneal limbus, which could be described as a corneal neo-limbus (the "arc shortening effect").[22] Moreover, the corneal ectasia, which is usually off-center, is shifted towards the center of this neo-limbus. This effect is even more pronounced on the posterior surface. The remodeling of the stromal thickness and the inflection of maximum curvature is reflected by the epithelial remodeling initially described by Reinstein (2001) on high-frequency ultrasound images; at the top of the implanted ICR, there is focal epithelial hypoplasia and epithelial hyperplasia in the areas juxtaposing the tunnel.[20] This observation is also visible in spectral domain–optical coherence tomography (SD–OCT).

The maximum curvature inflection is directly proportional to the thickness of the ICR and inversely proportional to its diameter.[24] The irregular arrangement of collagen fibers in KCN contributes to the uncertain outcomes of ICRs in a corneal flattening treatment. Additionally, the resulting impact on the cylinder is frequently less than the intended effect.[25,26] The flattening of the cone improves corneal asphericity (Q-index), which is considered one of the markers of visual quality. ICR induces a reduction in the anterior Q-index, which then approaches a more physiological value around −0.23 (over an optical zone of 4.5 mm),[27] reducing the excessive corneal prolaticity.[28–31] The modification of the asphericity is directly proportional to the thickness and the arc length of the ICR.[32]

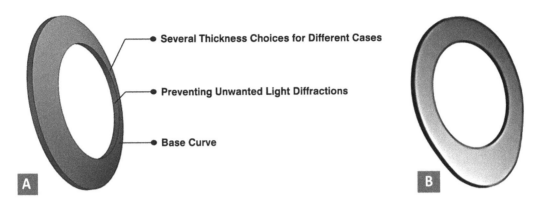

Figure 18.2 A: Symmetric annular intracorneal implant (AICI); Schematic view of different specifications. B: Schematic view of asymmetric AICI.

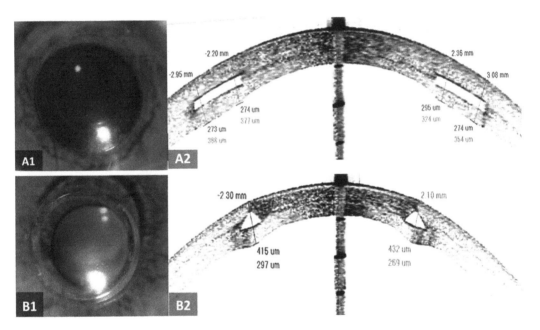

Figure 18.3 A comparison of annular intracorneal implant (AICI) and MyoRing into the stromal pocket; A: A1: Frontal view of an eye implanted with AICI. A2: Anterior-segment optical coherence tomography (AS-OCT) view of a cornea implanted with AICI. B: MyoRing; B1: Frontal view of an eye implanted with MyoRing. A2: AS-OCT view of a cornea implanted with MyoRing.

Refractive Action The refractive effects in corneal geometry by ICRs are multiple: the decrease in axial length and central corneal curvature reduces the spherical equivalent (defocus).[24,33] The amount of central flattening depends on the thickness of the ICR;[34]

the regularization of the asymmetry due to the ectasia allows the reduction of irregular astigmatism;[25]

the recentering of the ectasia on the visual axis limits the excess of high-order aberrations (HOAs), such as coma aberration and negative spherical aberration;[25,32]

the presence of transparent rings in the middle periphery of the cornea implies a redesign of the effective optical zone of the eye. It implies refractive effects at the edges of the ICRs, especially troublesome when they are small in diameter or interfere with an off-center or over-dilated pupil. The patient then perceives various degrees of light disturbances, possibly more disturbing for night driving.[35]

Table 18.1   Annular Intracorneal Implant (AICI) Ring Selection Criteria

Mean K-Reading	Cone Location	Spherical Equivalent	Ring
<48 D	Central and paracentral	<4 D, hyperopia	AICI 140
	Central and paracentral	<–2 D, myopia	Symmetric AICI 160
<48 D	Asymmetric	<–2 D, myopia	Asymmetric AICI 160
48–52 D	Central and paracentral	<–4 D, myopia	Symmetric AICI 180
48–52 D	Asymmetric	<–4 D, myopia	Asymmetric AICI 180
>52 D	Central and paracentral	<–6 to –8 D, myopia	Symmetric AICI 200
>52 D	Asymmetric	<–6 to –8 D, myopia	Asymmetric AICI 200

Biomechanical Action The ICRs cause a modest decrease in the depth of the anterior chamber due to the concentration of the tension of the lamellae in front of the ICRs, which is under the effect of the intraocular pressure.[36] Therefore, they redefine a biomechanical reinforcement zone and imply stress redistribution in the central zone.[36] This would have the virtue of limiting the progression of the KCN by reducing the stress localized at the top of the posterior surface of the ectasia. The biomechanical dimension is further illustrated by the slowly progressive nature of the effectiveness of the ICR over time.[37,38] Some authors have demonstrated functional and topographic improvements after more than 18 months of implantation.[39,40]

The refractive, topographical, aspherical, and aberrometric modifications induced by the ICR depend on the geometry of the keratoconus and the ring used. They are summarized in Table 18.2.

Indications, Contraindications, Preoperative Evaluation, and Prognostic Factors In order to ensure the success of intracorneal ring implantation, patient selection plays a crucial role.[41] A thorough clinical examination including biomicroscopy, measurement of visual acuity (corrected and uncorrected), corneal topography, and corneal pachymetry (in the form of a map) to assess thickness at the site of implantation, as well as aberrometry, must be performed.[7] To ensure the accuracy of corneal measurements, patients must abstain from wearing rigid gas-permeable contact lenses for a minimum of two weeks prior to ICR implantation surgery.

ICRs are proposed for patients over 18 years of age whose KCN is stable and who have poor visual acuity with spectacles and intolerance to contact lenses.[42] Pachymetry at ring insertion should be at least 400 µm. Most studies suggest that the best indication for implantation

Table 18.2   Specifications of the Most Commonly Used Intracorneal Ring Segments

Design	Keraring ± AS	Keraring SG	Intacs ± Sk	Ferrara	MyoRing
Manufacturer	Mediphacos (Belo Horizonte; Brazil)	Mediphacos (Belo Horizonte; Brazil)	Addition Technology (Sunnyvale, CA, USA)	Ferrara Ophtalmics (Belo Horizonte, Brazil)	Dioptex (Linz; Austria)
Arc length	Sl-5: 90, 120, 160, 210, 340° Sl-6: 90, 120, 150, 210, 340° AS: 160°	Sl-5: 160, 330°	Sl-5: 90. 130. 150°	Sl-5: 90, 120, 140, 150, 160, 180, 210, 320°	Sl-5: 360°
Profile	Prismatic	Double arch, curved	Hexagonal/ elliptical (Sk)	Triangular	Triangular
Thickness (µm)	150 to 350 µm (50 µm increments) AS: Variable clockwise or counterclockwise, 150 to 250 and 200 to 300 µm	NA Curvature between the two arches: 30. 35. 40 or 45D	Hexagonal/ elliptical (Sk) 210, 250 to 400 in 50 µm increments +500 (Sk)	150 to 350 50m steps	+77

AS: asymmetric; SI: optical zone; Sk: severe keratoconus; SG: second generation; NA: Not applicable

corresponds to stages II and III of the Amsler–Krumeich classification;[43,44] however, some studies increasingly extend the limit of maximum keratometry beyond 55 D.[45] It would seem that the results in patients with maximum keratometry of over 62 D are much less predictable.[46] Corrected pre-operative visual acuity of less than 0.6 on a decimal scale,[47,48] and alignment of the keratometric and refractive axes may be favorable prognostic factors.[26,49,50]

Manufacturers that produce ICRs have developed nomograms based on cohorts of treated patients.[10] These nomograms allow the surgeon to choose the most appropriate ring to correct the corneal ectasia. The disadvantage of nomograms is their empirical nature based on unpublished data and the absence of a mathematical model predicting their effect on the cornea. The interpretation of the topographic profiles from which the nomograms are derived is also subjective.[51]

The following factors should be considered systematically before a surgical procedure:

Subjective refractive sphere and cylinder as well as visual acuity

Mesopic pupillary diameter (if the selected ring diameter is 5 mm and the mesopic pupil has a diameter greater than 5 mm, the patient may present with post-operative halos)

Axis of the steepest meridian on an anterior sagittal topographic map

Type of KCN (defined by the anterior sagittal map and the posterior elevation map), such as nipple, bowtie, or crescent

Corneal asphericity (to determine the Q-index needed to bring the asphericity factor to almost normal values

Topographic astigmatism

Pachymetry at the incision and tunnel sites (to determine tunnel depth and maximum ring thickness).

KCN has three axes to be considered in the implantation procedure: the axis of the subjective clinical astigmatism, the axis of the coma, and the axis of the topographic steepest meridian. The latter is most often chosen as the incision axis.[10,28–30,45,49,52,53] However, the axis of the coma is generally unknown, and the axis of subjective clinical astigmatism is usually uncertain.

ICRs with a diameter of 5 mm are the most commonly used implant. Clinically, the smaller the diameter, the greater the flattening effect.[54] Some manufacturers use larger-diameter ICRs, especially when the KCN is in its early stages, the central cornea is not involved, and the central keratometry is less than 52 D.[18] There is a tendency to use a larger diameter ring when the mesopic pupillary diameter is greater than 5 mm to avoid disturbing halos and when the KCN is extended to the more peripheral areas (i.e., with an apex located more than 5 mm from the center).[18] Therefore, the segment thickness must be modified and increased when a 5-mm ICR is substituted for a 6-mm ICR.

The thickness of the implanted ICR is directly proportional to the degree of flattening effect desired.[32] In other words, if a greater flattening effect is desired, a thicker ring must be implanted. This correlation between ring thickness and its effect on keratometry and asphericity becomes less controlled in ring thicknesses of over 250 μm.[32,55,56] The ICR should not have a thickness that exceeds 50% of the total corneal thickness at the site where the segment is inserted. Otherwise, the risk of extrusion would be very high. Therefore, a ring should be chosen of lesser thickness and shorter arc length to allow the same effect, or with a diameter corresponding to a thicker corneal area.

The more advanced the stage of the KCN, the less predictable the effectiveness of the ICR.[53] In fact, a slightly opacified cornea, excessively deformed, thinned, and loose, will not respond favorably to the biomechanical demands of ICR. As a consequence, corneas with significant paracentral scarring, pronounced central astigmatism (greater than 5 D), thin central pachymetry (less than 350 μm), and high central simulated keratometry (SimKmax greater than 55 D) have a poorer prognosis.[57] Furthermore, the location of the ectasia defining the type of KCN also affects the prognosis. Centered forms (nipple cone) are more difficult to treat than decentered forms, which ICR can "recenter," or peripheral forms, which ICR can "exclude."

Histological, Refractive, Topographic, and Biomechanical Effects of Intracorneal Ring Implantation Surgery: Histological Reactions: The ICRs made of PMMA seem to have high long-term biocompatibility. However, some localized disorders of corneal metabolism have been described in front of the rings. These events have been expressed by the progressive accumulation of inert whitish deposits at the edges of the rings and by the reduction of the keratocyte density in front of and behind the rings.[58–60]

Refractive and Topographic Effects: Due to the wide variety of ectatic corneal disorders and the multiplicity of implantation methods, it is difficult to easily predict the efficacy of ICRs for a specific patient. However, several meta-analyses of the literature have identified trends in optimal outcomes.[61–64] The studies showed a decrease in spherical equivalent and keratometry that was relatively comparable and wasabout 4 ± 3 D. The reduction in astigmatism is less important and is found to be reduced by about 2 ± 2 D. The reduction of spherical and comatic aberrations had not been quantified because the rings compromise aberrometric measurements. However, the reduction of corneal asphericity (Q-index) or eccentricity and the decrease in the irregularity indices of the anterior surface is significant.[65,66] The progression of the KCN is usually halted, but a few studies ignored this point.[1,67,68] Compared with corrected visual acuity with spectacles, the improvement in uncorrected visual acuity with ICRs is limited, primarily attributed to the significant residual ametropia (approximately two logMAR lines). The quality of vision is also undoubtedly improved but is seldom evaluated.

Biomechanical Effects: The biomechanical effectiveness of ICRs was evaluated *in vivo* by the ocular response analyzer (ORA; Reichert, Buffalo, NY, USA).[23,38] No significant variation in biomechanical parameters was observed, but only changes in the profiles of the deformation curves.[18,23] However, this examination essentially analyzes the center of the cornea and may not "reflect" the changes induced by the ICR. The new interpretation software, which refines the analysis of the curves, could provide more relevant information.[36] Dynamic elastography technologies is also useful to learn more about the innermost mechanisms of ICR operation in the future.[69]

Surgical Technique: The surgical procedure is performed under topical anesthesia and does not require sutures.[50] The precision of the tunnel depth can be improved by utilizing the femtosecond laser (15% of the tunnels created manually are at the planned depth $\pm$ 10 μm, versus 67% with the femtosecond laser technique).[70] Although the implantation of the rings is now greatly facilitated by the use of femtosecond laser technology which allows the automated and secure creation of the tunnel and the opening incision,[7,45,52,53,68,70,71] several points are important for the success of the surgery:

verification of the suitability of the cutting parameters for the type of ICR chosen (depth, diameter, thickness of the tunnel, position of the incision)

the corneal marking of the patient's visual axis to find the centering of the laser incision when the cornea is flattened

the verification of the optimal depth of implantation (80%) on the tomographic maps and by ultrasound pachymetry at the point of implantation, supposed to be the finest on the path of the ring

the identification of the axis of the incision before the patient is positioned horizontally to prevent the natural cyclotorsion effect during the supine position and induced by the suction or involuntary rotation of the globe by the surgeon during the laser applanation

the insertion of the rings, respecting the epithelium as much as possible, and spacing the end of the segments sufficiently far from the incision zone.

In this surgery procedure, the center of the cornea will be marked before implanting the suction ring. The pressure, exerted during suction, flattens the cornea, which decenters inferotemporally and dilates the pupil, the center of which shifts nasally. These two factors contribute to decentering the treatment zone, which is more regularly observed when the cone is large.[72] Marking can be done with a slit lamp before installation or just before suctioning under the microscope in the supine position using a compass or the Purkinje reflex as a central point.[73]

Several parameters are to be programmed into the laser, depending on the ICR chosen. The incision axis is defined when choosing the ring. The manufacturer defines the optical zone and the internal and external diameters for each ICR but they can be modified by the surgeon according to their implantation scheme. The tunnel is made at a depth ranging from 70% to 80% of the total thickness of the cornea at the level of the thinnest point of the implantation zone. Highly superficial ICRs lead to more extrusion by anterior stromal compression and increased oxidative stress.[58,74] To comprehensively analyze corneal thickness at the tunnel level corresponding to the ring diameter, it is essential to perform a thorough corneal mapping of a 6- to 7-mm radius. This plan enables a complete assessment of the corneal thickness and facilitates accurate measurement of the tunnel depth. The energy delivered to create the tunnel depends on the laser used and is between 1.2 and 1.5 mJ.

At the end of the procedure, an anti-inflammatory and antibiotic eyedrop is administered to the cornea. An anti-inflammatory, antibiotic, and lubricant treatment is generally prescribed for 15 to 30 post-operative days. The patient is asked not to rub their eyes to avoid displacement of the ICR.

Combined Intracorneal Ring Implantation and Corneal Cross-Linking Procedures: ICRs do not slow the progression of KCN and should be applied to patients with non-progressive KCN. Corneal cross-linking (CXL) is the procedure that can halt the progression of KCN.[75,76] In recent years, scientists have been exploring various options for combined treatments to improve therapeutic outcomes and correct refractive anomalies in patients with corneal ectatic disorders. An example is a combination of ICR implantation and CXL.[77–81] This kind of combination not only has a therapeutic effect (improvement of biomechanical properties of the cornea) but also has corrective and refractive effects, allowing changes in the morphology of the cornea and flattening of its ectatic surface.[82–84]

This method is minimally invasive and effective in the treatment of corneal ectasia in the initial stages of the disease.[85] At the III–IV stages of KCN, CXL can be combined with the implantation of corneal segments, including MyoRing implants.[86] The combination of the two procedures (CXL plus) also allows for the implantation of progressive KCN.[87–91]

Previous research has suggested that combining CXL and ICR implantation might result in greater effectiveness than either procedure performed alone.[178790–95] Studies have also investigated the optimal treatment sequence for managing KCN through the following approaches: performing ICR before CXL in separate surgical sessions, ICR after CXL in separate surgical sessions, and simultaneous ICR and CXL in a single session. In a prospective comparative study, Coskunseven et al. found that conducting ICR (KeraRing) before CXL resulted in better outcomes than performing CXL before ICR.[87] The study involved two surgeries conducted at a mean interval of 7 months, followed by patient observation over a period averaging 13 months. The authors reported that patients who underwent CXL as their primary procedure had stiffer corneas compared with those who received CXL as a secondary intervention. This occasion could potentially lower the effectiveness of subsequent ICR implantations. Studies have also investigated the optimal treatment sequence for managing KCN through various approaches. Henriquez et al. found that performing CXL before ICR implantation (Ferrara) could reduce the rate of KCN progression.[96] In contrast, Legare et al. reported no significant difference in the progression of KCN between combined ICR (Intacs) and CXL versus CXL alone.[95] They hypothesized that the corneal biomechanical effects of the CXL technique could reduce the effectiveness of ICR. Simultaneous ICR and CXL may result in greater improvements due to the accumulation of vitamin B2 (riboflavin) in the corneal pockets created just before ICR implantation.[97] This could enhance the flattening effects of CXL and improve post-operative keratometric and refractive outcomes.[93,94] Hashemi et al. conducted a systematic review and meta-analysis on the procedure sequence in combined ICR and CXL and found that concurrent ICR and CXL resulted in superior keratometric outcomes to those from a sequential order.[93] Gouvea et al. reported that, whereas the combined ICR and CXL method had greater effects than standalone treatments, both ICR implantation alone and combined ICR and CXL, in any form, simultaneous or sequential, were successful in treating KCN patients who could not tolerate contact lenses.[98]

Clinical Post-Operative Outcomes: Numerous studies have evaluated the post-operative outcomes in patients who underwent ICR implantation with complete 360-degree rings. Daxer reported the results of a three-year follow-up of 22 patients (26 eyes) aged from 18 to 46 years who had KCN at stages I–IV according to the Amsler–Krumeich classification at the Congress of the European Society of Cataract and Refractive Surgeons in Milan (September 2012).[99] All patients had MyoRing implanted into the corneal pocket using the PocketMaker microkeratome. Post-operative follow-up was between 6 and 38 months. Patients were divided into three groups according to the mean value of keratometry (mean-K): Group 1 consisted of seven eyes with mean-K of 60 D or more, Group 2 consisted of ten eyes with mean-K from 50 to 59.99 D, while Group 3 consisted of nine eyes with mean-K less than 50 D. In 20 eyes, the cone apex was located inferiorly, and in six eyes, the cone was central. During three years of observation, the most significant results were seen in Group 1 with the mean-K of 60 D or more, with the value decreasing by 13.2 D. Groups 2 and 3 showed a reduction in mean-K of 5.1 and 3.1 D, respectively. In the post-operative period, all patients noticed a subjective improvement in their vision. The mean value of the best-corrected distance visual acuity (CDVA) in all groups showed different degrees of improvement: in the 1st group, by three lines; in the 2nd group, by 4,6 lines; and in the 3rd group, by 1,6 lines. However, refractive and visual stabilization occurred only by the 3rd to 4th month after surgery and persisted throughout the entire follow-up period. There were no intra- or post-operative complications. One MyoRing implant was removed at the patient's request due to insufficient improvement in uncorrected distance visual acuity (UDVA). One MyoRing implant was also removed due to patient complaints of glare and night vision problems.[99,100] Daxer et al. also conducted clinical studies of 15 eyes in 11 patients with KCN of stages I–IV according to Amsler–Krumeich classification.[16] The age of the patients was 22–66 years. The follow-up period was one year. All patients underwent intrastromal implantation of MyoRing using a PocketMaker microkeratome. A nomogram was used to calculate the size of MyoRing: mean-K less than 49.00 D: MyoRing 5/240; mean-K between 49.00 and 55.00 D: MyoRing 5/280; mean-K over 55.00 D: MyoRing 5/280 plus CXL. One month after surgery, the UDVA increased from 0.07 to 0.32, and after three months increased further to 0.56. Refractive and visual stabilization from months 3 to 12 remained unchanged. The value of the CDVA increased gradually over one year from 0.42 to 0.77. The mean-K value decreased from 48.96 to 43.20 D. The mean value of the spherical component changed from -5.13 ± 4.34 to $+0.1 \pm 3.2$ D, and of the cylindrical component from -3.50 ± 1.20 to -1.27 ± 0.75 D. There were no intra-operative complications. A diffuse corneal haze appeared in one eye the next day after MyoRing ring implantation combined with CXL but disappeared one month later as a result of standard post-operative therapy. Ring repositioning was performed in two eyes not included in the statistical analysis. Both rings were displaced to the zone of maximum corneal ectasia. Among side effects, the author observed glare and night vision problems in two cases, which he attributed to the smaller diameter of the MyoRing compared to the pupil diameter in mesopic conditions. This observation occurred mainly with a ring diameter of 5 mm. Daxer believed that this method provides an individual approach to each patient with KCN, as it allows changing all three parameters of the ring: diameter, height, and position.[99] In a short-term study by Khorrami-Nejad et al., significant improvement was observed in visual acuity, refractive error, and keratometry outcomes six months after MyoRing implantation surgery.[2] The authors concluded that the treatment was a secure and effective method for treating and stabilizing progressive KCN. In a prospective interventional study on 25 KCN patients, Hosny et al. compared preoperative values to four-week post-operative outcomes of complete and segmental ICRs (MyoRing versus KeraRing), both implanted using a femtosecond laser-assisted procedure.[101] According to the study, the two treatment methods yielded comparable results in terms of visual, refractive, and topographic outcomes, with the exception of Kmax, which was significantly reduced in the MyoRing group compared to the KeraRing group. The authors concluded that both treatment approaches were effective in improving visual acuity and corneal parameters in KCN patients. However, complete rings, such as MyoRing, may have a greater impact on reducing the anterior corneal curvature. Mohammadpour and colleagues conducted a cohort study wherein they observed significant alterations in the long-term post-operative visual, refractive, and corneal topographic data following the MyoRing implantation.[17]

In terms of AICI, Salamatrad et al. found that the implantation of AICI into rabbit eyes did not result in any changes in the density of corneal keratocytes compared with a control group.[14] Meanwhile, Jabbarvand et al. conducted the first human study on 34 KCN patients treated with AICI and observed significant improvements in visual functions and a reduction in the anterior surface of the cornea one year after implantation.[12] However, the long-term effects of combining AICI and A-CXL on visual, refractive, and tomographic measurements have yet to be investigated. Jabbarvand et al. conducted another study to assess the effectiveness and safety of AICI implantation in 95 patients with KCN.[13] The study compared the visual, refractive, aberrometric, and topographic outcomes of the patients before and one year after surgery. The results showed significant improvements in all parameters and the safety and efficacy indices of 1.8 and 1, respectively. These findings indicated 100% safety and 45% efficacy rates for the AICI implantation procedure.

Some studies suggested that thicker ring implants are more effective in flattening the cornea.[24] Given that MyoRing has a thicker profile (200–320 µm) than AICI (140–200 µm), it is expected to perform more effectively in patients with KCN. However, this effect may be influenced by other factors such as diameter, profile design, and degree of flexibility.[38] In practice, these factors balance the impact of both lenses on the corneal tissue, resulting in similar outcomes for corneas with KCN. Therefore, considering this compensational effect, AICI, which is available in thinner profiles, may be more appropriate for advanced cases of KCN, where the patients have thin corneas. Furthermore, a comparison of the aberrometric findings of the two ICRs showed that AICI resulted in lower higher-order aberration and spherical aberration values than MyoRing, which could be attributed to the difference in the cross-section design of the two ICRs (a rectangular shape for AICI compared with a trapezoidal shape for MyoRing), although this difference was not statistically significant.[78,102]

Creating stromal pockets during ICR can be done using a mechanical method or a femtosecond laser-assisted procedure. It is shown that using a femtosecond laser in the formation of the tunnel for corneal segments implantation leads to the improvement of biomechanical properties of the cornea, activation of reparative processes, and stromal thickening.[52,103,104] This technique is effective, safe, and predictable; however, it is used mainly to stabilize I–III stages of KCN and is limited by corneal thickness at the location of segment implantation.[105] According to Daxer, the major advantage of this technique, in comparison with other methods of KCN treatment, is the preservation of corneal biomechanical properties.[11,16] Corneal biomechanical stability characterizes the ability to resist the difference of forces between external and intraocular pressure. These forces generate tension within the cornea, and the stress lines tend to run along the orientation of the collagen fibrils. The PocketMaker microkeratome technology allows the formation of a pocket parallel to the collagen fibrils, thereby not disturbing the biomechanical properties of the cornea.[15,106]

Studies published before 2010 utilized mechanical methods for pocket creation, which were reported to have some intra- and post-operative complications, such as corneal epithelial damage, corneal perforation, and ICR dislocations.[107] Carrasquillo et al. conducted an early study comparing the effectiveness of femtosecond laser-assisted and mechanical procedures on post-operative outcomes 10.3 months after ICR implantation.[103] They reported that both methods were safe and had similar effects on post-operative outcomes. Subsequent studies conducted by Coskunseven et al.[62] and Ertan et al.[63] also reported similar conclusions regarding the safety and effectiveness of femtosecond laser-assisted pocket creation in KCN patients. Further studies have also shown that femtosecond laser-assisted procedures are safe and can improve post-operative outcomes due to their great precision in creating stromal channels.[108] Although minor complications have been reported, the incidence rate of sight-threatening complications is relatively insignificant.[108]

Comparison with Other Intracorneal Rings: There are some studies comparing the surgical outcomes of complete 360-degree ICRs versus segmental ICRs. For example, Janani et al. conducted a systematic review and meta-analysis evaluating the efficacy of a full-ring 360-degree implant (MyoRing) in treating KCN and found that complete ring implantation outperformed segmental ICRs one year after implantation.[109] In another study comparing segmented and complete 360-degree ICRs, Saleem investigated the efficacy and safety differences between KeraRing and MyoRing combined with CXL.[78] The author found that patients treated with MyoRing plus CXL experienced less myopia, while patients treated with KeraRing plus CXL had fewer astigmatic refractions six months after surgery. Similarly, previous reports had shown improvements in UDVA, CDVA, and refractive errors using complete 360-degree ICRs.[2,17,110] According to systematic reviews by Janani et al.[109] and Izquierdo Jr.,[111] MyoRing implantation is the most effective method for improving refractive, visual, and corneal curvature in patients with KCN. Complete ICR implants like MyoRing are more effective than incomplete ring segments in controlling KCN progression due to two mechanisms – corneal biomechanics and surgeon freedom.[11,38,112] Daxer et al. proposed the theory that the 360-degree design of a complete ring ICR acts as a second limbus, providing additional support to corneal biomechanical properties and strengthening its circumferences.[38] They also hypothesized that 360-degree ICRs provide three degrees of freedom for the surgeon, including implant thickness, diameter, and position, while segmental ICR implants only provide ring thickness as the sole degree of freedom.[11] Even minor misalignments of a segmented ICR could significantly reduce post-operative visual functions.[112] Similar to MyoRing's complete 360-degree ring, the visual and topographical improvement in KCN patients treated with AICI can also be attributed to biomechanical balance formation and relatively equal force distribution within the cornea.[109]

Complications, Adverse Effects, and Limitations

There are some complications, but rarely serious, due to the reversible and minimally invasive nature of ICR implantation surgery.[113] The overall complication rate is 5.7% (study of 850 operated eyes).[114] Intra-operatively, incomplete tunnel formation by the femtosecond laser (2.6%) or incomplete corneal incision (0.6%) requires manual completion of the tunnel, with a tunnel dissector or a surgical knife, for the incision.[114] Endothelial perforation (0.6%), characterized by the formation of an air bubble in the anterior chamber, requires discontinuation of the surgery. Loss of suction (0.1%) requires the same landmarks to be taken, and the procedure can be repeated immediately. Post-operatively, medical complications would be about 2.6%.[115] Displacement of the ICR (0.6%) can be corrected with a 10/0 monofilament suture.[114] Extrusion of the ICR is uncommon. It is accompanied by necrosis and neovascularization of limbal call localized around the incision. It is caused by inadequate incision, poor tunnel sizing, incisional damage, ocular rubbing, or excessively shallow implantation. Secondary migration and overlapping of the rings have also been documented.[116] When extrusion occurs, ring removal is necessary.[117] Generally, implantation at the correct depth avoids this complication. The excessive superficial placement of the ICR mainly causes stromal melting and corneal perforation (0.2%). In this case, ring removal is also necessary.[118] Perforation during implantation has become quite rare with the use of the femtosecond laser. Corneal edema (0.1%) occurs most often at the site of the ring incision. Infection in the tunnel is always possible and is potentially serious since it can lead to infectious uveitis and endophthalmitis.[114,119,120] Corneal neovascularization at the incision site may occur if the incision is made at midday in patients with a long history of contact lens wear, an allergic background, with pre-existing limbal vessels, or if the tunnel is excessively shallow.[121] Deposits in the tunnel may cause halos or stromal haze. They may resolve spontaneously.[122]

The occurrence of photophobia and decreased night vision have also frequently been noted in patients who were implanted with ICR.[18,110,123] The most frequent reason for this side effect is the reflection of light at the edges of the rings when the pupil interferes with their light transmission.[115] These phenomena represent 14% of the cases of ring removal.[118] Different ICR profiles (octagonal, triangular, or oval) or ICR coloring (yellow filter) do not seem to clearly alter the rate of glare perception reported by patients in scotopic conditions.[114] In contrast, the reduction in ICR diameter seems to correlate more significantly with the extent of functional impairment.

Over- or under-correction represent 23% of the total causes of ring removal, typically due to a bad implantation procedure or an implantation error (such as a ring implanted in the inferior nasal region).[118] In cases of over- or under-correction, to avoid ring removal, it is possible to perform complementary procedures if the pachymetry allows it (such as topo-guided or spherocylindrical PRK) or a lens prescription, if tolerated.[115]

Notably, the only limitation of MyoRing or AICI is pupil size. To prevent optical aberrations and night vision problems, implanting the MyoRing with a diameter no smaller than the pupil diameter under mesopic conditions is recommended.

CONCLUSION

ICRs have proven their effectiveness in the visual rehabilitation of KCN by improving the shape of the cornea and reducing refractive errors while having a low risk/benefit ratio. They are constantly being developed to enable an increasing number of KCN patients to be implanted. When indicated, combining procedures such as ICR implantation plus CXL allows further improvement of refractive and topographic parameters.

The choice of the different rings meets several rational criteria but suffers from uncertainty due to the lack of information on the biomechanical properties of every cornea and the multiplicity of cases encountered. Thus, several approaches generally tend to be possible for the same patient. Finally, implementing ICR for the management of KCN is currently considered part of a global corneoplastic approach combining different potentially synergistic and sequential technologies.

CXL COMBINED WITH COMPLETE RING

Several studies have reported CXL combined with complete (360°) intracorneal ring implantation. As shown in Table 18.3, to investigate the outcomes of same-day CXL surgery after MyoRing implantation, Studeny et al. have reported UDVA, CDVA, mean-K, sphere, cylinder, and SE improvements following surgery.[124] Mohammadpour et al. (2016, 2020, 2021) and Bikbova et al. (2018) have evaluated this combination simultaneously.[17,84,97,125] All studies have demonstrated improvements in refractive and keratometric values. Mohammadpour et al. and Bikbova et al. have divided patients into two groups: ICR or MyoRing implantation alone and in combination with CXL.[17,84] The improvements were better in the second group in the Mohammadpour et al. studies. In 2016, Nobari et al. compared the outcomes of MyoRing implantation after CXL and MyoRing implantation alone.[126] They have reported that most of the parameters improved similarly in both groups, such as UDVA, spherical equivalent, refractive astigmatism, and mean keratometric values, although there was greater improvement of CDVA in the MyoRing alone group than in the other one.

Another study μm was carried out by Emin et al. (2017) on 39 progressive (grade II–III) KCN. Patients had MyoRing implantation combined with CXL. At the 36-month follow-up, significant increases in UDVA and CDVA and a decrease in keratometry (mean reduction 9.43 D), SE (from 9.43 D to 6.25 D), and corneal thickness (from 426.93 ± 46.58 μm to 401.24 ± 39.12 μm) were

Table 18.3   Summary of Results for CXL Combined with Complete (360°) Intracorneal Ring Implantation

Reference	Sample Size	Follow-Up Period	Additional Explanation(s)	Outcome(s)
			Sequence: Complete Intraorneal Ring Implantation before CXL	
Studeny et al. (2014)[124]	22	12 months (1, 3, 6, 12, and 24 months)	Clinical results after same-day MyoRing implantation and CXL in an intrastromal pocket (CXL after MyoRing)	Increase in UDVA (6 lines) and CDVA (2.5 lines) Decrease in mean-K, sphere, cylinder, and spherical equivalents
			Sequence: Simultaneous Complete Intraorneal Ring Implantation and CXL	
Mohammadpour et al. (2016)[125]	A 23-year-old female	2 years	Progressive KCN A novel surgical technique Femtosecond laser-assisted MyoRing implantation and accelerated CXL with dextran and free riboflavin	Cornea was clear Decrease in central keratometry Increase in UDVA and CDVA
Bikbova et al. (2018)[128]	80	12, 24, and 36 months	Progressive KCN stage II–III according to Amsler–Krumeich classification Two groups: Group 1: MyoRing implantation alone (41) Group 2: MyoRing implantation combined with CXL (39) (In three patients: MyoRing was implanted 2 days after surgery)	Increase in UDVA, and CDVA (better improvements after 12 months in the first group, but no difference after 36 months between groups) Decrease in mean keratometry (to 8.45 D vs 9.43 D), spherical equivalent (to 7.72 D vs 6.25 D), cylinder (to 3.33 D vs 3.31 D) in first and second group, respectively Nearly unchanged corneal thickness
Mohammadpour et al. (2020)[79]	60	10 months	Progressive KCN, contact lens intolerance, and CCT > 380 μm Two groups: Group 1: MyoRing alone (28) Group 2: femtosecond laser-assisted MyoRing implantation with CXL simultaneously (19) 47 eyes available at the end of the study	Increase in UDVA and CDVA (no significant difference between groups at 10 months) Decrease in SE from −6.51 ± 3 to −1.80 ± 2 in the first group after 10 months and from −6.63 ± 2.5 to −1.7 ± 2 in the second group. Significant decrease in K_{max} (in the second group) and mean-Km (in both groups) Decrease in mean RMS (0.55 μm) and horizontal coma in the second group (significantly lower than in first group) Increase in mean RMS in the first group (0.95 μm), mean RMS HOA in the first (0.71 μm) and second (0.01 μm) group. No complications post-operatively
Mohammadpour et al. (2021)[17]	35	5 years	Progressive KCN Two groups: First group (14 eyes): ICR implantation only Second group (21 eyes): 360-degrees ICR implantation combined with CXL	Increase in UDVA, CDVA after implantation of ICR (more marked in the second group) Decrease in flat-K, steep K, mean-K and astigmatism Better results of tomographic and biomechanical index in patients of the second group

(Continued)

Table 18.3 (Continued) Summary of Results for CXL Combined with Complete (360°) Intracorneal Ring Implantation

Reference	Sample Size	Follow-Up Period	Additional Explanation(s)	Outcome(s)
			Sequence: Complete Intracorneal Ring Implantation after CXL	
Nobari et al. (2016)[126]	33	1 year	A retrospective study Keratoconus stages II and III according to the Amsler–Krumeich classification Two groups: Group 1: CXL-MyoRing (MyoRing 12 months after CXL) Group 2: MyoRing alone	Increase in UDVA and CDVA in both groups (no significant difference between groups of UDVA, although greater improvement of CDVA in group 2 than 1) Decrease in spherical equivalent error, refractive astigmatism, and mean keratometric values in both groups (with no significant difference between groups)

ICR: Intracorneal rings, CXL: Corneal cross-linking, CDVA: Best-corrected distance visual acuity in the LogMar system, UDVA: Uncorrected distance visual acuity in the LogMar system, KCN: Keratoconus, flat-K: flat keratometry, steep-K: steep keratometry, mean-K: mean keratometry, RMS: root mean square, D: diopter.

observed. The authors determined that, in addition to being effective for KCN treatment, the combination of CXL and MyoRing implantation delayed the progress of the disease.[127]

In addition, another recent article, by Mohammadpour et al. (2020),[79] again divided patients into two groups of MyoRing and MyoRing + CXL and evaluated the effectiveness of femtosecond laser-assisted MyoRing implantation combined with CXL. According to the results, this combination is a safe and efficacious procedure for KCN treatment and the results were generally better in the MyoRing + CXL group. In contrast, horizontal coma was notably lower in this group than in the other.

Moreover, there are several studies that have assessed the proper combination of these surgeries; in the following, the most popular ones are presented.

Table 18.3 is a summary of recently published results for CXL combined with complete (360°) intracorneal ring implantation.

REFERENCES

1. Alió JL, Shabayek MH, Artola A. Intracorneal ring segments for keratoconus correction: long-term follow-up. *Journal of Cataract & Refractive Surgery.* 2006;32(6):978–85.

2. Khorrami-Nejad M, Aghili O, Hashemian H, Aghazadeh-Amiri M, Karimi F. Changes in corneal asphericity after MyoRing implantation in moderate and severe keratoconus. *Journal of Ophthalmic & Vision Research.* 2019;14(4):428.

3. Cochener B, Savary-LeFloch G, Colin J. Effect of intrastromal corneal ring segment shift on clinical outcome: one year results for low myopia. *Journal of Cataract & Refractive Surgery.* 2000;26(7):978–86.

4. Naderi M, Karimi F, Jadidi K, Mosavi SA, Ghobadi M, Tireh H, et al. Long-term results of MyoRing implantation in patients with keratoconus. *Clinical and Experimental Optometry.* 2021;104(4):499–504.

5. Khosravi B, Khorrami-Nejad M, Rajabi S, Amiri M, Hashemian H, Khodaparast M. Characteristics of astigmatism after myoring implantation. *Medical Hypothesis, Discovery and Innovation in Ophthalmology.* 2017;6(4):130.

6. Fleming JF, Reynolds A, Kilmer L, Burris TE, Abbott RL, Schanzlin DJ. *The intrastromal corneal ring: two cases in rabbits.* SLACK Incorporated Thorofare, NJ; 1987. p. 227–32.

7. Colin J, Cochener B, Savary G, Malet F. Correcting keratoconus with intracorneal rings. *Journal of Cataract & Refractive Surgery.* 2000;26(8):1117–22.

8. Fleming JF, Lovisolo CF. *Intrastromal corneal ring segments in a patient with previous laser in situ keratomileusis.* Slack Incorporated Thorofare, NJ; 2000. p. 365–7.

9. Burris TE. Intrastromal corneal ring technology: results and indications. *Current Opinion in Ophthalmology.* 1998;9(4):9–14.

10. Giacomin NT, Mello GR, Medeiros CS, Kiliç A, Serpe CC, Almeida HG, et al. Intracorneal ring segments implantation for corneal ectasia. *Journal of Refractive Surgery.* 2016;32(12):829–39.

11. Daxer A. Adjustable intracorneal ring in a lamellar pocket for keratoconus. *Journal of Refractive Surgery.* 2010;26(3):217–21.

12. Jabbarvand M, Khodaparast M, Jamali A, Ahmadzadeh H, Bordbar S. Changes in the optical corneal densitometry, visual acuity, and refractive error after the annular intracorneal inlay implantation. *Journal of Current Ophthalmology.* 2021;33(1):23.

13. Jabbarvand M, Ahmadzadeh H, Khodaparast M, Jamali A, Aghamirsalim M. Clinical outcomes of a new type of continuous intrastromal corneal ring for treatment of keratoconus. *Cornea*. 2021.

14. Salamatrad A, Jabbarvand M, Hashemian H, Khodaparast M, Askarizadeh F. Histological and confocal changes in rabbit cornea produced by an intrastromal inlay made of hexafocon A. *Cornea*. 2015;34(1):78–81.

15. Daxer A, Fratzl P. Collagen fibril orientation in the human corneal stroma and its implication in keratoconus. *Investigative Ophthalmology and Visual Science*. 1997;38(1):121–9.

16. Daxer A, Mahmoud H, Venkateswaran RS. Intracorneal continuous ring implantation for keratoconus: one-year follow-up. *Journal of Cataract & Refractive Surgery*. 2010;36(8):1296–302.

17. Mohammadpour M, Khoshtinat N, Khorrami-Nejad M. Comparison of visual, tomographic, and biomechanical outcomes of 360 degrees intracorneal ring implantation with and without corneal crosslinking for progressive keratoconus: a 5-year follow-up. *Cornea*. 2021;40(3):303–10.

18. Alio JL, Piñero DP, Daxer A. Clinical outcomes after complete ring implantation in corneal ectasia using the femtosecond technology: a pilot study. *Ophthalmology*. 2011;118(7):1282–90.

19. Mohammadpour M, Heirani M, Khoshtinat N, Khorrami-Nejad M. Comparison of two different 360-degree intrastromal corneal rings combined with simultaneous accelerated-corneal cross-linking. *European Journal of Ophthalmology*. 2023:11206721231171420.

20. Reinstein DZ, Srivannaboon S, Holland SP. *Epithelial and stromal changes induced by intacs examined by three-dimensional very high-frequency digital ultrasound*. Slack Incorporated Thorofare, NJ; 2001. p. 310–8.

21. Lai MM, Tang M, Andrade EM, Li Y, Khurana RN, Song JC, et al. Optical coherence tomography to assess intrastromal corneal ring segment depth in keratoconic eyes. *Journal of Cataract & Refractive Surgery*. 2006;32(11):1860–5.

22. Silvestrini T. A geometric model to predict the change in corneal curvature from the intrastromal corneal ring (ICR). *Invest Ophthalmol & Vis Sci*. 1994;35(4):S309.

23. Dauwe C, Touboul D, Roberts CJ, Mahmoud AM, Kérautret J, Fournier P, et al. Biomechanical and morphological corneal response to placement of intrastromal corneal ring segments for keratoconus. *Journal of Cataract & Refractive Surgery*. 2009;35(10):1761–7.

24. Burris TE, Baker PC, Ayer CT, Loomas BE, Mathis ML, Silvestrini TA. Flattening of central corneal curvature with intrastromal corneal rings of increasing thickness: an eye-bank eye study. *Journal of Cataract & Refractive Surgery*. 1993;19:182–7.

25. Piñero DP, Alió JL, Teus MA, Barraquer RI, Michael R, Jiménez R. Modification and refinement of astigmatism in keratoconic eyes with intrastromal corneal ring segments. *Journal of Cataract & Refractive Surgery*. 2010;36(9):1562–72.

26. Alfonso JF, Lisa C, Merayo-Lloves J, Cueto LF-V, Montés-Micó R. Intrastromal corneal ring segment implantation in paracentral keratoconus with coincident topographic and coma axis. *Journal of Cataract & Refractive Surgery*. 2012;38(9):1576–82.

27. Holmes-Higgin DK, Baker PC, Burris TE, Silvestrini TA. *Characterization of the aspheric corneal surface with intrastromal corneal ring segments*. Slack Incorporated Thorofare, NJ; 1999. p. 520–8.

28. Ferrara G, Torquetti L, Ferrara P, Merayo-Lloves J. Intrastromal corneal ring segments: visual outcomes from a large case series. *Clinical & Experimental Ophthalmology*. 2012;40(5):433–9.

29. Torquetti L, Cunha P, Luz A, Kwitko S, Carrion M, Rocha G, et al. Clinical outcomes after implantation of 320-arc length intrastromal corneal ring segments in keratoconus. *Cornea*. 2018;37(10):1299–305.

30. Lisa C, Cueto LF-V, Poo-López A, Madrid-Costa D, Alfonso JF. Long-term follow-up of intrastromal corneal ring segments (210-degree arc length) in central keratoconus with high corneal asphericity. *Cornea*. 2017;36(11):1325–30.

31. Sandes J, Stival LR, de Ávila MP, Ferrara P, Ferrara G, Magacho L, et al. Clinical outcomes after implantation of a new intrastromal corneal ring with 140-degree of arc in patients with corneal ectasia. *International Journal of Ophthalmology*. 2018;11(5):802.

32. Torquetti L, Ferrara P. Corneal asphericity changes after implantation of intrastromal corneal ring segments in keratoconus. *Journal of Emmetropia: Journal of Cataract, Refractive and Corneal Surgery*. 2010;1(4):178–81.

33. Schanzlin DJ, Asbell PA, Burris TE, Durrie DS. The intrastromal corneal ring segments: phase ii results far the correction of myopia. *Ophthalmology*. 1997;104(7):1067–78.

34. Asbell PA, Uçakhan ÖÖ, Durrie DS, Lindstrom RL. *Adjustability of refractive effect for corneal ring segments. Journal of Refractive Surgery*. 1999;15(6):627–31.

35. Schanzlin DJ. Studies of intrastromal corneal ring segments for the correction of low to moderate myopic refractive errors. *Transactions of the American Ophthalmological Society*. 1999;97:815.

36. Vinciguerra R, Fernández-Vega-Cueto L, Poo-Lopez A, Eliasy A, Merayo-Lloves J, Elsheikh A, et al. The effect of intracorneal ring segments implantation for keratoconus on in vivo corneal biomechanics assessed with the Corvis ST. *Journal of Refractive Surgery*. 2022;38(4):264–9.

37. Pinero DP, Alio JL, Barraquer RI, Michael R. Corneal biomechanical changes after intracorneal ring segment implantation in keratoconus. *Cornea*. 2012;31(5):491–9.

38. Daxer A. Biomechanics of corneal ring implants. *Cornea*. 2015;34(11):1493.

39. Torquetti L, Berbel RF, Ferrara P. Long-term follow-up of intrastromal corneal ring segments in keratoconus. *Journal of Cataract & Refractive Surgery*. 2009;35(10):1768–73.

40. Villanueva JLG, Palau MM, Salinas C, Amat DE, Castellón OG, Manero F. Four-year follow-up of intrastraomal corneal ring segments in patients with keratoconus. *Journal of Emmetropia: Journal of Cataract, Refractive and Corneal Surgery*. 2010;1(1):9–15.

41. Sakellaris D, Balidis M, Gorou O, Szentmary N, Alexoudis A, Grieshaber MC, et al. Intracorneal ring segment implantation in the management of keratoconus: an evidence-based approach. *Ophthalmology and Therapy*. 2019;8:5–14.

42. Al-Tuwairqi WS, Osuagwu UL, Razzouk H, AlHarbi A, Ogbuehi KC. Clinical evaluation of two types of intracorneal ring segments (ICRS) for keratoconus. *International Ophthalmology*. 2017;37:1185–98.

43. Rabinowitz YS. INTACS for keratoconus and ectasia after LASIK. *International Ophthalmology Clinics*. 2013;53(1):27.

44. Gauthier A, Friot M, Montard R, Saleh M, Delbosc B. Femtosecond-assisted Ferrara intrastromal corneal ring implantation for treatment of keratoconus: functional outcomes at one year. *Journal Francais D'ophtalmologie*. 2016;39(5):428–36.

45. Fahd DC, Alameddine RM, Nasser M, Awwad ST. Refractive and topographic effects of single-segment intrastromal corneal ring segments in eyes with moderate to severe keratoconus and inferior cones. *Journal of Cataract & Refractive Surgery.* 2015;41(7):1434–40.

46. Zare MA, Mehrjardi HZ, Afarideh M, Bahrmandy H, Mohammadi S-F. Visual, keratometric and corneal biomechanical changes after intacs SK implantation for moderate to severe keratoconus. *Journal of Ophthalmic & Vision Research.* 2016;11(1):17.

47. Vega-Estrada A, Alio JL, Brenner LF, Javaloy J, Puche ABP, Barraquer RI, et al. Outcome analysis of intracorneal ring segments for the treatment of keratoconus based on visual, refractive, and aberrometric impairment. *American Journal of Ophthalmology.* 2013;155(3):575–84.e1.

48. Guyot C, Libeau L, Vabres B, Weber M, Lebranchu P, Orignac I. Refractive outcome and prognostic factors for success of intracorneal ring segment implantation in keratoconus: a retrospective study of 75 eyes. *Journal Francais D'ophtalmologie.* 2019;42(2):118–26.

49. Peña-García P, Alió JL, Vega-Estrada A, Barraquer RI. Internal, corneal, and refractive astigmatism as prognostic factors for intrastromal corneal ring segment implantation in mild to moderate keratoconus. *Journal of Cataract & Refractive Surgery.* 2014;40(10):1633–44.

50. Vega-Estrada A, Alio JL. The use of intracorneal ring segments in keratoconus. *Eye and Vision.* 2016;3:1–7.

51. Piñero DP, Alio JL. Intracorneal ring segments in ectatic corneal disease–a review. *Clinical & Experimental Ophthalmology.* 2010;38(2):154–67.

52. Piñero DP, Alio JL, El Kady B, Coskunseven E, Morbelli H, Uceda-Montanes A, et al. Refractive and aberrometric outcomes of intracorneal ring segments for keratoconus: mechanical versus femtosecond-assisted procedures. *Ophthalmology.* 2009;116(9):1675–87.

53. Zare MA, Hashemi H, Salari MR. Intracorneal ring segment implantation for the management of keratoconus: safety and efficacy. *Journal of Cataract & Refractive Surgery.* 2007;33(11):1886–91.

54. Jabbarvand M, SalamatRad A, Hashemian H, Mazloumi M, Khodaparast M. Continuous intracorneal ring implantation for keratoconus using a femtosecond laser. *Journal of Cataract & Refractive Surgery.* 2013;39(7):1081–7.

55. Ferrara P, Torquetti L. Clinical outcomes after implantation of a new intrastromal corneal ring with a 210-degree arc length. *Journal of Cataract & Refractive Surgery.* 2009;35(9):1604–8.

56. Lyra D, Ribeiro G, Torquetti L, Ferrara P, Machado A, Lyra JM. Computational models for optimization of the intrastromal corneal ring choice in patients with keratoconus using corneal tomography data. *Journal of Refractive Surgery.* 2018;34(8):547–50.

57. Alió JL, Shabayek MH, Belda JI, Correas P, Feijoo ED. Analysis of results related to good and bad outcomes of Intacs implantation for keratoconus correction. *Journal of Cataract & Refractive Surgery.* 2006;32(5):756–61.

58. Ruckhofer J, Böhnke M, Alzner E, Grabner G. Confocal microscopy after implantation of intrastromal corneal ring segments. *Ophthalmology.* 2000;107(12):2144–51.

59. Ly LT, McCulley JP, Verity SM, Cavanagh HD, Bowman RW, Petroll WM. Evaluation of intrastromal lipid deposits after intacs implantation using in vivo confocal microscopy. *Eye & Contact Lens.* 2006;32(4):211–5.

60. Samimi S, Leger F, Touboul D, Colin J. Histopathological findings after intracorneal ring segment implantation in keratoconic human corneas. *Journal of Cataract & Refractive Surgery*. 2007;33(2):247–53.

61. Ertan A, Kamburoğlu G, Bahadır M. Intacs insertion with the femtosecond laser for the management of keratoconus: one-year results. *Journal of Cataract & Refractive Surgery*. 2006;32(12):2039–42.

62. Coskunseven E, Kymionis GD, Tsiklis NS, Atun S, Arslan E, Jankov MR, et al. One-year results of intrastromal corneal ring segment implantation (KeraRing) using femtosecond laser in patients with keratoconus. *American Journal of Ophthalmology*. 2008;145(5):775–9.e1.

63. Ertan A, Kamburoğlu G. Intacs implantation using a femtosecond laser for management of keratoconus: comparison of 306 cases in different stages. *Journal of Cataract & Refractive Surgery*. 2008;34(9):1521–6.

64. Colin J. European clinical evaluation: use of Intacs for the treatment of keratoconus. *Journal of Cataract & Refractive Surgery*. 2006;32(5):747–55.

65. Utine CA, Ayhan Z, Engin CD. Effect of intracorneal ring segment implantation on corneal asphericity. *International Journal of Ophthalmology*. 2018;11(8):1303.

66. Mousa RM. Corneal asphericity changes after implantation of intracorneal ring segment (kerarings) in the treatment of Keratoconus. *NILES Journal for Geriatric and Gerontology*. 2021;4:68–77.

67. Park SE, Tseng M, Lee JK. Effectiveness of intracorneal ring segments for keratoconus. *Current Opinion in Ophthalmology*. 2019;30(4):220–8.

68. Ertan A, Colin J. Intracorneal rings for keratoconus and keratectasia. *Journal of Cataract & Refractive Surgery*. 2007;33(7):1303–14.

69. Tanter M, Touboul D, Gennisson J-L, Bercoff J, Fink M. High-resolution quantitative imaging of cornea elasticity using supersonic shear imaging. *IEEE Transactions on Medical Imaging*. 2009;28(12):1881–93.

70. Monteiro T, Alfonso JF, Franqueira N, Faria-Correia F, Ambrósio Jr R, Madrid-Costa D. Predictability of tunnel depth for intrastromal corneal ring segments implantation between manual and femtosecond laser techniques. *Journal of Refractive Surgery*. 2018;34(3):188–94.

71. Kanellopoulos AJ, Lawrence HP, Perry HD, Donnenfeld ED. Modified intracorneal ring segment implantations (INTACS) for the management of moderate to advanced keratoconus: efficacy and complications. *Cornea*. 2006;25(1):29–33.

72. Ertan A, Kamburoğlu G. Analysis of centration of Intacs segments implanted with a femtosecond laser. *Journal of Cataract & Refractive Surgery*. 2007;33(3):484–7.

73. Coskunseven E, Jankov MR, Grentzelos MA, Plaka AD, Limnopoulou AN, Kymionis GD. Topography-guided transepithelial PRK after intracorneal ring segments implantation and corneal collagen CXL in a three-step procedure for keratoconus. *Journal of Refractive Surgery*. 2013;29(1):54–8.

74. Gorgun E, Kucumen RB, Yenerel NM, Ciftci F. Assessment of intrastromal corneal ring segment position with anterior segment optical coherence tomography. *Ophthalmic Surgery, Lasers and Imaging Retina*. 2012;43(3):214–21.

75. Wollensak G. Crosslinking treatment of progressive keratoconus: new hope. *Current Opinion in Ophthalmology*. 2006;17(4):356–60.

76. Wollensak G, Iomdina E. Biomechanical and histological changes after corneal cross-linking with and without epithelial debridement. *Journal of Cataract & Refractive Surgery.* 2009;35(3):540–6.

77. Janani L, Jadidi K, Mosavi SA, Nejat F, Naderi M, Nourijelyani K. MyoRing implantation in keratoconic patients: 3 years follow-up data. *Journal of Ophthalmic & Vision Research.* 2016;11(1):26.

78. Saleem MIHA. Combined cross-linking with femtosecond laser myoring implantation versus combined cross-linking with femtosecond laser keraring implantation in the treatment of keratoconus. *Journal of the Egyptian Ophthalmological Society.* 2015;108(3):140.

79. Mohammadpour M, Masoumi A, Dehghan M, Hashemian MN, Karami SA, Mahmoudi A. Myoring implantation with and without corneal collagen crosslinking for the management of keratoconus. *Journal of Ophthalmic & Vision Research.* 2020;15(4):486.

80. Busin M, Santorum P, Barbara R. Combined tissue excision and corneal tuck for the surgical treatment of extremely advanced pellucid marginal corneal degeneration. *Cornea.* 2013;32(12):1628–30.

81. Kubaloglu A, Sari ES, Cinar Y, Koytak A, Kurnaz E, Piñero DP, et al. A single 210-degree arc length intrastromal corneal ring implantation for the management of pellucid marginal corneal degeneration. *American Journal of Ophthalmology.* 2010;150(2):185–92.e1.

82. Abad JC. Paradoxical central corneal steepening after collagen crosslinking in a case with intrastromal corneal ring segments. *Journal of Cataract & Refractive Surgery.* 2012;38(10):1879–80.

83. Abdelmassih Y, El-Khoury S, Dirani A, Antonios R, Fadlallah A, Cherfan CG, et al. Safety and efficacy of sequential intracorneal ring segment implantation and cross-linking in pediatric keratoconus. *American Journal of Ophthalmology.* 2017;178:51–7.

84. Bikbova G, Kazakbaeva G, Bikbov M, Usubov E. Complete corneal ring (MyoRing) implantation versus MyoRing implantation combined with corneal collagen crosslinking for keratoconus: 3-year follow-up. *International Ophthalmology.* 2018;38:1285–93.

85. Wollensak G, Spörl E, Seiler T. Treatment of keratoconus by collagen cross linking. *Der Ophthalmologe: Zeitschrift der Deutschen Ophthalmologischen Gesellschaft.* 2003;100(1):44–9.

86. Wollensak G, Spoerl E, Seiler T. Stress-strain measurements of human and porcine corneas after riboflavin–ultraviolet-A-induced cross-linking. *Journal of Cataract & Refractive Surgery.* 2003;29(9):1780–5.

87. Coskunseven E, Jankov II MR, Hafezi F, Atun S, Arslan E, Kymionis GD. Effect of treatment sequence in combined intrastromal corneal rings and corneal collagen crosslinking for keratoconus. *Journal of Cataract & Refractive Surgery.* 2009;35(12):2084–91.

88. El-Raggal TM. Sequential versus concurrent KERARINGS insertion and corneal collagen cross-linking for keratoconus. *British Journal of Ophthalmology.* 2011;95(1):37–41.

89. Saelens IE, Bartels MC, Bleyen I, Van Rij G. Refractive, topographic, and visual outcomes of same-day corneal cross-linking with Ferrara intracorneal ring segments in patients with progressive keratoconus. *Cornea.* 2011;30(12):1406–8.

90. Hersh PS, Issa R, Greenstein SA. Corneal crosslinking and intracorneal ring segments for keratoconus: A randomized study of concurrent versus sequential surgery. *Journal of Cataract & Refractive Surgery.* 2019;45(6):830–9.

91. Kankariya VP, Dube AB, Grentzelos MA, Kontadakis GA, Diakonis VF, Petrelli M, et al. Corneal cross-linking (CXL) combined with refractive surgery for the comprehensive management of keratoconus: CXL plus. *Indian Journal of Ophthalmology*. 2020;68(12):2757.

92. Kremer I, Aizenman I, Lichter H, Shayer S, Levinger S. Simultaneous wavefront-guided photorefractive keratectomy and corneal collagen crosslinking after intrastromal corneal ring segment implantation for keratoconus. *Journal of Cataract & Refractive Surgery*. 2012;38(10):1802–7.

93. Hashemi H, Alvani A, Seyedian MA, Yaseri M, Khabazkhoob M, Esfandiari H. Appropriate sequence of combined intracorneal ring implantation and corneal collagen cross-linking in keratoconus: a systematic review and meta-analysis. *Cornea*. 2018;37(12):1601–7.

94. Saleem MIH, Ibrahim Elzembely HA, AboZaid MA, Elagouz M, Saeed AM, Mohammed OA, et al. Three-year outcomes of cross-linking PLUS (combined cross-linking with femtosecond laser intracorneal ring segments implantation) for management of keratoconus. *Journal of Ophthalmology*. 2018;2018.

95. Legare ME, Iovieno A, Yeung SN, Lichtinger A, Kim P, Hollands S, et al. Intacs with or without same-day corneal collagen cross-linking to treat corneal ectasia. *Canadian Journal of Ophthalmology*. 2013;48(3):173–8.

96. Henriquez MA, Izquierdo Jr L, Bernilla C, McCarthy M. Corneal collagen cross-linking before Ferrara intrastromal corneal ring implantation for the treatment of progressive keratoconus. *Cornea*. 2012;31(7):740–5.

97. Mohammadpour M, Farhadi B, Mirshahi R, Masoumi A, Mirghorbani M. Simultaneous photorefractive keratectomy and accelerated collagen cross-linking in high-risk refractive surgery (Tehran protocol): 3-year outcomes. *International Ophthalmology*. 2020;40(10):2659–66.

98. Gouvea L, Rocha KM, Dickson D, Waring IV GO. Combined intracorneal ring segments and corneal-collagen crosslinking. *WJOVR MS ID*. 2019;510.

99. Daxer A. Intracorneal ring in pocket shows promise for treatment of keratoconus. *Journal of Refractive Surgery*. 2009;32:17.

100. Fratzl P, Daxer A. Structural transformation of collagen fibrils in corneal stroma during drying. An x-ray scattering study. *Biophysical Journal*. 1993;64(4):1210–4.

101. Hosny M, El–Mayah E, Sidky MK, Anis M. Femtosecond laser-assisted implantation of complete versus incomplete rings for keratoconus treatment. *Clinical Ophthalmology (Auckland, NZ)*. 2015;9:121.

102. Coşkunseven E, Ambrósio R, Smorádková A, León FS, Sahin O, Kavadarli I, et al. Visual, refractive and topographic outcomes of progressive thickness intrastromal corneal ring segments for keratoconic eyes. *International Ophthalmology*. 2020;40(11):2835–44.

103. Carrasquillo KG, Rand J, Talamo JH. Intacs for keratoconus and post-LASIK ectasia: mechanical versus femtosecond laser-assisted channel creation. *Cornea*. 2007;26(8):956–62.

104. Rabinowitz YS, Li X, Ignacio TS, Maguen E. *INTACS inserts using the femtosecond laser compared to the mechanical spreader in the treatment of keratoconus*. Slack Incorporated Thorofare, NJ; 2006. p. 764–71.

105. Kwitko S, Severo NS. Ferrara intracorneal ring segments for keratoconus. *Journal of Cataract & Refractive Surgery*. 2004;30(4):812–20.

106. Colin J, Velou S. Implantation of Intacs and a refractive intraocular lens to correct keratoconus. *Journal of Cataract & Refractive Surgery*. 2003;29(4):832–4.

107. Ruckhofer J, Stoiber J, Alzner E, Grabner G. One year results of European multicenter study of intrastromal corneal ring segments: part 2: complications, visual symptoms, and patient satisfaction. *Journal of Cataract & Refractive Surgery*. 2001;27(2):287–96.

108. Monteiro T, Alfonso JF, Freitas R, Franqueira N, Faria-Correira F, Ambrósio R, et al. Comparison of complication rates between manual and femtosecond laser-assisted techniques for intrastromal corneal ring segments implantation in keratoconus. *Current Eye Research*. 2019;44(12):1291–8.

109. Janani L, Tanha K, Najafi F, Jadidi K, Nejat F, Hashemian SJ, et al. Efficacy of complete rings (MyoRing) in treatment of Keratoconus: a systematic review and meta-analysis. *International Ophthalmology*. 2019;39(12):2929–46.

110. Daxer A, Ettl A, Hörantner R. Long-term results of MyoRing treatment of keratoconus. *Journal of Optometry*. 2017;10(2):123–9.

111. Izquierdo Jr L, Mannis MJ, Mejías Smith JA, Henriquez MA. Effectiveness of intrastromal corneal ring implantation in the treatment of adult patients with keratoconus: a systematic review. *Journal of Refractive Surgery*. 2019;35(3):191–200.

112. Shetty R, D'Souza S, Ramachandran S, Kurian M, Nuijts RM. Decision making nomogram for intrastromal corneal ring segments in keratoconus. *Indian Journal of Ophthalmology*. 2014;62(1):23.

113. Ferrer C, Alió JL, Montañés AU, Pérez-Santonja JJ, del Rio MAD, de Toledo JA, et al. Causes of intrastromal corneal ring segment explantation: clinicopathologic correlation analysis. *Journal of Cataract & Refractive Surgery*. 2010;36(6):970–7.

114. Coskunseven E, Kymionis GD, Tsiklis NS, Atun S, Arslan E, Siganos CS, et al. Complications of intrastromal corneal ring segment implantation using a femtosecond laser for channel creation: a survey of 850 eyes with keratoconus. *Acta Ophthalmologica*. 2011;89(1):54–7.

115. Kugler LJ, Hill S, Sztipanovits D, Boerman H, Swartz TS, Wang MX. Corneal melt of incisions overlying corneal ring segments: case series and literature review. *Cornea*. 2011;30(9):968–71.

116. Colin J, Buestel C, Touboul D. Unusual secondary displacement of Intacs segments—superimposition of distal ends. *Journal of Refractive Surgery*. 2010;26(12):924–5.

117. Gharaibeh AM, Sana'M M, AbuKhader IB, Ababneh OH, Abu-Ameerh MA, Albdour MD. KeraRing intrastromal corneal ring segments for correction of keratoconus. *Cornea*. 2012;31(2):115–20.

118. Nguyen N, Gelles JD, Greenstein SA, Hersh PS. Incidence and associations of intracorneal ring segment explantation. *Journal of Cataract & Refractive Surgery*. 2019;45(2):153–8.

119. Shihadeh WA. Aspergillus fumigatus keratitis following intracorneal ring segment implantation. *BMC Ophthalmology*. 2012;12:1–4.

120. Chalasani R, Beltz J, Jhanji V, Vajpayee RB. Microbial keratitis following intracorneal ring segment implantation. *British Journal of Ophthalmology*. 2010;94(11):1541.

121. Kymionis GD, Kontadakis GA, editors. *Severe corneal vascularization after intacs implantation and rigid contact lens use for the treatment of keratoconus. Seminars in ophthalmology*; 2012. Taylor & Francis.

122. Kaufman MB, Dhaliwal DK. Spontaneous improvement of channel deposits following Intacs implantation. *Journal of Refractive Surgery.* 2011;27(4):303–5.

123. Jabbarvand M, Hashemi H, Mohammadpour M, Khojasteh H, Khodaparast M, Hashemian H. Implantation of a complete intrastromal corneal ring at 2 different stromal depths in keratoconus. *Cornea.* 2014;33(2):141–4.

124. Studeny P, Krizova D, Stranak Z. Clinical outcomes after complete intracorneal ring implantation and corneal collagen cross-linking in an intrastromal pocket in one session for keratoconus. *Journal of Ophthalmology.* 2014;2014. https://doi.org/10.1155/2014/568128

125. Mohammadpour M, Hahemi H, Jabbarvand M. Technique of simultaneous femtosecond laser assisted Myoring implantation and accelerated intrastromal collagen cross-linking for management of progressive keratoconus: a novel technique. *Contact Lens and Anterior Eye.* 2016;39(1):9–14.

126. Nobari SM, Villena Cepeda C, Jadidi K. Myoring implantation alone versus corneal collagen cross-linking following myoring implantation for management of keratoconus: 1 year follow up. *Acta Medica Mediterranea.* 2016;32(2):1077–85.

127. Emin U, Mukharram B, Gyulli K, Guzel B. Complete corneal ring (MyoRing) implantation combined with corneal collagen crosslinking in keratoconus treatment. *Acta Ophthalmologica.* 2017;95. https://doi.org/10.1111/j.1755-3768.2017.0s033

128. Bikbova G, Kazakbaeva G, Bikbov M, Usubov E. Complete corneal ring (MyoRing) implantation versus MyoRing implantation combined with corneal collagen crosslinking for keratoconus: 3-year follow-up. *International Ophthalmology.* 2018;38(3):1285–93.

19 Phakic IOLs in Keratoconus

Mohammad-Reza Sedaghat and Javad Sadeghi

INTRODUCTION

Keratoconus is a common disorder in which the cornea undergoes progressive thinning. Its prevalence was estimated at 1 per 2000,[1] while recent studies reported higher prevalence rates. Hashemi et al. reported a 2.5% frequency of keratoconus in Mashhad, Iran.[2] Keratoconus is associated with myopia and keratorefractive procedures are not recommended. Therefore, phakic intraocular lenses (IOLs) are considered a suitable refractive procedure without the risk of corneal ectasia.

Corneal surgery and IOLs are recommended to correct refractive errors. In keratorefractive surgeries, normal corneas with proper thickness and biomechanics are required. Therefore, the use of this method is limited in patients with keratoconus, thin cornea, and high myopia. Clear lens extraction (CLE) with IOL is another refractive surgery that is sufficiently effective, predictable, and stable. However, the loss of accommodation (in young people) and the risk of complications, such as retinal detachment (especially in myopic patients), restrict the use of this method. The third refractive procedure is phakic IOLs, with the following advantages:

1. Save the accommodation in young patients.

2. Lower risk of retinal detachment, compared to CLE.

3. The lens is removable and exchangeable.

4. The result is predictable and immediately stable.

TYPES OF PHAKIC INTRAOCULAR LENSES

The phakic intraocular lenses (IOLs) are divided into three categories, based on their fixation points:

1. Anterior chamber phakic IOLs

2. Anterior-posterior phakic IOLs

3. Posterior chamber phakic IOLs

Anterior Chamber Phakic IOLs

Angle-fixated and iris-supported lenses are included in this group.

Angle-fixated IOLs were initially introduced to correct aphakia. Afterward, they were also used to correct myopia in phakic patients. The challenge with these lenses is choosing the appropriate size to reduce complications, such as endothelial cell loss, uveitis, hyphema, increased intraocular pressure, peripheral synechia, and iris atrophy, which limit the use of these lenses. Recently, the foldable form of these lenses has become available, which can be inserted through a small corneal incision.[3,4]

Iris-claw IOLs are the most-available iris-supported lenses. They were initially used for aphakia but, since 1986, they have also been utilized to correct myopia (Fechner–Worst lens). They also have possible complications, including endothelial cell loss, pigment dispersion, cataracts, irregular pupils, and visual symptoms, such as glare/halo. Recent studies show that intra-operative endothelial cell loss after iris-claw IOLs is similar to cataract surgery. Additionally, over time, cell change does not seem significantly greater than the natural loss (0.6% annually).[5] The greatest advantage of iris-claw phakic IOLs is that "one size fits all"; therefore, it is easy and inexpensive to use them. Artisan lens (Ophtec, Groeningen, the Netherlands) is one of the most popular iris-claw phakic IOLs, and the foldable type of these IOLs (Artiflex) is inserted through a small corneal incision.[6,7]

Anterior-Posterior Phakic IOLs

These lenses were not very popular due to their many complications, but studying them became the basis for the production of the posterior chamber (PC) phakic IOLs.[3]

Posterior Chamber (PC) Phakic IOLs

Different models of PC phakic IOLs have been introduced. The new generation of these lenses is covered with a collagen polymer (Collamer) layer to increase biocompatibility. STAAR (Monrovia,

DOI: 10.1201/9781003371601-19

CA, USA) patented this material for implantable contact lenses (ICLs). The range of correction for the ICL is from +10 D to −20 D, with cylindrical correction up to 6 D, and it is available in four sizes, namely 12.1, 12.6, 13.2, and 13.7 mm. Initially, under-correction was the main problem with these lenses; however, regression analysis formulae solved this problem, and currently, IOL sizing is the biggest challenge in using these lenses.[8] Phakic refractive lens (PRL; Carl Zeiss Meditec, Jena, Germany) is another PC phakic IOL available.

Best Phakic IOL for Keratoconus

The selection of appropriate lenses in keratoconus (KCN) patients is challenging, especially in patients with low spherical and high cylindrical refractive errors. Different phakic IOL models are used for these patients to correct these errors.

Leccisotti and Fields evaluated angle-fixated IOLs in KCN patients with high myopia. The spherical refractive errors corrected ±1D, but the magnitude of astigmatism did not significantly improve. Most patients were satisfied; however, in patients with low myopia, residual astigmatism restricted visual outcomes.[9]

We have already reported the visual outcome of phakic Artisan and phakic toric Artisan lenses in stable keratoconus patients. The improvements in the corrected and uncorrected distance visual acuity were statistically significant. We suggested that keratoconic patients who have good preoperative visual acuity and a high spherical-to-cylindrical ratio are good candidates for the implantation of phakic Artisan lenses.[10]

Alio et al.[11] and Alfonso et al.[12] confirmed the safety, efficacy, stability, and predictability of ICL implantation to correct myopia and astigmatism in eyes with keratoconus. The widely available range of ICL power, especially in cylindrical correction, makes it an appropriate lens for keratoconus.

PRE-OPERATIVE CONSIDERATIONS

IOL Power Calculation

Phakic IOL implantation is considered to be a refractive surgery with the minimum accepted refractive error. The refractive outcome should be ±1D from the attempted refraction. Axial length, lens thickness, and vitreous chamber length remained completely unchanged after surgery and are not determined.

For anterior chamber (AC) phakic IOLs (angle-fixated and iris-claw), the Van der Heijde formula is recommended. In this formula, refraction, anterior chamber depth (ACD), and keratometric values are used for calculation.[13,14] Moreover, a free online Ophtec calculator (ARTICALC) is available to calculate Artisan and Artiflex. The simulation and calculation of iris-claw phakic IOLs are considered in OCULUS Pentacam AXL.

Many methods have been introduced to calculate the ICL power, including the STAAR Surgical Online Calculation and Ordering System software (OCOS), JPhakic software, Olsen–Feingold formula, Holladay formula, and Linz–Homburg–Castrop (LHC) formula. Recent studies demonstrated that the Olsen–Feingold formula achieved a significantly higher refractive error than other methods. However, the OCOS software and JPhakic software, as well as the Holladay and LHC formulae, showed similar results and can be cross-checked.[15]

IOL Sizing

Getting the right size remains the main problem in using phakic IOLs. Two reasons play a major role in this challenge.

First, it is not clear which parameter can better calculate the IOL size. Several parameters, such as ACD, white-to-white (WTW), sulcus-to-sulcus (STS), and angle-to-angle (ATA), were measured by many devices and used for IOL sizing. Reinstein et al. have shown that STS is a better predictor for ICL sizing and achieves a suitable post-operative vault height.[16]

The second reason is the limited range of available standard sizes of IOLs. Currently, ICL is available in four sizes, namely 12.1, 12.6, 13.2, and 13.7 mm. Table 19.1 shows recommended ICL sizes according to WTW and ACD.

The wrong size increases complications. A larger phakic IOL leads to a high vault and increases pigment dispersion syndrome, endothelial cell damage, and raised intraocular pressure. Smaller

Table 19.1 FDA-Recommended Diameter of ICL According to WTW and ACD Measurements for STAAR ICL[17]

WTW (mm)	ACD (mm)	Recommended ICL length
<10.50	All	Not recommended
10.5–10.6	≤3.5	Not recommended
10.5–10.6	>3.5	12.1
10.7–11.0	All	12.1
11.1	≤3.5	12.1
11.1	>3.5	12.6
11.2–11.4	All	12.6
11.5–11.6	≤3.5	12.6
11.5–11.6	>3.5	13.2
11.7–12.1	All	13.2
12.2	≤3.5	13.2
12.2	>3.5	13.7
12.3–12.9	All	13.7
≥13	All	Not recommended

ICL: Implantable contact lens, WTW: White-to-white, ACD: Anterior chamber depth

size, on the other hand, leads to a low vault and increases the risk of cataract formation and post-operative IOL rotation.[17]

Calculating ICL size in keratoconus patients will be more difficult. The discrepancy between the measured WTW and the actual sulcus diameter may be due to corneolimbal stretching, making the IOL size calculations difficult. It seems that STS is a better predictor in keratoconus patients.[18]

Patient Selection

Detailed pre-operative examinations are necessary to reduce complications and improve visual outcomes. It is also crucial to perform accurate manifest and cycloplegic refraction and the evaluation of the best spectacle-corrected visual acuity (BSCVA). In all patients, stable refraction changes of less than 0.50 D in six to 12 months are necessary. Moreover, due to the progressive feature of keratoconus, a longer follow-up period is needed.[19]

The anterior segment should be evaluated carefully by slit-lamp biomicroscopy and imaging instruments. The perception of cataracts, glaucoma, ocular hypertension, uveitis, and iris abnormalities in slit-lamp examination and tonometry can prevent surgery. It is also essential to measure the central corneal thickness (CCT), axial length, endothelial cell count, keratometric values, and mesopic pupil diameter. Gonioscopy and the evaluation of the anterior chamber angle configuration are important, and ACD, WTW, ATA, STS, as well as crystalline lens rise (CLR), should also be measured.

Indirect ophthalmoscopy, with a careful peripheral retinal examination, is essential, especially in the myopic fundus. In most patients, consultation with a retina surgeon is recommended to reduce the risk of retinal detachment. Macular optical coherence tomography (OCT) is also recommended.

The evaluation of the endothelium is necessary because the loss of endothelial cells occurs during the operation and in the years after. It seems that intra-operative cell loss is similar to that during cataract surgery, and, over time, cell loss is similar to natural loss. However, phakic IOL implantation is performed at a younger age than cataract surgery. Therefore, the minimum pre-operative endothelial cell count is required (according to the patient's age) to provide added safety for long-term corneal clarity.[20,21] At 20 years of age, at least 2,500 cells/mm², and at 40 years, more than 2,000 cells/mm² must be present.[3]

The ACD is an important parameter to improve long-term safety of this operation. Previous studies found a significant correlation between lower ACDs and endothelial cell loss.[22] Moreover, the implantation of phakic IOLs in eyes with a narrow angle and a shallow anterior chamber increases the risk of cataracts, glaucoma, and pigment dispersion. The minimum ACD for phakic IOL eligibility is generally 3.0 mm for ICL and 3.2 mm for iris-claw lenses, as measured between the central anterior lens capsule and the endothelium. Iris configuration and anterior chamber angle are other parameters to be considered.[19] Angle should be at least a Shaffer grade of 3 and 4. Structural iris abnormalities are more problematic in iris-claw IOLs, but iris posterior bowing may increase the risk of pigment dispersion after ICL implantation (Figure 19.1).

Crystalline lens rise (CLR), which is the distance between the anterior pole of the crystalline lens and the line connecting the 3 o'clock to 9 o'clock angle recess, is measured by the anterior segment OCT (Figure 19.2). Post-operative lens vault, the distance between the ICL and anterior pole of the crystalline lens, is affected by ACD, WTW, and CLR. A higher CLR reduces the lens vault and increases the risk of cataract formation (Figure 19.3).[23] Acceptable CLR for ICL implantation

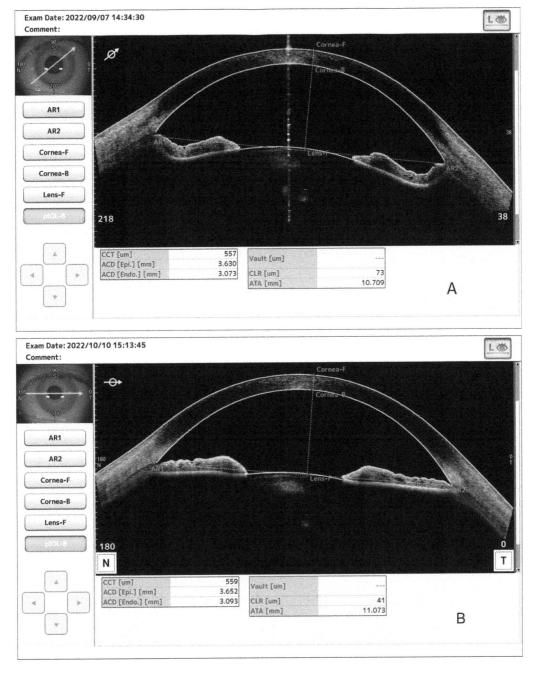

Figure 19.1 A. Iris posterior bowing in myopic patients, B. Resolved iris bowing after laser peripheral iridotomy.

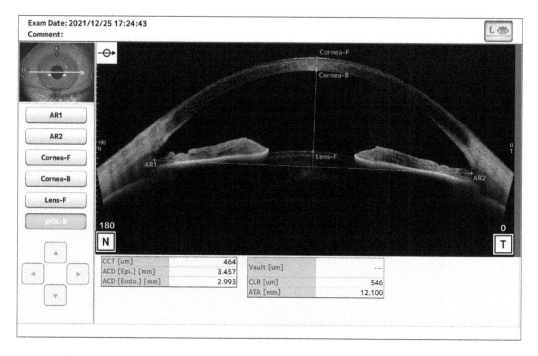

Figure 19.2 Crystalline lens rise.

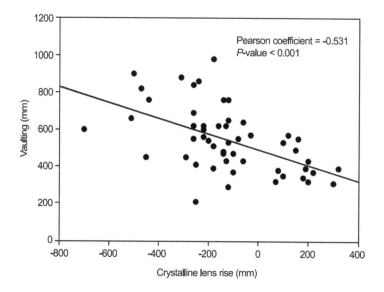

Figure 19.3 Correlation between crystalline lens rise and the central vaulting of the implantable contact lens.

depends on age. It is better to have less than 600 CLR at the age of 40. Optimal vault after ICL implantation is considered to be between 250 and 750 μm (Figures 19.4 and 19.5).[24]

We summarize the accepted criteria for implanting phakic IOLs in Table 19.2.

Considering that phakic IOLs in keratoconus patients are associated with more challenges, progressive characteristics and irregular astigmatism in these patients restrict visual outcomes. We classify keratoconus treatments into three categories: stabilizing procedure, regularizing procedure, and refractive procedure. Phakic IOLs belong to the refractive procedure category; therefore, before this operation, the cornea should be stabilized and regularized. Corneal cross

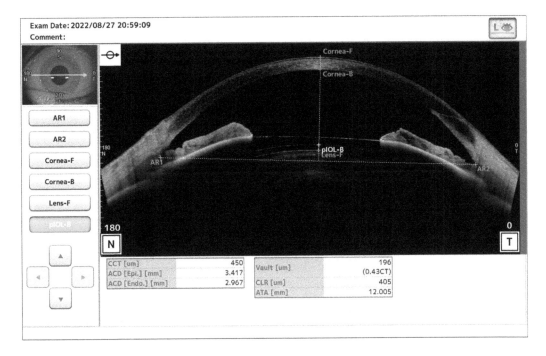

Figure 19.4 Low vault after implantable contact lens.

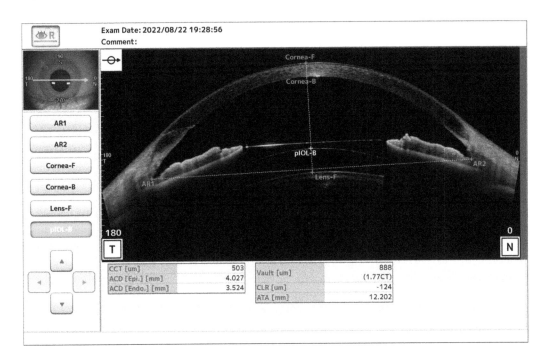

Figure 19.5 High vault after implantable contact lens.

linking (CCL) is the most common stabilizing procedure. Refractive errors should remain stable within two years of follow-up. Furthermore, corneal irregularities should be treated before phakic IOL implantation. The BSCVA is a good indicator of corneal regularity. If BSCVA is good, corneal irregularity is avoidable, and phakic IOLs can be considered. On the other hand, in patients with a low BSCVA, as well as a high corneal curvature and irregularity, regularizing procedures are

Table 19.2 Accepted Criteria for Implanting Phakic IOLs

Ages 21 to 45

Stable manifest refraction

ACD: more than 3.00 mm for ICL
ACD: more than 3.2 mm for iris-claw

Irido-corneal angle aperture: Shaffer grade 3 and 4

Endothelial cell count: ≥2,500 cells/mm² at 20 years
Endothelial cell count: ≥2,000 cells/mm² at 40 years

No ocular pathology (corneal disorders, glaucoma, uveitis, cataract, and maculopathy)

No previous ocular surgery

IOL: Intraocular lens, ACD: Anterior chamber depth
ICL: Implantable contact lens

Table 19.3 Practice Pattern in KCN Patients

	Stable Refraction	Unstable Refraction
Regular Cornea	Phakic IOL	CCL + Phakic IOL
Irregular Cornea	ICRS + Phakic IOL	ICRS + CCL + Phakic IOL

IOL: Intraocular lens, CCL: Corneal cross linking, ICRS: Intra-corneal ring segment

necessary, which include intra-stromal ring segment, photorefractive keratectomy (PRK) plus CCL, and keratoplasty. We summarize our practice pattern for phakic IOL implantation in KCN patients in Table 19.3.

INTRA-OPERATIVE CONSIDERATIONS

Surgical Techniques

For iris-claw IOLs, it is better to constrict the pupil with miotic drops. If possible, a limbal or corneal incision is made in the steepest corneal meridian. The incision size is approximately equal to the lens optic diameter. The IOL is pushed to the anterior chamber under the ophthalmic viscosurgical device (OVD). A suitable iris fold and enclavation allow the long-term stability of IOL. Intra-operative or pre-operative peripheral iridectomy is necessary. At the end of the surgery, OVD should be removed, and the corneal incision for Artisan needs to be sutured, but Artiflex is inserted through a 3.2-mm self-sealing incision.

For patients who are candidates for ICL, the pupil is dilated with mydriatic drops, and the procedure can be performed under topical anesthesia. A 3.2-mm temporal clear corneal incision is created, and the anterior chamber is filled with OVD. The ICL is then injected in the anterior chamber, parallel to the iris plane, and gently pushed beneath the iris. The new generation of ICL has a central hole, so peripheral iridectomy is not necessary. We must be careful not to put the ICL in upside down.

POSTOPERATIVE CONSIDERATIONS

Follow-Up

After the phakic IOL implantation, patients should be followed up carefully. Examinations are scheduled for one day, one week, one month, three months, six months, one year, and then annually. In the first days after the operation, the patient should be examined for infection, the appropriate position of the lens, and the lens vault. The accurate measurement of intraocular pressure is also very important. Uncorrected visual acuity (UCVA) and BCVA, as well as dry and cycloplegic refraction, help to understand the efficacy of IOLs and the residual refractive error. One month after surgery, a fundus examination with a dilated pupil is necessary to evaluate the peripheral retina. In long-term follow-ups, endothelial cell count should be evaluated yearly. If there is an annual endothelial cell loss rate of more than 1% per year, then implant removal may be considered.[25]

Outcome

Large numbers of studies have demonstrated that all three types of phakic IOLs have excellent results. Safety and efficacy are two indicators with which to evaluate IOL outcomes. The safety index is the ratio of post-operative BCVA/pre-operative BCVA (indicates the risk of vision loss), and the efficacy index is the ratio of post-operative UCVA/pre-operative BCVA (the ability to achieve acceptable correction).[26]

Safety

Safety is still one of the main concerns related to phakic IOLs, which is affected by intra-operative and post-operative complications. Today, the improved quality of materials, lens design, and surgeons' skills have reduced intra-operative complications. Some post-operative complications have also been reduced for the same reasons, but long-term complications may affect phakic IOL outcomes.[27]

Phakic IOL implantation is an intraocular surgery with a potential risk for the development of post-operative endophthalmitis. One case of post-operative endophthalmitis by β-hemolytic strep-tococci has been reported.[28]

Glare and Halos. Optic diameter is one of the factors affecting glare and halos. Larger optical diameters are associated with less visual disturbance. Therefore, Artisan (especially with a 6-mm optical diameter) produces less glare than ICL (with an optical diameter of up to 5.5 mm) and PRL (with an optical diameter of up to 5 mm).[29,30] Decentration is another factor that causes more glare and halos in the PC phakic IOLs.[31] In the first months after the operation, the amount of glare and halos is higher, but in the following months, it gradually decreases.[32] Studies also demonstrated that Artisan IOLs do not change contrast sensitivity and high-order aberrations.[21,33]

Surgically Induced Astigmatism. Artisan is made of non-foldable materials (PMMA) and is inserted through a large corneal incision. This incision can induce astigmatism and affect visual outcomes. On the other hand, Artiflex and ICL are inserted through a small corneal incision and cause less astigmatism.[21]

Loss of Corneal Endothelial Cells. Intra-operative direct trauma, post-operative inflamma-tion, toxicity, and the contact between IOLs and the cornea cause endothelial cell loss (ECL). This damage is more common in the first months after surgery but decreases in the following months.[34] Endothelial cell loss was reported to be between 0.7% and 4.8% three years after the Artisan implantation[7,21] and about 3.7% four years after the ICL implantation.[35] There is a significant nega-tive correlation between ECL and ACD. The distance between the edge of Artisan and the endo-thelium also affects the loss of endothelial cells. It is thus recommended that this distance be at least 1.5 mm.[22,36,37]

Less corneal ECL was reported with PC phakic IOLs than AC IOLs. The safety of angle-sup-ported phakic IOLs was impacted by significant ECL (more than 1% per year), and this type of phakic IOLs will leave the market.[38–40] However, Artisan and Visian ICL are safe and approved by the FDA.

Pigment Dispersion. In the early months after the Artisan implantation, pigments are depos-ited on IOL and cleared in the following months.[21,41] However, in the case of ICL implantation, the continuous contact between the IOL and pigment epithelium of the iris developed constant pigment dispersion.[42] High vault and high CLR increase the risk of pigment dispersion. Studies indicated that a CLR of less than 600 μm is associated with a lower risk of pigment dispersion.[43]

Intraocular Pressure Elevation. Spikes of intraocular pressure (IOP) elevation occurred in the early days after surgery, but studies demonstrated that long-term IOP elevation did not happen.[44] The ICL implantation is associated with more iris contact but the Collamer material is similar to a lens capsule and does not induce pigmentary glaucoma.[20,35]

Cataract Formation. Cataract formation is one of the remaining challenges of phakic IOLs. The risk of cataract formation of ICL is more than for Artisan because of the ICL contact with the crystalline lens in the mid periphery. The prevalence of cataract formation after myopic Artisan implantation is 1.1%, of which nuclear cataract is the most common type. Cataracts are observed in 8.5% of patients after ICL implantation, and anterior subcapsular cataract is the most common type.[45,46] The new design of ICL in the V4 type decreases the risk to 2.1%.[47] Getting the right size will result in the right vault after the operation and is mandatory to minimizing the risk of crystal-line lens contact and preventing cataract formation.

Retinal Detachment. Retinal complications, especially retinal detachment (RD), are an impor-tant problem associated with high myopia. The RD rate after Artisan implantation is 0.3% per year and is similar to the RD rate of high myopic patients without operation.[21] The prevalence of RD after ICL implantation is 0.5%, and RDs are part of the natural characteristics of the myopic fundus.[48] Detailed pre-operative and post-operative retinal examination is mandatory to perform laser photocoagulation, if required.

In keratoconus patients, phakic IOLs are safe, and because of the high ACD of these patients, endothelial cell loss is less worrying. However, the discordance between WTW and STS in these patients increases the risk of wrong sizing and can lead to cataracts or pigment dispersion. Improper vault size is more common in keratoconus patients than myopic patients.[49] Some keratoconic patients, who are candidates for phakic IOLs, have a high corneal curvature with a smaller axial length; therefore, they are associated with a lower risk of retinal detachment.

Efficacy

Previous studies demonstrated that there is no significant difference in visual acuity improvement between the Artisan and Visian ICLs.[41] In FDA trials, Artisan showed a good visual outcome and had high safety and efficacy in myopic patients. Six months' follow-up showed that 83% of patients achieved UCVA of ≥20/40, and 90% of patients were within 1 D of the intended correction. Long-term studies also found stable refraction. After three years of follow-up, 84%, and after 10 years, 82% of patients had UCVA of ≥20/40.[6,7,21,50,51]

Keratoconic patients with stable refraction and contact lens intolerance can be candidates for phakic IOLs. Fischinger et al. indicated that Artisan/Artiflex is a suitable refractive procedure in patients with keratoconus. This study demonstrated that the UCVA after IOL implantation is equal to or better than the pre-operative BCVA in 71% and better in 34% of patients. Patients with a pellucid marginal degeneration-like pattern and those with low astigmatism have better results. On the other hand, patients with higher Amsler–Krumeich stage and advanced keratoconus were correlated with a worse post-operative UCVA.[52]

ICL implantation is another appropriate refractive procedure for keratoconus patients, which has an acceptable correction of spherical and cylindrical refractive errors and good visual outcome. Fairaq et al. found that 93% of keratoconus patients maintained or gained lines of BCVA after the ICL implantation; however, 18% were unsatisfied with the quality of vision, and one out of 32 patients had to explant the ICL due to residual refractive errors.[53] Alfonso et al. reported that 97% of keratoconus patients maintained or gained multiple lines of BCVA after surgery.[12] Hashemian et al. indicated that the efficacy and safety index of ICL implantation after a five-year follow-up were 1.328 and 1.58, respectively. In this study, safety and efficacy indexes were more than others because milder keratoconus patients were included.[54]

In progressive keratoconus, CCL is necessary to stabilize the disease, and phakic IOL implantation should be considered after a delay. Some authors suggested waiting three to six months after CCL before IOL implantation.[55,56] In the study of Antonios et al., the ICL was inserted six months after CCL. The visual outcome was acceptable after two years, but a small hyperopic shift was observed.[57] We recommend at least one year of follow-up to achieve the maximum flattening effect of CCL and confirm the stability of refraction.

In patients with moderate keratoconus, the intracorneal ring segment can be considered a regularizing procedure to reduce keratometry, refraction, and corneal astigmatisms. After six months, residual refractive errors can be corrected by phakic IOLs.[58,59] The effective correction of residual refractive errors after topo-guided PRK + CCL by phakic IOL has recently been reported.[60]

We recommend phakic IOLs as a refractive procedure to correct refractive errors of stable as well as mild to moderate keratoconus patients with low aberrations. Patients with non-coincidental cylinder axis at refraction and topography may be less satisfied after this surgery.

REFERENCES

1. Rabinowitz YS. Keratoconus. *Survey of Ophthalmology*. 1998;42(4):297–319.

2. Hashemi H, Khabazkhoob M, Yazdani N, Ostadimoghaddam H, Norouzirad R, Amanzadeh K, et al. The prevalence of keratoconus in a young population in Mashhad, Iran. *Ophthalmic and Physiological Optics*. 2014;34(5):519–27.

3. Lovisolo CF, Reinstein DZ. Phakic intraocular lenses. *Survey of ophthalmology*. 2005;50(6):549–87.

4. Pérez-Santonja JJ, Iradier MT, Sanz-Iglesias L, Serrano JM, Zato MA. Endothelial changes in phakic eyes with anterior chamber intraocular lenses to correct high myopia. *Journal of Cataract & Refractive Surgery*. 1996;22(8):1017–22.

5. Bourne WM, Nelson LR, Hodge DO. Central corneal endothelial cell changes over a ten-year period. *Investigative Ophthalmology & Visual Science*. 1997;38(3):779–82.

6. Alexander L, John M, Cobb L, Noblitt R, Barowsky RT. US clinical investigation of the Artisan myopia lens for the correction of high myopia in phakic eyes. Report of the results of phases 1 and 2, and interim phase 3. *Optometry (St Louis, Mo)*. 2000;71(10):630–42.

7. Budo C, Hessloehl JC, Izak M, Luyten GP, Menezo JL, Sener BA, et al. Multicenter study of the Artisan phakic intraocular lens. *Journal of Cataract & Refractive Surgery*. 2000;26(8):1163–71.

8. Zaldivar R, Oscherow S, Ricur G. The STAAR posterior chamber phakic intraocular lens. *International Ophthalmology Clinics*. 2000;40(3):237–44.

9. Leccisotti A, Fields SV. Angle-supported phakic intraocular lenses in eyes with keratoconus and myopia. *Journal of Cataract & Refractive Surgery*. 2003;29(8):1530–6.

10. Sedaghat M, Ansari-Astaneh M-R, Zarei-Ghanavati M, Davis SW, Sikder S. Artisan Iris-supported Phakic IOL implantation in patients with keratoconus: a review of sixteen eyes. *Journal of Refractive Surgery*. 2011;27(7):489–493. https://doi.org/10.3928/1081597x-20110203-01

11. Alió JL, Peña-García P, Zein G, Abu-Mustafa S. Comparison of iris-claw and posterior chamber collagen copolymer phakic intraocular lenses in keratoconus. *Journal of Cataract & Refractive Surgery*. 2014;40(3):383–94.

12. Alfonso JF, Fernández-Vega L, Lisa C, Fernandes P, González-Méijome JM, Montés-Micó R. Collagen copolymer toric posterior chamber phakic intraocular lens in eyes with keratoconus. *Journal of Cataract & Refractive Surgery*. 2010;36(6):906–16.

13. Fechner PU, van der Heijde GL, Worst JG. The correction of myopia by lens implantation into phakic eyes. *American Journal of Ophthalmology*. 1989;107(6):659–63.

14. Van der Heijde G. Some optical aspects of implantation of an IOL in a myopic eye. *European Journal of Implant and Refractive Surgery*. 1989;1(4):245–8.

15. Wendelstein JA, Hinterberger S, Hoffmann PC, Hirnschall N, Koss MJ, Langenbucher A, et al. Evaluation of phakic IOL power calculation using the new LHC formula and comparison with four conventional methods. *Journal of Cataract & Refractive Surgery*. 2022:10.1097.

16. Reinstein DZ, Lovisolo CF, Archer TJ, Gobbe M. Comparison of postoperative vault height predictability using white-to-white or sulcus diameter–based sizing for the visian implantable collamer lens. *Journal of Refractive Surgery*. 2013;29(1):30–5.

17. Deshpande K, Shroff R, Biswas P, Kapur K, Shetty N, Koshy AS, et al. Phakic intraocular lens: Getting the right size. *Indian Journal of Ophthalmology*. 2020;68(12):2880.

18. Arora R, Manudhane A, Jain P, Goyal JL, Jain P. Implantable collamer lens (ICL) sizing in advanced keratoconus. *The Official Scientific Journal of Delhi Ophthalmological Society*. 2016;27(1):38–40.

19. Huang D, Schallhorn SC, Sugar A, Farjo AA, Majmudar PA, Trattler WB, et al. Phakic intraocular lens implantation for the correction of myopia: a report by the American Academy of Ophthalmology. *Ophthalmology*. 2009;116(11):2244–58.

20. Jiménez-Alfaro I, del Castillo JMBt, García-Feijoó J, de Bernabé JGG, de la Iglesia JMS. Safety of posterior chamber phakic intraocular lenses for the correction of high myopia: anterior segment changes after posterior chamber phakic intraocular lens implantation. *Ophthalmology*. 2001;108(1):90–9.

21. Stulting RD, John ME, Maloney RK, Assil KK, Arrowsmith PN, Thompson VM, et al. Three-year results of Artisan/Verisyse phakic intraocular lens implantation: results of the United States Food and Drug Administration clinical trial. *Ophthalmology*. 2008;115(3):464–72.e1.

22. Saxena R, Boekhoorn SS, Mulder PG, Noordzij B, van Rij G, Luyten GP. Long-term follow-up of endothelial cell change after Artisan phakic intraocular lens implantation. *Ophthalmology*. 2008;115(4):608–13.e1.

23. Kwak AY, Ryu IH, Kim JK, Im Kim T, Ha BJ. Effect of preoperative crystalline lens rise on vaulting after implantable collamer lens implantation. *Journal of the Korean Ophthalmological Society*. 2012;53(12):1749–55.

24. Montés-Micó R, Ruiz-Mesa R, Rodríguez-Prats JL, Tañá-Rivero P. Posterior-chamber phakic implantable collamer lenses with a central port: a review. *Acta Ophthalmologica*. 2021;99(3):e288–e301.

25. MacRae S, Holladay JT, Hilmantel G, Calogero D, Masket S, Stark W, et al. Special report: American Academy of Ophthalmology Task Force Recommendations for specular micros-copy for phakic intraocular lenses. *Ophthalmology*. 2017;124(1):141–2.

26. Jonker SM, Berendschot TT, Saelens IE, Bauer NJ, Nuijts RM. Phakic intraocular lenses: an overview. *Indian Journal of Ophthalmology*. 2020;68(12):2779.

27. Kohnen T, Kook D, Morral M, Güell JL. Phakic intraocular lenses: part 2: results and complications. *Journal of Cataract & Refractive Surgery*. 2010;36(12):2168–94.

28. Pérez-Santonja JJ, Ruíz-Moreno JM, de la Hoz F, Giner-Gorriti C, Alió JL. Endophthalmitis after phakic intraocular lens implantation to correct high myopia. *Journal of Cataract & Refractive Surgery*. 1999;25(9):1295–8.

29. Maroccos R, Vaz F, Marinho A, Guell J, Lohmann C. Glare and halos after" phakic IOL". Surgery for the correction of high myopia. *Der Ophthalmologe: Zeitschrift der Deutschen Ophthalmologischen Gesellschaft*. 2001;98(11):1055–9.

30. Hoyos JE, Dementiev DD, Cigales M, Hoyos-Chacón J, Hoffer KJ. Phakic refractive lens experience in Spain. *Journal of Cataract & Refractive Surgery*. 2002;28(11):1939–46.

31. Menezo JL, Peris-Martínez C, Cisneros A, Martínez-Costa R. *Posterior chamber phakic intra-ocular lenses to correct high myopia: a comparative study between Staar and Adatomed models*. Slack Incorporated Thorofare, NJ; 2001. p. 32–42.

32. Moshirfar M, Holz HA, Davis DK. Two-year follow-up of the Artisan/Verisyse iris-supported phakic intraocular lens for the correction of high myopia. *Journal of Cataract & Refractive Surgery*. 2007;33(8):1392–7.

33. Chung S-H, Lee SJ, Lee HK, Seo KY, Kim EK. Changes in higher order aberrations and contrast sensitivity after implantation of a phakic artisan intraocular lens. *Ophthalmologica*. 2007;221(3):167–72.

34. Menezo JL, Cisneros AL, Rodriguez-Salvador V. Endothelial study of iris-claw phakic lens: four year follow-up. *Journal of Cataract & Refractive Surgery*. 1998;24(8):1039–49.

35. Kamiya K, Shimizu K, Igarashi A, Hikita F, Komatsu M. Four-year follow-up of posterior chamber phakic intraocular lens implantation for moderate to high myopia. *Archives of Ophthalmology*. 2009;127(7):845–50.

36. Doors M, Berendschot TT, Webers CA, Nuijts RM. Model to predict endothelial cell loss after iris-fixated phakic intraocular lens implantation. *Investigative Ophthalmology & Visual Science*. 2010;51(2):811–5.

37. Doors M, Cals DW, Berendschot TT, de Brabander J, Hendrikse F, Webers CA, et al. Influence of anterior chamber morphometrics on endothelial cell changes after phakic intraocular lens implantation. *Journal of Cataract & Refractive Surgery*. 2008;34(12):2110–8.

38. Knorz MC, Lane SS, Holland SP. Angle-supported phakic intraocular lens for correction of moderate to high myopia: three-year interim results in international multicenter studies. *Journal of Cataract & Refractive Surgery*. 2011;37(3):469–80.

39. Kohnen T, Maxwell WA, Holland S. Correction of moderate to high myopia with a foldable, angle-supported phakic intraocular lens: results from a 5-year open-label trial. *Ophthalmology*. 2016;123(5):1027–35.

40. Ostovic M, Hofmann C, Klaproth OK, Kohnen T. Corneal decompensation and angle-closure glaucoma after upside-down implantation of an angle-supported anterior chamber phakic intraocular lens. *Journal of Cataract & Refractive Surgery*. 2013;39(5):806–9.

41. Menezo JL, Peris-Martínez C, Cisneros AL, Martínez-Costa R. Phakic intraocular lenses to correct high myopia: adatomed, staar, and artisan. *Journal of Cataract and Refractive Surgery*. 2004;30(1):33–44.

42. García-Feijoó J, Alfaro IJ, Cuiña-Sardiña R, Méndez-Hernandez C, Del Castillo JM, García-Sánchez J. Ultrasound biomicroscopy examination of posterior chamber phakic intraocular lens position. *Ophthalmology*. 2003;110(1):163–72.

43. Baïkoff G, Bourgeon G, Jodai HJ, Fontaine A, Lellis FV, Trinquet L. Pigment dispersion and Artisan phakic intraocular lenses: crystalline lens rise as a safety criterion. *Journal of Cataract & Refractive Surgery*. 2005;31(4):674–80.

44. Yamaguchi T, Negishi K, Yuki K, Saiki M, Nishimura R, Kawaguchi N, et al. Alterations in the anterior chamber angle after implantation of iris-fixated phakic intraocular lenses. *Journal of Cataract & Refractive Surgery*. 2008;34(8):1300–5.

45. Chen L-J, Chang Y-J, Kuo JC, Rajagopal R, Azar DT. Metaanalysis of cataract development after phakic intraocular lens surgery. *Journal of Cataract & Refractive Surgery*. 2008;34(7):1181–200.

46. Menezo JL, Peris-Martínez C, Cisneros-Lanuza AL, Martínez-Costa R. *Rate of cataract formation in 343 highly myopic eyes after implantation of three types of phakic intraocular lenses.* Slack Incorporated Thorofare, NJ; 2004. p. 317–24.

47. in Treatment TICL. US Food and Drug Administration clinical trial of the Implantable Contact Lens for moderate to high myopia. *Ophthalmology*. 2003;110(2):255–66.

48. Group IiToMS. United States Food and Drug Administration clinical trial of the Implantable Collamer Lens (ICL) for moderate to high myopia: three-year follow-up. *Ophthalmology*. 2004;111(9):1683–92.

49. Alhamzah A, Alharbi SS, Alfardan F, Aldebasi T, Almudhaiyan T. Indications for exchange or explantation of phakic implantable collamer lens with central port in patients with and without keratoconus. *International Journal of Ophthalmology*. 2021;14(11):1714.

50. Tahzib NG, Nuijts RM, Wu WY, Budo CJ. Long-term study of Artisan phakic intraocular lens implantation for the correction of moderate to high myopia: ten-year follow-up results. *Ophthalmology.* 2007;114(6):1133–42.

51. Senthil S, Reddy KP. A retrospective analysis of the first Indian experience on Artisan phakic intraocular lens. *Indian Journal of Ophthalmology.* 2006;54(4):251–5.

52. Fischinger IR, Wendelstein J, Tetz K, Bolz M, Tetz MR. Toric phakic IOLs in keratoconus—evaluation of preoperative parameters on the outcome of phakic anterior chamber lens implantation in patients with keratoconus. *Graefe's Archive for Clinical and Experimental Ophthalmology.* 2021;259:1643–9.

53. Fairaq R, Almutlak M, Almazyad E, Badawi AH, Ahad MA. Outcomes and complications of implantable collamer lens for mild to advance keratoconus. *International Ophthalmology.* 2021;41:2609–18.

54. Hashemian SJ, Saiepoor N, Ghiasian L, Aghai H, Jafari ME, Alemzadeh SP, et al. Long-term outcomes of posterior chamber phakic intraocular lens implantation in keratoconus. *Clinical and Experimental Optometry.* 2018;101(5):652–8.

55. Izquierdo Jr L, Henriquez MA, McCarthy M. Artiflex phakic intraocular lens implantation after corneal collagen cross-linking in keratoconic eyes. *Journal of Refractive Surgery.* 2011;27(7):482–7.

56. Güell JL, Morral M, Malecaze F, Gris O, Elies D, Manero F. Collagen crosslinking and toric iris-claw phakic intraocular lens for myopic astigmatism in progressive mild to moderate keratoconus. *Journal of Cataract & Refractive Surgery.* 2012;38(3):475–84.

57. Antonios R, Dirani A, Fadlallah A, Chelala E, Hamade A, Cherfane C, et al. Safety and visual outcome of visian toric ICL implantation after corneal collagen cross-linking in keratoconus: up to 2 years of follow-up. *Journal of Ophthalmology.* 2015;2015.

58. Dirani A, Fadlallah A, Khoueir Z, Antoun J, Cherfan G, Jarade E. Visian toric ICL implantation after intracorneal ring segments implantation and corneal collagen crosslinking in keratoconus. *European Journal of Ophthalmology.* 2014;24(3):338–44.

59. Abdelmassih Y, El-Khoury S, Chelala E, Slim E, Cherfan CG, Jarade E. Toric ICL implantation after sequential intracorneal ring segments implantation and corneal cross-linking in keratoconus: 2-year follow-up. *Journal of Refractive Surgery.* 2017;33(9):610–6.

60. Sakla HF, Altroudi W, Sakla YF, Muñoz G, Pineza C. Visual and refractive outcomes of toric implantable collamer lens implantation in stable keratoconus after combined topography-guided PRK and CXL. *Journal of Refractive Surgery.* 2021;37(12):824–9.

20 Corneal Transplantation in Keratoconus

Mohammad Soleimani and Ahmad Masoumi

INTRODUCTION

Historically, penetrating keratoplasty (PKP) was considered the only treatment option for patients with advanced keratoconus (KCN). However, thanks to the improvement of equipment and advances in surgical techniques, deep anterior lamellar keratoplasty (DALK) gradually replaced PKP as the most common corneal transplantation technique for advanced KCN.[1,2] The cornea is considered an "immune privileged site" and therefore the host and donor tissue do not need to be matched. Corneal transplantation (either PKP or DALKP) is indicated in eyes with advanced KCN. There are several classification schemes that define the stage of KCN based on corneal curvature, corneal thickness, and visual acuity (including Amsler–Krumeich and the ABCD grading system). However, recent studies found that there is little agreement between the grade of KCN and the impact of the disease on a patient's life.[3] Therefore, most authors now agree that corneal transplantation is indicated in patients with KCN when visual acuity has declined to unacceptable levels, spectacle correction is not sufficient, and contact lens wear is intolerable. The technique of corneal transplantation as a result of KCN does not differ significantly from keratoplasty performed for other etiologies. However, several pre-operative and intra-operative factors need to be taken into account when considering surgery for these patients.

MENTAL DISABILITY

Corneal surgeons are often consulted to manage KCN in a patient with mental disability. This is a rather common situation, due to high association of KCN and Down syndrome.[4] Patients with mental retardation tend to have a worse outcome after corneal transplantation, mostly due to higher incidences of post-operative complications.[5] These patients may frequently rub their eyes and they have a higher incidence of ocular self-trauma. This may lead to suture problems and increases the risk of infectious keratitis.DALK does not compromise the structure of the cornea as much as PKP; therefore, it seems to be more suitable for patients with mental retardation. Moreover, faster wound healing in DALK allows earlier suture removal that decreases the risk of corneal infection.[6]

MAXIMUM CORNEAL STEEPNESS (K_{MAX})

K_{max} is not believed to affect the outcome of PKP for KCN. However, there is growing evidence that eyes with K_{max}>60 D fare worse after DALK, due to Descemet's membrane (DM) folds that may develop in the visual axis after surgery.[7] These folds arise from the mismatch between the Descemet's membrane of the host and donor tissue. The stretched DM in a cornea with KCN has greater surface area compared with the posterior surface of the donor cornea. DM folds may resolve spontaneously one to two years after surgery.[7]

CORNEAL THICKNESS

Eyes with KCN need to be examined carefully for peripheral corneal thinning before planning for surgery. These eyes may need an oversized graft that may increase the risk of complications, including allograft rejection. In eyes with significant corneal thinning, a modified technique (tuck-in lamellar keratoplasty) provides tectonic support to the central and peripheral cornea. Moreover, peripheral corneal thinning is associated with DM fragility that increases the risk of DM perforation during a DALK procedure, especially if an "Anwar big bubble technique" is used. Therefore, "Melles manual dissection" may be the preferred technique for these eyes.

PRE-EXISTING CORNEAL SCAR

DALK can be successfully tried in corneal scars that do not involve DM. However, if the corneal scar reaches DM, the risk of perforation increases, especially if the "Anwar big bubble technique" is employed. Corneal hydrops may lead to corneal scars in eyes with advanced KCN. DM may be incorporated in the corneal scar and therefore many surgeons opt to proceed with PKP in these eyes. However, it has been shown that the corneal endothelium is healthy in eyes with a history of hydrops,[8] and therefore PKP should not be considered the only treatment option if a corneal scar is present in a patient with KCN. Eyes with a history of hydrops might especially benefit

DOI: 10.1201/9781003371601-20

from the lower risk of rejection in a DALK procedure, as PKP outcomes tend to be poorer in these eyes.[9] Several studies have demonstrated an increased risk of rejection in corneas with previous hydrops. It is postulated that the increased risk of allograft rejection is due to a higher prevalence of corneal neovascularization.[10,11] Moreover, allergic eye disease is more common in these eyes, leading to frequent eye rubbing and ocular surface disease. Anwar big bubble technique should not be tried in eyes with a corneal scar as the formation of a big bubble may lead to DM rupture. Melles manual dissection technique is the preferred approach for DALK in eyes with a corneal scar.

DONOR SIZE

In patients with KCN, the cone should be fully removed to circumvent the problem of recurrent disease. Therefore, the surgeon needs to define the cone location, which is usually displaced inferiorly. Slit-lamp examination and identification of Fleicher's iron ring can be very helpful for this goal. The host trephine is usually centered on the optical axis. The horizontal corneal diameter determines the size of the trephine used (normally 7.5 to 8.5 mm). The donor corneal button is approximately 0.25–0.5 mm less in diameter when it is punched from the endothelial surface, compared with epithelial surface. Therefore, using the current techniques, the donor button needs to be 0.25 to 0.50 mm larger than the host trephine.[12] Some surgeons prefer to undersize the donor button in patients with KCN to reduce post-operative myopia which means they use same size punching from the endothelial side. Every 0.25 mm reduction in the size of donor button creates a 2-D hyperopic shift.[13] However, one must be wary in this regard, as undersizing the donor button may circumvent the creation of a watertight wound closure.

SUTURING TECHNIQUE

Non-absorbable 10-0 nylon sutures are usually used to close the wound. The needle needs to be passed at approximately 90% of the depth of the donor tissue and then passed through the host cornea. The needle should engage the same amount of tissue in order to properly approximate the Bowman's membrane of the host and donor tissue. The first cardinal suture is placed at the 12 o'clock position. The second cardinal suture is placed at 6 o'clock position, 180° away from the first one. The second suture determines the final graft position. It needs to be placed in a position that divides the cornea in two equal halves so that the remaining sutures can be placed more symmetrically. Inappropriate positioning of this suture results in graft misalignment and increases post-operative astigmatism. The surgeon might choose one of these suturing techniques depending on his/her preference: interrupted sutures, combined interrupted and continuous sutures, single continuous sutures, or double continuous sutures. The frequency of post-operative astigmatism is similar in all these techniques.[14] The post-operative appearances of DALK and PKP procedures are shown in Figures 20.1 (A) and 20.1 (B), respectively.

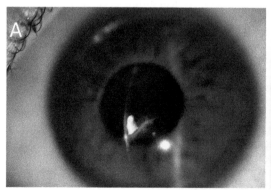
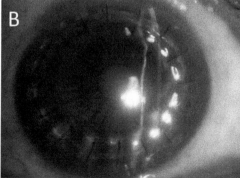

Figure 20.1 A: Post-operative day 3 after DALK in a patient with KCN. B: Three months after PKP in another patient with KCN.

SURGICAL TECHNIQUES FOR DALK

Anwar Big Bubble Method

Anwar and Teichman described the big bubble technique in 2002.[15] They observed that intrastromal injection of air creates cleavage planes just above the DM. Cornea is trephined at approximately 300–400 μm depth. A 27- or 30-gauge needle is then bent to 30–40° at 5 mm from its tip. The needle is advanced with the bevel facing down through the trephination groove and air is forcibly injected into the corneal stroma to detach the DM from the corneal stroma. The stromal tissue above the DM is then removed cautiously, avoiding the inadvertent perforation of DM at this stage. The DM and endothelium is removed from the donor tissue, and it is sutured to the host using one of the techniques described previously.

MELLES MANUAL METHOD

The anterior chamber is filled with air. A stromal pocket is then created using a superior scleral incision. A series of blunt spatulas are used to dissect the stromal tissue from the underlying DM. The surgeon judges the depth of stromal dissection by observing the distance from the tip of the instrument to a light reflex that is created by the difference in refractive indices of the intracameral air and the cornea. The host is then trephined and the donor button is sutured to the recipient cornea.

FEMTOSECOND LASER-ASSISTED KERATOPLASTY

Femtosecond laser-assisted keratoplasty was first introduced in 2006 as a new modification of the conventional corneal transplantation. The femtosecond laser is an infrared laser that delivers energy in very short pulses to create cuts in the cornea.[16,17] The laser-assisted keratoplasty involves several straight incisions that need to interact with each other in order to create a continuous wound that is easy to dissect. This new technology offers the possibility of creating customized cuts in donor and recipient corneas, that result in the perfect matching of donor and host corneas. Several configurations have been tried for donor and recipient corneas in laser- assisted keratoplasty, including top hat and mushroom configurations. In a top hat-based edge profile, the software creates a larger posterior diameter of the tissue compared with the anterior surface.[18] A mushroom-based edge profile is essentially the inverted version of top hat. This profile consists of a wider anterior side cut compared with the posterior side cut, which makes it suitable for anterior surface surgery, including KCN.

OUTCOMES

About 40% of patients with advanced KCN that undergo PKP reach a final uncorrected visual acuity (UCVA) of 20/40 or better.[19,20] Irregular astigmatism may arise in the graft in the long term which limits the ability of spectacles to correct vision. DALK, if performed properly, has the same visual outcome.[21,22] Residual stromal tissue on the DM as a result of incomplete stromal dissection limits the visual improvement after DALK. Moreover, large intra-operative DM perforations are associated with a worse visual outcome. Visual recovery seems to be quicker after DALK compared with PKP, due to earlier suture removal. DALK eliminates the risk of endothelial rejection, although it seems that the risk of graft failure is almost twice as high in DALK compared with PKP.[23] Endothelial cell loss (ECL) is much lower in DALK than in PKP. One study found that ECL is as high as 34.6% after PKP, compared with 13.9% after DALK.[24]

REFERENCES

1. Boimer C, Lee K, Sharpen L, Mashour RS, Slomovic AR. Evolving surgical techniques of and indications for corneal transplantation in Ontario from 2000 to 2009. *Canadian Journal of Ophthalmology*. 2011;46:360–6.

2. Reddy JC, Hammersmith KM, Nagra PK, Rapuano CJ. The role of penetrating keratoplasty in the era of selective lamellar keratoplasty. *International Ophthalmology Clinics*. 2013;53:91–101.

3. Sahebjada S, Fenwick EK, Xie J, Snibson GR, Daniell MD, Baird PN. Impact of keratoconus in the better eye and the worse eye on vision-related quality of life. *Investigative Ophthalmology & Visual Science*. 2014;55:412–6.

4. Wroblewski KJ, Mader TH, Torres MF, Parmley VC, Rotkis WM. Long-term graft survival in patients with down syndrome after penetrating keratoplasty. *Cornea*. 2006;25:1026–8.

5. García GPG, Martínez JB. Outcomes of penetrating keratoplasty in mentally retarded patients with keratoconus. *Cornea*. 2008;27:980–7.

6. Haugen OH, Høvding G, Eide GE, Bertelsen T. Corneal grafting for keratoconus in mentally retarded patients. *Acta Ophthalmologica Scandinavica*. 2001;79:609–15.

7. Mohamed S, Manna A, Amissah-Arthur K, McDonnell P. Non-resolving Descemet folds 2 years following deep anterior lamellar keratoplasty: the impact on visual outcome. *Contact Lens and Anterior Eye*. 2009;32:300–2.

8. Alsuhaibani AH, Al-Rajhi AA, Al-Motowa SM, Wagoner MD. Corneal endothelial cell density and morphology after acute hydrops in keratoconus. *Cornea*. 2008;27:535–8.

9. Maharana PK, Sharma N, Vajpayee RB. Acute corneal hydrops in keratoconus. *Indian Journal of Ophthalmology*. 2013;61:461.

10. Maurice D, Zauberman H, Michaelson I. The stimulus to neovascularization in the cornea. *Experimental Eye Research*. 1966;5:168-IN8.

11. Rowson NJ, Dart J, Buckley RJ. Corneal neovascularisation in acute hydrops. *Eye*. 1992;6:404–6.

12. Olson RJ. Variation in corneal graft size related to trephine technique. *Archives of Ophthalmology*. 1979;97:1323–5.

13. Wilson SE, Bourne WM. Effect of recipient-donor trephine size disparity on refractive error in keratoconus. *Ophthalmology*. 1989;96:299–305.

14. Javadi MA, Naderi M, Zare M, Jenaban A, Rabei HM, Anissian A. Comparison of the effect of three suturing techniques on postkeratoplasty astigmatism in keratoconus. *Cornea*. 2006;25:1029–33.

15. Anwar M, Teichmann KD. Big-bubble technique to bare Descemet's membrane in anterior lamellar keratoplasty. *Journal of Cataract & Refractive Surgery*. 2002;28:398–403.

16. Price Jr FW, Price MO. Femtosecond laser shaped penetrating keratoplasty: one-year results utilizing a top-hat configuration. *American Journal of Ophthalmology*. 2008;145:210–4.e2.

17. Peng W-y, Tang Z-m, Lian X-f, Zhou S-y. Comparing the efficacy and safety of femtosecond laser-assisted vs conventional penetrating keratoplasty: a meta-analysis of comparative studies. *International Ophthalmology*. 2021;41:2913–23.

18. Bahar I, Kaiserman I, Srinivasan S, Berger Y, McAllum P, Slomovic A, et al. Manual top hat wound configuration for penetrating keratoplasty. *Cornea*. 2008;27:521–6.

19. Sutton G, Hodge C, McGhee CN. Rapid visual recovery after penetrating keratoplasty for keratoconus. *Clinical & Experimental Ophthalmology*. 2008;36:725–30.

20. Javadi MA, Motlagh BF, Jafarinasab MR, Rabbanikhah Z, Anissian A, Souri H, et al. Outcomes of penetrating keratoplasty in keratoconus. *Cornea*. 2005;24:941–6.

21. Fontana L, Parente G, Sincich A, Tassinari G. Influence of graft–host interface on the quality of vision after deep anterior lamellar keratoplasty in patients with keratoconus. *Cornea*. 2011;30:497–502.

22. Funnell C, Ball J, Noble B. Comparative cohort study of the outcomes of deep lamellar kerato-plasty and penetrating keratoplasty for keratoconus. *Eye*. 2006;20:527–32.

23. Jones MN, Armitage WJ, Ayliffe W, Larkin DF, Kaye SB. Penetrating and deep anterior lamel-lar keratoplasty for keratoconus: a comparison of graft outcomes in the United Kingdom. *Investigative Ophthalmology & Visual Science*. 2009;50:5625–9.

24. Zhang Y-m, Wu S-q, Yao Y-f. Long-term comparison of full-bed deep anterior lamellar kera-toplasty and penetrating keratoplasty in treating keratoconus. *Journal of Zhejiang University SCIENCE B*. 2013;14:438–50.

21 Femtosecond Laser-Assisted Penetrating Keratoplasty in Keratoconus

Hassan Hashemi and Saeid Shahhosseini

INTRODUCTION

Penetrating keratoplasty is the last but the best approach to the treatment of advanced KCN and has been well established for more than one century.[1,2] As the last shot, the more accurate and precise the procedure, the better the result. Despite the refinement of surgical tools and techniques, this procedure is still mostly performed manually by trephining the recipient's cornea and punching the donor's one, then suturing in different ways. Apart from graft rejection, induced corneal irregular astigmatism is the main obstacle to achieving the best possible vision. Although the skill and experience of the surgeon are very important factors, the irregular cut edges due to manual cutting are a serious factor in this issue. Furthermore, tight sutures for preventing leakage in such mismatched and irregular cut edges make the situation worse. On the other hand, the stability and the wound strength in a butt-joint-shaped interface in the conventional method are compromised and vulnerable, even in not-so-serious traumas. Thus, creating a regular, precise, and patterned cutting-edge would theoretically improve and (relatively) solve these problems in achieving a good and stable vision.

The femtosecond laser is an infrared laser with pulses of femtosecond duration. Its fine, focused, and contiguous pulses can create a very precise, accurate, and reproducible cut in a desired orientation and depth of the cornea, leaving surrounding tissue unaffected and undamaged.[3,4] By performing the first femtosecond laser-enabled keratoplasty (FLEK) (also named laser-assisted keratoplasty (FLAK)) in 2005, in which both recipient and donor corneas were prepared by laser, a new and promising window was opened in corneal grafting.[5,6]

PATIENT SELECTION AND PROCEDURE

Regarding the limitation of laser penetration, ducking, and suction during laser procedure, patients with significant and dense corneal scars and opacities at the laser zone, considerable surface irregularities, elevated filtering blebs or shunts, deep-set eyes with small orbits and also impending perforation eyes should be excluded. In addition, due to IOP rising during laser, the retina should be examined carefully before planning.

In conventional penetrating keratoplasty (CPKP), the axial and radial forces during mechanical cutting cause rough and irregular edges, especially when cutting of the donor button is performed from the endothelial side. So, the donor button size should be considered 0.25–0.50 mm larger than the recipient trephination size to compensate for the eventual mismatch. But, with the use of the femtosecond laser, both recipient and donor corneas are accurately lasered and cut from the epithelial side and therefore the donor tissue could be oversized by only 0.1 mm.[7]

The donor cornea may be prepared in two ways. If we have a whole globe, first, the IOP should be optimized by injecting balanced salt situation (BSS) or saline into the vitreous and, after wrapping in a sterile gauze and fixing it with a clamp, carry out the lasering. In the case of the precut cornea, it should be assembled on the artificial chamber for being lasered (Figure 21.1).

After 2005 and applying femtosecond laser in PKP, several laser machines have been equipped with relevant software to perform FLEK. Intralase, FEMTEC, VisuMax, FemtoLDV, Wavelight FS200, and VICTUS platforms have this ability with their own nomograms and profiles. Apart from the straight cut (butt-joint), which has the benefit of accuracy compared with the conventional technique, the main advantage of FLEK is in its patterned cuts. By femtosecond laser, we can create a posterior side cut, a lamellar cut, and an anterior side cut with desired angles to each other, in both the host and donor corneas. The various combinations of those cuts create different patterns for shaped keratoplasty depending on the femtosecond machine and its software. The theoretical superiority of these patterns is to enhance wound integrity and matching, so that less suture tension would be needed. The most common ones are the top hat, mushroom, zig-zag, and Christmas tree patterns (Figure 21.2). Although all these patterns make more wound surface area, integrity, and strength, depending on the special characteristics of each one, they have their own applications and uses. The mushroom-shaped incision pattern may be superior in KCN by covering a greater anterior surface, while the top hat-shaped incision pattern has an advantage in endothelial disease by providing more endothelial cells. All in all, among these patterns, the zig-zag seems to be more practical and effective with fewer complications, according to the reports. The

DOI: 10.1201/9781003371601-21

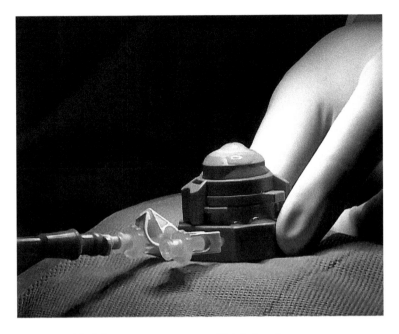

Figure 21.1 An assembled donor cornea on an artificial chamber.

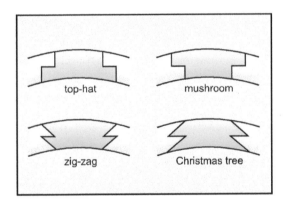

Figure 21.2 The most common laser patterns.

zig-zag profile improves wound opposition and healing by increasing the donor–recipient contact area. It consists of a horizontal lamellar cut with two side cuts oriented at 30°, so that sutures could easily be placed at approximately 50% depth at the outer tip of the Z (Figure 21.3). The top hat profile has technical difficulties in deep suturing through the posterior wing of the donor tissue to avoid posterior wound gape. The mushroom pattern has the risk of protrusion of the anterior wing between sutures and subsequent surface problems.[4,8–12]

An accurate pachymetry is necessary before laser application. Preparing a pachymetry map could be done by anterior OCT, Pentacam, or ultrasound in at least four quadrants of the laser zone. Then, according to the considered profile and nomogram of each machine, the pattern of laser and depth, diameter, and angle of each cut would be designed. In order to prevent wound leakage and infection, the laser cut in the recipient's cornea in the laser room should not be complete and an uncut bridge at the posterior side cut is crucial (approximately 70–75 μm) (Figure 21.4). Then, this uncut bridge could be easily dissected with a knife and the anterior chamber would be opened in a sterile situation in the operating room. As the laser begins from the posterior to the anterior of the cornea, the appearance of air bubbles in the anterior chamber is a sign of a too-deep posterior side cut which should be immediately corrected. In the operating room, the donor cornea is first separated and removed from the whole globe or the artificial chamber by gentle and blunt

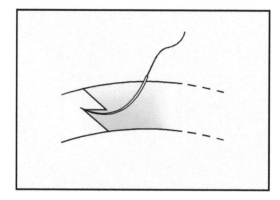

Figure 21.3 The suturing of the zig-zag pattern cut.

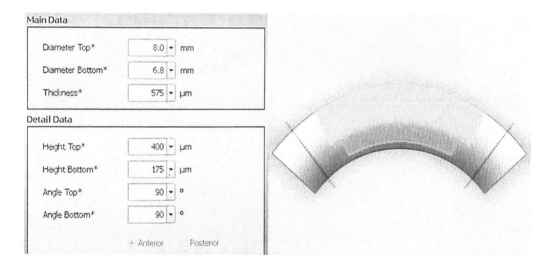

Figure 21.4 An uncut bridge in patient cornea.

dissection. After making sure that it is perfect, it is time to dissect and cut the uncut bridge of the patient's cornea (Figure 21.5). Suturing techniques are like conventional PKP, although regarding the patterned cut edge, as mentioned before, good apposition is crucial in achieving optimum results and preventing complications (Figure 21.6).

BENEFITS AND DRAWBACKS

Theoretically, FLEK should have many advantages over the CPKP, such as faster suture removal, faster visual recovery, lower post-operative astigmatism, more wound stability, and fewer complications. In the first decade after introducing FLEK to the world of ophthalmology, the studies mentioned some advantages of it. In most of them, faster suture removal, reduced astigmatism, better BCVA, lower risk of graft rejection, and lower rates of endothelial cell loss were reported compared with CPKP.[11,13–16] But, with more studies, as cases and follow-up time increased, the results turned out to be different. Although incisions made by laser are precise and regular, post-operative astigmatism and BCVA are also associated with many other factors. A recent meta-analysis showed that FLEK may not be superior to CPKP in decreasing post-operative topographic astigmatism and reported comparable spherical equivalent, graft rejection/ graft failure and complications between them.[17] Another, more recent meta-analysis revealed that there is no significant long-term visual disparity between FLEK and CPKP, although FLEK may be superior during the early six months post-operatively.[18]

In terms of laser equipment and logistical issues, costs, and risk of possible immune reaction from the femtosecond laser, it seems to be logical to select FLEK, regarding the patient's demands

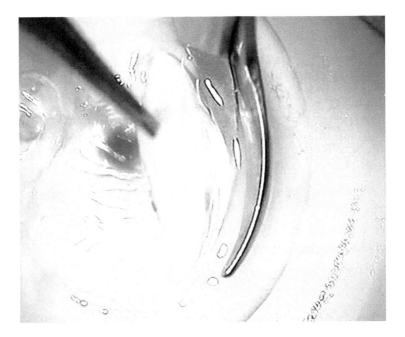

Figure 21.5 Scissoring the uncut bridge in the operating room.

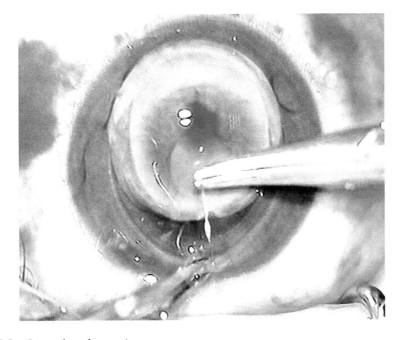

Figure 21.6 Corneal graft suturing.

and economic situation. According to our limited experience and also available studies, it seems reasonable to choose FLEK (especially zig-zag or even butt-joint patterns) only in selected KCN cases until well-designed prospective randomized controlled trials reveal more facts.

REFERENCES

1. Elschnig A. Keratoplasty. *Arch Ophthalmol*. 1930; 4: 165–173.

2. Moffatt SL, Cartwright VA, Stumpf TH. Centennial review of corneal transplantation. *Clin Exp Ophthalmol.* 2005; 33: 624–657.

3. Juhasz T, Djotyan G, Loesel FH, Kurtz RM, Horvath C, Bille JF, et al. Application of femtosecond lasers in corneal surgery. *Laser Phys.* 2000; 10: 495–500.

4. Mian SI, Shtein RM. Femtosecond laser-assisted corneal surgery. *Curr Opin Ophthalmol.* 2007; 18(4): 295–299.

5. Farid M, Steinert RF. Femtosecond laser-assisted corneal surgery. *Curr Opin Ophthalmol.* 2010; 21(4): 288–292.

6. Slade SG. Applications for the femtosecond laser in corneal surgery. *Curr Opin Ophthalmol.*2007; 18(4): 338–341.

7. Deshmukh R, Stevenson LJ. Vajpayee RB. Laser-assisted corneal transplantation surgery. *Surv Ophthalmol.* 2021, Sep-Oct; 66(5): 826–837.

8. Asota I, Farid M, Garg S, Steinert RF. Femtosecond Laser- enabled keratoplasty. Int Ophthalmol Clin. 2013 Spring; 53(2): 103–114.

9. Buratto L, Bohm E. The use of the femtosecond laser in penetrating keratoplasty. *Am J Ophthalmol.* 2007; 143: 737–742.

10. Birnbaum F, Wiggermann A, Major PC, et al. Clinical results of 123 femtosecond laser-assisted penetrating keratoplasty. *Graefes Arch Clin Exp Ophthalmol.* 2012.

11. Bahar I, Kaiserman I, Lange AP, et al. Femtosecond laser versus manual dissection for top-hat penetrating keratoplasty. *Br J Ophthalmol.* 2009; 93: 73–78.

12. Price FW, Price MO. Femtosecond laser shaped penetrating keratoplasty: one- year results utilizing a top- hat configuration. *Am J Ophthalmol.* 2008; 145: 210–214.

13. Chamberlin WD, Ruck SW, Mathers WD, Cabezas M, Fraunfelder FW. Comparison of femtosecond Laser- assisted keratoplasty versus conventional penetrating keratoplasty. *Ophthalmology.* 2011; 118(3): 486–491.

14. Daniel MC, Böheringer D, Maier P, Eberwein P, Birnbaum F, Reinhard T. Comparison of long-term outcomes of femtosecond laser-assisted keratoplasty with conventional keratoplast. *Cornea.* 2016; 35(3): 293–298.

15. Levinger E, Trivizki O, Levinger S, Kremer I. Outcome of mushroom pattern femtosecond laser-assisted keratoplasty versus conventional penetrating keratoplasty in patients with keratoconus. *Cornea.* 2014; 33(5): 481–485.

16. Kamiya K, Kabashi H, Shimizu K, Igarashi A. Clinical outcomes of penetrating keratoplasty performed with the VisuMax femtosecond Laser system and comparison with conventional penetrating keratoplasty. *PLoS One.* 2014; 9(8): e105464.

17. Liu Y, Li W, Jiu X, Tian M. Systematic review and meta-analysis of femtosecond Laser-enabled keratoplasty versus conventional penetrating keratoplasty. *Eur J Ophthalmol.* 2021 May; 31(3): 976–987.

18. Peng WY, Tang ZM, Lian XF, Zhou SY. Comparing the efficacy and safety of femtosecond laser-assisted vs. conventional penetrating keratoplasty: a meta-analysis of comparative studies. *Int Ophthalmol.* 2021 Aug; 41(8): 2913–2923.

22 Femtosecond Laser-Assisted Deep Anterior Lamellar Keratoplasty

Ramin Salouti and M. Hossein Nowroozzadeh

INTRODUCTION

A femtosecond laser emits laser energy bursts at an extremely fast rate, making it an optical system with remarkable precision and predictability for creating surgical incisions in transparent tissues, surpassing manual techniques. The femtosecond laser was first introduced in the United States during the early portion of the 1990s, following its development by Prof. Ron M. Kurtz at the University of Michigan. In 2001, the femtosecond laser attained approval from the US Food and Drug Administration for utilization in laser-assisted *in-situ* keratomileusis, or LASIK eye surgery.[1] With later advancements, femtosecond laser systems became capable of more complex tasks and were integrated into cataract surgery and keratoplasty platforms.[2]

One of the primary advantages of using femtosecond lasers in keratoplasty is the ability to custom-create various rim shapes, which provide better vertical and rotational stability of the graft compared to manual trephination. Moreover, due to the larger surface area of the graft–host interface, femtosecond lasers are associated with more rapid wound healing.[3–6] In this chapter, we will focus on the most widely-used techniques for femto-assisted deep anterior lamellar kerato-plasty (DALK).

PHYSICAL PROPERTIES

As ophthalmologists, it's crucial for us to understand the underlying physics of femtosecond lasers to optimize surgical outcomes and stay up-to-date with technological advancements. Femtosecond lasers emit ultrashort pulses of light, lasting about 10^{-15} second (a femtosecond). These pulses are generated using a process called mode-locking, which synchronizes the phases of multiple longitudinal modes within a laser cavity, resulting in constructive interference and the formation of ultrashort pulses. The most commonly used femtosecond laser type in ophthalmology is the solid-state, Ti: sapphire laser, which offers a broad tuning range, high peak powers, and excellent beam quality.[7–9]

The interaction between femtosecond laser pulses and ophthalmic tissue is characterized by a process called nonlinear multiphoton absorption. In this process, the high peak intensity of the ultrashort pulse allows for the simultaneous absorption of multiple photons, leading to the generation of a free electron. Subsequent collisions between the free electron and other atoms within the tissue cause localized ionization, creating a plasma. The rapid expansion and collapse of this plasma generate an acoustic shock wave, which mechanically disrupts the tissue, resulting in a precise and localized photodisruption effect. This process minimizes collateral thermal damage to surrounding tissue, making femtosecond lasers ideal for delicate ophthalmic procedures.[10]

PRE-OPERATIVE EVALUATION

In DALK, the primary indication is a diseased cornea with a healthy endothelium. The pre-operative assessment should include a comprehensive ocular examination, with special attention paid to the retina, optic nerve, and lens status. A detailed slit-lamp examination of the cornea should be performed to detect Fuchs' endothelial dystrophy, posterior polymorphous dystrophy, irido-corneal endothelial syndrome, and any breaks in Descemet's membrane (DM). Corneal imaging, including corneal tomography, is essential to determine the severity of the disease and locate the cone in keratoconus eyes for preparation of the femtosecond setting.

Specular microscopy is necessary to objectively evaluate the endothelial cells, while anterior segment optical coherence tomography (OCT) may be required to determine the depth of the opacity and pathology. Measuring the best-corrected visual acuity with rigid gas-permeable lenses is crucial in order to obtain the most accurate post-operative vision measurement and detect any amblyopia or functional component.

SURGICAL TECHNIQUES

The femto-assisted DALK operation consists of two main stages. The first stage is the laser treatment for making proper corneal incisions in donor and recipient tissues, which is typically performed under topical anesthesia. The second stage, the main transplant operation, is usually accomplished under general anesthesia (or local anesthesia) in an operating room.

DOI: 10.1201/9781003371601-22

Femtosecond Laser Treatment

Several femtosecond laser platforms have been successfully used for laser-assisted keratoplasty. Although some energy settings and corneal rim shape patterns may differ between devices, the main surgical concept is similar. Therefore, if one has learned to do surgery with one platform, you can easily do it with other systems by using minor modifications in the device's setting. The most femto-DALK experiences of the main author of this chapter (RS) were with the VICTUS™ platform (software version 3.4.1.7; TECHNOLAS Perfect Vision, Bausch & Lomb, Munich, Germany). The VICTUS femtosecond laser is a versatile platform that consists of a pulsed solid laser with a repetition rate of 80–160 kHz that emits laser radiation with a wavelength of 1040 ± 25 nm and features a pulse duration of 290–550 fs. It also integrates swept-source (2S) OCT technology for online, continuous viewing of the entire keratoplasty procedures.

Femtosecond Laser Setting

Proper femtosecond laser settings are crucial for successful femto-assisted DALK. All femtosecond platforms have fixed characteristics regarding the laser wavelength, pulse duration, pulse frequency, and power output, which are not intended to be manipulated by the operator. However, there are two other classes of laser settings that can be adjusted.

The first is energy settings plus spacings of laser bursts within the corneal bed and rim, which help for smooth and effective tissue dissection. Other settings related to the graft–host interface geometry, such as rim shape, depth, cutting angle, outer radius, diameter, and length, all affect one another, and their manipulation will determine the results. We should also consider the disease to be treated and the ocular characteristics of the recipient (e.g., corneal diameter, pachymetry, etc.) when finalizing the laser settings.

Laser Energy Settings

The laser energy settings are similar for donor and recipient tissue. For the purpose of side cut, we set laser energy at 1.3 to 1.5 μJ, with spot spacing at 5.0 μm and line spacing equal to 2.0 μm. The top bonus of 100 microns is optimal to ensure full thickness cut. The arc length is a 360-degree corneal incision and could be started from any angle (usually set at 180 degrees). For the purpose of bed preparation in lamellar keratoplasty, the energy is set at 0.9 to 1.0 μJ, with both spot spacing and line spacing at 5.0 μm. The required energy may be influenced by machine/environmental factors and differs slightly according to the optical clarity of the tissue.

Rim Shape

The rim shape can be selected as circular (round) vs. polygonal (decagonal). The round rim shape is similar to manual trephination and is the most widely used method. The decagonal rim shape has the ability to finely respect and follow the topographic position of the donor on the recipient. The angles may also resist graft rotation. The exact value of the decagonal rim shape is yet to be determined.

Side Cut Shape

The side cut can be straight (conventional) or stepped (Figure 22.1). The decagonal rim shape can only accept a straight side cut, but the round rim shape can accept all figures. Compared with straight rim cuts, stepped rim cuts increase the surface of the donor-recipient interface and are claimed to enhance the wound healing process after keratoplasty.[3] They may also improve the initial wound seal and prevent the long-term risk of post-operative graft rotation.

A mushroom side cut can be applied for a variety of corneal diseases, especially keratoconus. The midplane depth is set to half of the pachymetry value and is typically smaller than the anterior diameter of the graft. The optimal side cut angle at the top and bottom incisions is 90 degrees.[6,11] The mushroom pattern is ideal for anterior corneal disorders, such as keratoconus and pellucid marginal degeneration (PMD) because a greater area of superficial cornea is transplanted compared with deep cornea. This configuration also allows for more direct visualization of deeper corneal tissue, which is useful in the Big Bubble technique (Figure 22.1). The anvil pattern resembles the mushroom, but the posterior edge of the upper side cut slants outward. In this method, the femtosecond laser creates a precise incision in the cornea in the shape of an inverted "V." The incision is made at a depth of approximately 90% of the corneal thickness and is followed by the removal of the diseased corneal tissue.[12–14] This pattern allows for a larger healing surface of grafted tissue.

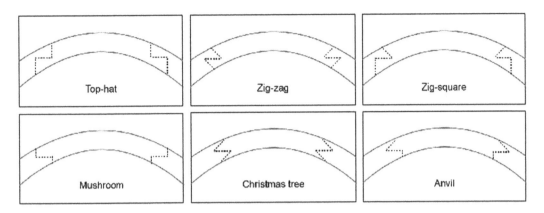

Figure 22.1 Different configurations of the side-cut.

The zig-zag-shaped side cut is more complex than other rim patterns and offers more biomechanical strength and the largest wound healing area. This profile has slanted anterior and posterior side cuts that are connected by a ring lamellar cut in the half-pachymetry value. If the side cut angle is set at 120 degrees, the midplane diameter is larger than the anterior diameter (typical zig-zag), and, if the side cut is set at 60 degrees, the midplane diameter is smaller than the anterior diameter (the Christmas tree pattern). The zig-zag pattern may be useful for various cornea disorders where rapid healing is the main concern (Figure 22.1).[15,16]

The top-hat side cut is the reverse of the mushroom pattern, so the midplane diameter is larger than the anterior diameter. This configuration is usually recommended for posterior corneal diseases such as Fuchs' endothelial dystrophy or bullous keratopathy. In a typical top-hat, the angulation of vertical side cuts is 90 degrees. If the posterior edge of the upper side cut slants inward, it again adds more wound strength and healing surface and is named the flask profile (or zig-square) (Figure 22.1).[17,18]

Cutting Angle

The projection of the laser beam onto the corneal surface can be deviated from 90 degrees. According to the cutting angle, the projected arc length will differ for the various depths of tissue, and, consequently, the achieved diameter will vary.

The cutting angle is defined as the angle between the corneal surface tangent and the incision plane (Figure 22.2). In the VICTUS system, increasing the cutting angle (from 80 or 90 towards 120 degrees) of a straight side cut (with either a round or decagonal rim shape) will increase the

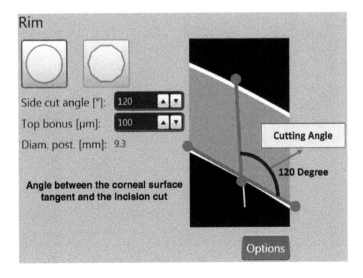

Figure 22.2 The definition of the cutting angle in the VICTUS platform.

posterior diameter of the graft (in either donor or recipient) compared with the anterior diameter, and vice versa. Decreasing the side cut angle below 90 degrees leads to a larger anterior than posterior diameter. For example, if the anterior diameter of the cornea is set at 9.30 mm with a cutting angle of 80 degrees, the actual posterior diameter of the graft will be calculated as 8.50 mm (about 0.8 mm smaller). If the anterior diameter of the cornea is set at 9.30 mm with a cutting angle of 120 degrees, the posterior diameter of the graft is about 9.40 mm (approximately 0.1 mm larger). In our experience with VICTUS, the cutting angle of 120 degrees provides an excellent donor-recipient interface for most indications. Please note that the cutting angle should be the same for the donor and recipient.

Diameter of the Graft

The anterior diameter of the recipient is determined by the white-to-white (WTW) distance and the space of about 1.5 mm required for suturing around the graft: diameter of recipient = WTW – (1.5 mm × 2). To calculate the anterior diameter of the donor cornea, add 0.2 mm disparity to the recipient diameter. The posterior diameter of the recipient or donor is automatically calculated by your recommended cutting angle (or side cut pattern). In the VICTUS platform, the anterior and posterior graft diameters are almost the same when you pick up the cutting angle of 120 degrees (which is recommended by the author).

Pachymetry is related to the thickness of the corneal bottom at the determined diameter. Cutting depth is measured by tissue swelling plus a bonus at the bottom and top for cutting the whole depth of the donor (30 to 40% of pachymetry). The posterior diameter of the donor is automatically calculated by your recommended cutting angle (Figure 22.3).

Pachymetry is related to the thickness of the recipient at the determined diameter. Cutting depth is determined by the technique of your surgery. In the Melles technique, the cutting depth is set at 310 μm as default, and the ratio according to the pachymetry is calculated (Figure 22.3).

Different Techniques

Femto-assisted DALK can be accomplished via two main techniques: the Melles or the Big Bubble techniques. The laser setting of the Melles technique is similar to penetrating keratoplasty (PKP) (with all straight and stepped rim cut configurations) except for the pachymetry setting, which should be set at 310 μm. In the Big Bubble technique, you can use one of the two femtosecond laser settings: the conventional method, which only uses lamellar keratoplasty with a depth of 300 μm or more (considering the thinnest pachymetry value), and the DALK Incision technique (which will be explained later in this chapter).

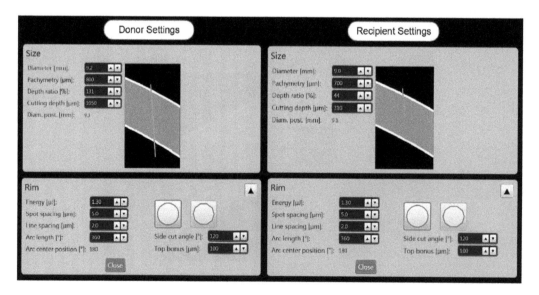

Figure 22.3 Illustration of the optimal donor and recipient laser settings for femto-assisted DALK with the Melles technique, using the VICTUS system.

There is no consensus regarding which laser treatment should be performed first: the donor or the recipient? We prefer to do laser cuts on the recipient tissue first because of the unplanned modifications and customizations that may be required on the recipient cornea. Then, we can make adjustments on the donor cornea to match the recipient. This approach, however, demands another corneal bottom in reserve.[5,19]

Different Methods for Recipient Bed Preparation

Melles Technique

Laser Room Procedures

In this technique, recipient tissue preparation is performed under local anesthesia in a dust-free, dry operating room using the following steps:

Guide and inform the patient to lie down on the femtosecond laser bed, and ensure that the patient's legs are not crossed. Secure and fix the patient's head in the molded headrest with fine adjustments in order that the cornea is placed in the horizontal plane position.

After prep and drape, both eyes of the patient are anesthetized using topical 0.5% tetracaine hydrochloride, and the lid speculum is inserted. After confirming the setting of the femtosecond for the recipient, the patient's interface kit plastic bag is opened. Then, the suction clip is also opened and placed centrally over the eye, respecting the geometrical center of the cornea (Videos 1–3).

In the next step, the vacuum of the suction clip is activated. The patient's bed slowly moves upward, and docking of the eye to the space cone is accomplished by perpendicular applanation using X, Y, and Z plane adjustments, and closing of the suction clip by pressing the ends of the clip (Video 4).

The achievement of a perfectly symmetrical position of the cornea is observed using OCT live video while dealing with cone positioning (Video 5). The exact central location of the corneal incision in respect to the geometrical center of the cornea and pupil position is guaranteed with a three-click centration button or aligning the treatment area to the pupil or the limbus manually by dragging and dropping the circle of treatment in the correct position.

At this point, the start button is pressed, and then the PROCEDURE footswitch is activated to start the laser treatment. After complete corneal laser dissection, the suction is turned off, and the fixation ring and patient interface are removed. Next, the eye is protected by a shield and patch, and the patient is transferred to the main operating room for the following steps of the procedure.

Donor tissue preparation is performed in the same setting immediately after the recipient cornea is prepared. All donor tissues are stored in cold storage medium (Optisol) and are received from the Eye Bank as corneoscleral buttons. The corneoscleral size should be at least 17 to 18 mm to prevent leakage and ensure appropriate engagement within the artificial chamber. As previously mentioned, another donor tissue should be available as a reserve for safeguarding against any unpredictable event.

The donor cornea is mounted on a Barron artificial anterior chamber (Katena, Denville, NJ, USA) filled with a dispersive viscoelastic material (Coatel, Bausch & Lomb, Waterford, Ireland) or balanced salt solution (BSS), and the pressure is raised to achieve a proper condition. Then, the cornea is repositioned to lay center in the artificial chamber, the corneal epithelium is removed using a cellulose sponge, and the head of the cone is applanated over the geometrical center of the cornea. The donor laser setting is similar to the recipient regarding the rim profile or stepped rim configuration, except for the donor size, which is larger (our suggestion for donor–recipient disparity is 0.2 to 0.5 mm).

After further adjustments of corneal incision centration using OCT live video, the position of the corneal incision is manually verified, and laser shooting is started (Video 6). At the conclusion of the procedure, the applanation cone is removed, and the donor cornea is transferred to the main operating room.

Manual Surgical Procedures

The procedure is started under local or general anesthesia (the latter being preferred by the surgeon and patient) by rechecking the centration of the femtosecond corneal incision (Video 7). The superior rectus muscle is secured with a stay suture (Video 8), and a limbus-based localized peritomy is created in the supratemporal area of the bulbar conjunctiva (Video 9). To begin deep layer dissection within the cornea, a scleral incision (4-mm length and 310-μm depth) is created 1.5 mm behind the limbus using a diamond knife (Video 10). Deep corneal dissection is started through the scleral incision using a diamond or metal crescent knife up to 1 mm inside the cornea (Video 11). At this point, a self-sealing side port incision is made in the supratemporal (right eye) or supranasal (left eye) quadrant (Video 12), and the aqueous humor is aspirated and replaced with air (Video 13).

The most critical point of the Melles technique is to begin with dissection at a proper depth, deeply in the pre-Descemet area using a special corneal splitter (deep lamellar corneal dissector, 6–607; Duckworth & Kent). To achieve that goal, there are four steps. In the first step, using the semi-sharp end of the spatula, deep dissection of the cornea is started at a 45-degree angle to the corneal surface (Video 14). The dissection is advanced in the same manner until the dark area around the leading edge of the spatula becomes thinner. This dark band represents a non-reflective area between the specular light reflex of the cornea and the bright tip of the spatula and represents approximately half of the real non-incised corneal tissue at the back (Figure 22.4). By gauging this dark band, a proper plane could be found, and progress with steps 2–4 can be made.

The second step is deep dissection of the left third of the cornea (for a right-handed surgeon). It is practical to frequently check the plane depth during the dissection by pressing the spatula over the remaining stroma (and assessing the dark band width) (Video 15). The next step of the pre-Descemet dissection is continued on the right one-third of the cornea up to the limbus (Video 16). The last step is accomplished on the middle one-third of the cornea by severing the remaining bridges between the nasal and temporal dissections (Video 17).

After complete dissection of the cornea from limbus to limbus, the scleral tunnel is closed with a 10–0 Nylon suture (Video 18), and the air is removed from the anterior chamber (Video 19). Then, the created corneal pocket is filled with viscoelastic material (Video 20), and the

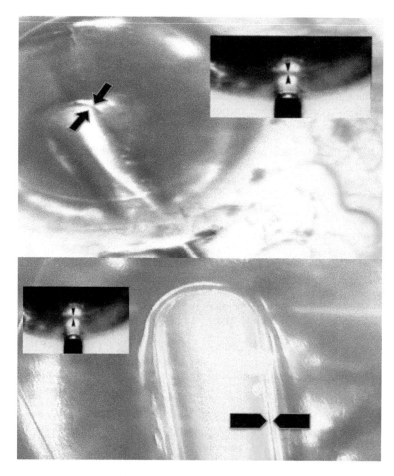

Figure 22.4 Illustrates the dark band or non-reflective area between the specular light reflex of the cornea and the bright tip of the spatula (between arrows), which approximately represents one-half of the real non-incised corneal tissue at the back of the cornea.

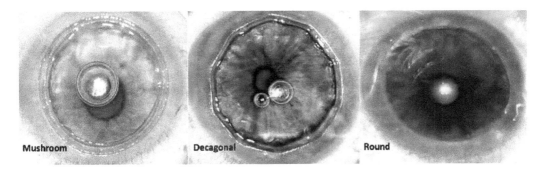

Figure 22.5   Illustration of different rim shapes that are possible using the VICTUS system.

femtosecond-crafted anterior corneal side-cut is loosened with a Sinskey hook and opened using a sharp 15° metal knife (Video 21). Finally, the posterior side-cut incisions are released using curved corneal scissors (Video 22), and the anterior corneal cap is removed (Video 23) (Figure 22.5).

The same procedure is performed on the donor cornea while mounting over the artificial chamber to open the anterior and posterior side cuts using a Sinskey hook. The corneal graft is irrigated to clean remaining viscoelastic materials (Video 24). It is optional to remove the endothelium from the donor cornea or leave it in place. We prefer to remove the donor DM and endothelium with a dry cellulose sponge and smooth tooth forceps (Video 25).

At this point, we proceed with the final stages of transplantation. The recipient bed is vigorously irrigated with balanced salt solution to clear all viscoelastic and cell debris from the corneal bed (Video 26). Then, the donor button is transferred to the recipient stromal bed (Video 27) and sutured with 10–0 monofilament Nylon sutures (Video 28).

There are different accepted patterns for corneal graft suturing, including interrupted sutures, running (continuous) method, or a combination thereof. The running sutures could have a rotational predilection and are classified into anti-torque, torque, or no-torque. Our preference is interrupted sutures (eight evenly distributed for round and ten for decagonal [one at each angle]) combined with two rows of no-torque running sutures (Figure 22.6). In the mushroom side-cut configuration, the interrupted sutures are placed and advanced to a depth of 310 μm (touching the outer step of the mushroom-shaped dissection).

Big Bubble Technique

There are two types of femto-assisted DALK using the Big Bubble technique: the conventional method and the DALK incision method.

The conventional method starts with measuring the thinnest point at 6 mm off the corneal center and setting the pachymetry of lamellar dissection at 70% of this value, ensuring that the dissection is not closer than 100 to 125 μm to the endothelial side. All settings for energy, centration, rim pattern, and side cut profiles are the same as previously recommended for the Melles technique. The donor preparation is also the same.

The DALK incision variation of the Big Bubble technique involves creating a tunnel incision into the deep part of the corneal stroma to facilitate the achievement of a true Big Bubble pneumo-dissection.[20] You can use the following recommendations to perform DALK incision surgery with the VICTUS platform (software version 3.4.1.7), using one license without repeated docking. The DALK incision dialog box is opened and all the parameters required for DALK incision are set (Figure 22.7).

After completing the DALK incision requirements, the anterior lamellar dissection is set to 65 to 70% of the thinnest pachymetry at the determined local thickness and the depth of incision adjusted while viewing the online video to set it at 100 to 125 microns from the endothelial side (Figure 22.7). The energy for treating the bed should be set at 0.9 to 1.0 μJ, and the energy for the rim incision should be 130 to 140 μJ.

Under the view of online OCT, the corneal incision is centered with the three-click centration button and refined manually. By clicking the start button, the DALK incision is initially created, followed by the lamellar corneal incision. Then, the anterior lamellar cut is removed, and a 23-gauge needle (or Foglas cannula) is inserted into the angulated DALK incision plane 1 and inserted up to the end through the length of plane 2. After reaching the end of the tunnel and

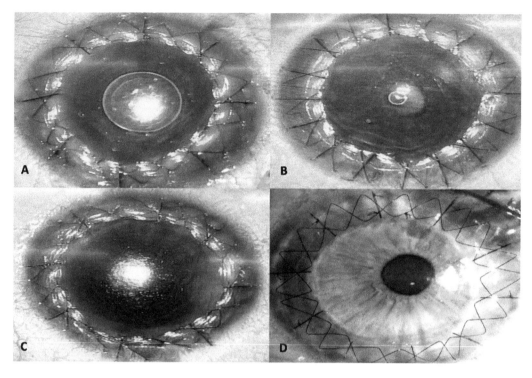

Figure 22.6 A) Round rim shape with interrupted plus no-torque running sutures. B) Round rim shape with interrupted plus torque running sutures. C) The same as A. D) Decagonal rim shape with interrupted plus no-torque running sutures.

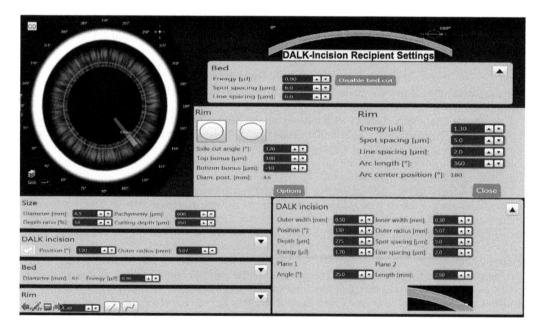

Figure 22.7 Recipient settings of the DALK incision method, using VICTUS platform.

Table 22.1 Femtosecond Specific Laser Settings of the DALK Incision Technique

Axial position of DALK incision	130-degree (for a right-handed surgeon)
Entrance distance of incision from treatment center	4.5 to 5 mm
Width at the entry of the incision	0.5 to 0.6 mm[a]
Width at the endpoint of the incision	0.4 to 0.5 mm[b]
Angle of first plane (plane 1) at the entry of incision	25 to 45 degrees
Length of posterior plane (plane 2) incision.[c]	0.5 mm to 2 mm
Depth of incision	100–125 μm from the endothelial side

[a] About the size of the canula used for air injection.
[b] Smaller than the size of the canula used for air injection.
[c] Parallel to the posterior part of the cornea

finding the final resistance, air is injected with a 5-mL syringe to form the Big Bubble. Table 22.1 summarizes the optimized laser settings for the DALK incision technique.

It has been claimed that the femtosecond laser enhances the achievement of the Big Bubble compared to the manual technique, and the DALK incision method may further improve the success rate of Big Bubble formation, particularly the type 1 bubble (with a lower risk of perforation).

The donor preparation for the Big Bubble technique is the same as previously described for the Melles technique. The diameter of the donor cornea should be at least 0.2 mm larger than the recipient cornea, and the cutting depth should be about 30 to 40% of the measured pachymetry at the incision site (Figure 22.8).

POST-OPERATIVE CONSIDERATIONS

The major concern during the early post-operative period is rapid epithelial healing and prevention of infection. Bandage contact lenses are the gold standard in promoting the epithelial healing process in every case. Topical antibiotics are started the day after surgery every four hours for one week and then tapered over one month or more based on the corneal epithelial healing process. Topical steroids are started the day after surgery every four hours and then slowly tapered over four months to reach the final once-daily dose, which is continued until sutures are to prevent the risk of stromal rejection.

IOP monitoring and regular checks for loose sutures (to prevent interface vascularization) are other important post-operative care steps. Three months after surgery, selective removal of

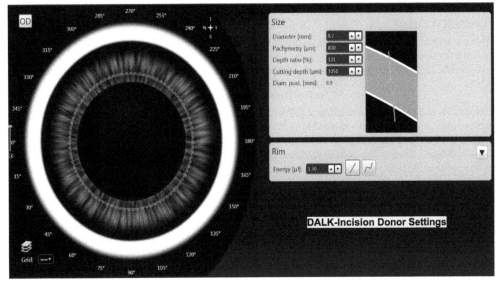

Figure 22.8 Donor settings of the DALK incision method, using VICTUS system.

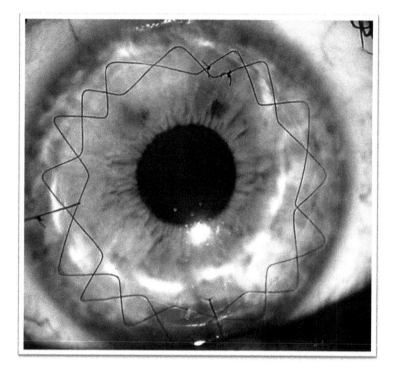

Figure 22.9 This figure shows an eye that underwent femto-assisted DALK, wherein selective suture removal of the interrupted sutures was performed in multiple sessions to minimize post-operative astigmatism.

interrupted sutures (at the steep axis) is performed to minimize astigmatism (Figure 22.9). At the same time, spectacles or contact lenses could be prescribed to restore vision. The eyes should be regularly monitored for any new epithelial defect, loose sutures, suture-related inflammation/infection, and herpes simplex activation. All sutures could be removed at two to three years after the surgery.

COMPLICATIONS

There is an acceptable rate of overall complications in both manual and femto-assisted DALK, making these techniques the first choice in corneal diseases with normal and healthy endothelial cells (Table 22.2). These complications are classified as intra-operative and post-operative.

Intra-Operative Complications

Perforation of Descemet's membrane (DM) is the most common and yet the most important complication during femto-assisted DALK with a reported rate of 4% to 39% with the manual Big Bubble technique. This complication has occurred less frequently in the manual Melles technique (0.2% to 8%).[21-23] In the Big Bubble method, the risk of DM perforation is related to the level of dissection within the cornea. DM perforation is more common in type 2 bubbles (dissection over the DM) than in type 1 (dissection over the Dua layer). As previously mentioned, the DALK incision method increases the likelihood of type 1 bubble formation and hence decreases the overall risk of DM perforation.

Management of DM perforation depends on the method used and the size of the perforation. With the Melles technique, if macro-perforation occurs with a large DM rupture, conversion into PKP is recommended. If micro-perforation develops in the far periphery of the cornea, the anterior chamber should be filled with air, and all but the area over the perforation should be gently dissected with a Melles spatula. At this point, the scleral tunnel is sutured, the air is aspirated from the anterior chamber, and viscoelastic is injected into the dissected pocket. Then, the corneal cap is removed, and open dissection is performed over the area of DM perforation in a more superficial plane. Finally, the corneal donor is placed over the dissected bed, four cardinal sutures are tied,

Table 22.2   Intra- and Post-Operative Complications after Femto-Assisted DALK, Reported in a Previous Large-Scale Study

Study	Salouti et al. N = 391 Keratoconus Patients
Intra-operative	
DM perforation	0.0%
Decentration	1.5%
Suction loss	1.0%
Post-operative	
Persistent epithelial defect	1.0%
Epithelial rejection	2.0%
Stromal rejection	1.0%
Persistent IOP elevation	0.8%
Urrets–Zavalia syndrome	not reported
Epithelial herpetic keratitis	0.3%

DM, Descemet's membrane; IOP, intraocular pressure.

and an air bubble is injected into the anterior chamber to adhere the DM to the overlying layers, and the surgery is continued.

If micro-perforation occurs in the early stages of the dissection (steps 1 or 2), there are two options. The first option is to suture the scleral tunnel and initiate the surgery in another location (temporal) and continue dissection with particular caution in the superior part of the cornea (the area of DM perforation). The other option is to create another more anterior scleral dissection (closer to the limbus) at 300 μm depth instead of the previous 310 μm plane and continue the procedure to the end.

In the Big Bubble technique, the perforation during femtosecond trephination is relatively rare compared with the manual method.[24,25] If perforation occurs during the surgery, it is recommended to continue dissecting the stroma to remove the corneal cap, lower the intraocular pressure (to prevent enlargement of the perforation), and try to dissect peripheral stromal tissue off from the DM (stromectomy). The site of the perforation should be dissected lastly. As mentioned before, air injection is recommended to reattach the DM after placing four cardinal sutures between the donor and recipient corneas.

In cases where there is a large perforation during the femto-assisted Big Bubble technique, it is recommended to attempt stromectomy. If possible, the leaking aqueous humor should be dried using the Weck-Cel cellulose sponge, and the DM should be unrolled to its normal position. Afterward, the donor cornea should be secured with four cardinal sutures and air injected into the anterior chamber through paracentesis, far from the site of the perforation. If the anterior chamber is formed and the DM is attached in the proper position, the surgery should be continued by completing the suturing. If not, the procedure should be converted to PKP. It should be noted that the rate of Urrets–Zavalia syndrome is generally estimated to be between 0.2% and 4%, and it is higher in cases of DM rupture compared with uncomplicated DALK. Therefore, prophylactic inferior peripheral iridotomy, vigilant monitoring of postoperative intraocular pressure, and the use of brimonidine eye drops are useful measures for preventing IOP rise and restoring pupil configuration.[26–28]

Decentration of femtosecond trephination with modern femto-machines is uncommon, and the average incidence of decentration is 5.5%, with a range of 0% to 27.3%. The chance of this complication occurring is more common in manual DALK, where human errors can occur. If the decentration of the incision was minimal, completing the surgery is recommended as the graft will cover the pupil completely. However, if the decentration was substantial, the femtosecond trephination of the donor cornea should be aborted. To prevent this complication and save donor corneas, we suggest performing laser incisions of the recipient first.[29,30]

Occasionally, thick remaining stroma may occur with the Melles technique, especially in the hands of novice surgeons. This complication may compromise long-term visual performance and should be avoided. During lamellar dissection, if the dark band around the spatula tip is thick (a sign that shows that the remaining stroma is thick), the surgeon should stop further dissection and redo the dissection from the scleral entry within a deeper plane.

Suction loss is an uncommon complication during surgery, and the incidence of suction loss during femtosecond DALK is reported to be around 1–2% in the literature. The major cause is usually an uncooperative patient or unintentional eye and head movement during laser surgery. If this event occurs in the early phase of corneal incision (less than 10% of incisions), it is recommended to re-attempt for re-docking and proceed with the rest of the surgery. Otherwise, it is reasonable to switch to manual DALK to prevent tissue damage during the second attempt at femto-dissection.[1,31,32]

Post-Operative Complications

Double anterior chamber is a more common complication with the Big Bubble method than with the Melles technique. This complication is due to (missed) intra-operative Descemet's membrane (DM) rupture. Corneal edema and associated low vision are the major consequences of this complication. Because there is a high possibility of fibrosis within the detached DM, long-term observation is not reasonable, and early intervention (air injection) for rapid recovery of visual acuity is recommended.[33–35]

Urrets–Zavalia syndrome is a relatively uncommon complication in keratoconus patients who underwent DALK with or without DM rupture. This complication may be induced by repeated anterior chamber air injections during or at the end of the surgery. The air may cause pupillary block and increased intraocular pressure (IOP), which can result in irreversible iris sphincter damage, persistent mydriasis, posterior synechia, anterior subcapsular cataract, and pigment dusting on the lens and posterior surface of the corneal graft. This complication could be prevented by avoiding repeated injection of large air bubbles into the anterior chamber and closely monitoring immediate post-operative IOP.[26–28]

Stromal rejection after DALK has a lower incidence than PKP, and the main pathophysiology is immunologic rejection of stromal tissue. Clinical signs include corneal stromal infiltrates, vascularization, and edema that are restricted to the donor cornea. This complication should be differentiated from herpetic stromal keratitis. The treatment is intense topical steroids in combination with subconjunctival anti-vascular endothelial growth factor (VEGF) therapy (if vascularization has occurred).[36–38]

The corneal epithelial regeneration process after DALK is relatively similar to PKP and is directly related to the status of the ocular surface and tear production. Because of the preparation method of the donor cornea in femto-assisted DALK, all epithelium over the cornea is removed, so epithelial healing may be more prolonged than in PKP. Proper donor and recipient apposition is crucial for normal epithelial migration in femto-assisted DALK, and any interface mismatch may predispose to persistent epithelial defects. Meibomian gland dysfunction, blepharitis, and dry eye associated with corneal diseases, such as keratoconus and allergic conjunctivitis, may interfere with epithelial healing. Donor abnormalities such as basement membrane dystrophy and long-term storage are also linked to this entity. Reactivation of herpes simplex keratitis should be considered as a cause in any persistent epithelial defect after DALK.

Treatment of the persistent epithelial defect starts with the management of any underlying disease (e.g., dry eye and ocular surface abnormality). Using a soft therapeutic contact lens after keratoplasty for several weeks will promote epithelial regeneration and prevent desiccation. If the epithelial defect persists, temporary punctal occlusion is the next step. Lateral tarsorrhaphy is reserved as the last option for the most resistant cases.[39–42]

High corneal astigmatism is a fairly common complication after uneventful corneal transplantations. This complication can be predisposed by several factors such as donor- or recipient-related corneal abnormalities, improper trephination of the donor or recipient corneas, incorrect graft size, bad wound apposition, inappropriate suturing techniques, exuberant wound healing or inflammation, type of post-operative medications, and so on. To minimize high astigmatism, the risk factors should be managed peri-operatively. Three months after the operation, suture adjustment should be considered (especially removal of single interrupted sutures) to reduce corneal astigmatism below three diopters.[43–45] Then, the patient should be observed for evaluation of graft survival. Final suture removal is usually at two to three years after surgery, depending on the remaining astigmatism. There are two further options for significant residual astigmatism: femtosecond-assisted astigmatic keratotomy (FSAK) for mixed astigmatism with a spherical equivalent of near zero and laser vision correction for compound myopic astigmatism.

Several studies showed lower astigmatism (especially at six to 12 months after surgery) in femto-assisted DALK compared with manual techniques.[21,46] This finding may be attributed to the more fine and predictable trephinations in femto-assisted DALK.

Descemet's fold or interface wrinkling is not common after DALK, with an incidence ranging from 2% to 14%. They may be fine or coarse, and transient or persistent. Most cases will disappear over time (usually at one to two years after surgery), but some cases may persist for several years. The peripheral folds (more common) usually have no impact on visual function, but central folds (less common) may impair vision. The two main underlying causes are the severity of baseline corneal disorders (particularly advanced ectasia) and insufficient donor–recipient disparity. To avoid this complication, a disparity of at least 200 μm should be adopted, and, in high-risk cases, corneal massage (with a spatula, from the center to the periphery) should be applied at the conclusion of the surgery in an eye maintained with high-normal IOP (by injecting BSS).[47–49]

DALK VERSUS PKP

Penetrating keratoplasty has been accepted as a definitive treatment for several disorders such as very advanced cases of keratoconus (with or without central hydrops), poor endothelial cell count of the recipient, and diseases that affect both the stroma and the endothelium. Visual outcomes after PKP have been promising, but the procedure could be associated with some serious intra- or post-operative complications. Progressive endothelial cell loss in the graft (graft failure) and endothelial rejection are the two most worrisome complications of PKP that could be largely prevented by choosing DALK in proper cases. In comparison to PKP, DALK preserves the patient's own endothelium, is less invasive (and thus prevents open sky complications such as expulsive hemorrhage), is associated with less anterior segment inflammation and fewer cases of endophthalmitis, preserves more corneal biomechanical strength, and demands less steroid dependency with a lower chance of resultant glaucoma or cataract. It should be noted that the flattening of the posterior cornea in advanced cases of keratoconus after DALK can interfere with the correct evaluation of endothelial cells. In some extreme cases, we may encounter an apparent increase in endothelial cell counts.[50] There are also more appropriate donors for DALK than PKP (corneas with lower cell counts are included). Therefore, it is reasonable to choose DALK over PKP in any patient who is eligible for both procedures.[51–55]

FEMTO-ASSISTED VERSUS MANUAL DALK

Visual Outcomes

Previous studies have reported similar or better visual outcomes for femto-assisted DALK compared with manual methods. Sharma et al. reported better post-operative visual acuity in the femto-assisted DALK subgroup.[51] Other investigators reported a more rapid visual recovery at three to six months after surgery for femto-assisted DALK. A few other studies on patients with keratoconus also concluded that there was a better visual outcome in the femto-assisted DALK subgroup.[46,56,57]

In our retrospective study of patients with keratoconus, 391 underwent femto-assisted DALK, and 469 underwent manual DALK (both with the Melles technique). We found no significant difference in best-corrected visual acuity in either the 12-month or 24-month post-operative results [21].

Overall, these studies suggest that both techniques significantly improve vision in patients with corneal disorders. Whether the femto-assisted technique offers any advantage over the manual method remains to be determined in future prospective trials.

Refractive Outcomes

There is some evidence to suggest that the refractive outcome is generally better with femtosecond-assisted DALK than with the manual technique. The laser-assisted approach has been linked to less residual myopia, lower mean and apical keratometry, lower keratometric astigmatism and HOAs (especially coma, trefoil, and spherical aberration), and a more prolate corneal shape.[21,58,59]

Complications

As noted earlier, a key benefit of femto-assisted DALK over the manual technique is that it can decrease the risk of DM perforation using the Big Bubble method. In our study, which employed the Melles technique, the occurrence of DM perforation was very low in both groups (0/391 in femto-assisted DALK and 1/469 in manual DALK).[21] However, it should be noted that the risk of DM perforation in the Melles technique depends largely on the surgeon's experience and skill.

In conclusion, the more precise corneal incisions in femto-assisted DALK may be associated with better refractive and visual outcomes. However, currently, there is no solid evidence to support these claims, and well-designed long-term prospective studies are required to critically test the hypothesis. In addition, the femto-assisted Big Bubble method (and, particularly, the DALK-incision technique) enhances the chance of successful bubble formation, with lower risk of DM perforation compared with the manual technique. There are some features, such as diverse rim shapes and side-cut configurations, adjustable cutting angles, and customized trephination and disparity sizes, that are only possible by using a femtosecond laser. The clinical relevance of these features is yet to be determined.

CLINICAL PEARLS

- Patient selection is a key point in femto-assisted DALK. All patients with healthy endothelium and without significant deep scarring may be good candidates for this procedure.

- The surgeon should carefully plan the incision and dissection to ensure complete removal of the diseased cornea and proper alignment of the corneal incision in the donor tissue and recipient to achieve the best possible outcome.

- Selection of proper femtosecond laser settings is crucial for a proper outcome in femto-assisted DALK.

- Precise donor tissue preparation, including the selection of disparity and cutting angle, is essential for optimized visual and refractive results.

- Femtosecond-assisted DALK provides improved precision, an increased chance of Descemet's membrane baring, preservation of eye integrity, shorter recovery time, full customization of surgical technique, greater predictability, and ultimately a promising visual outcome.

- Vigilant post-operative care, patient monitoring, and close observation for signs of rejection or infection are mandatory for favorable results.

REFERENCES

1. Soong HK, Malta JB: Femtosecond lasers in ophthalmology. *Am J Ophthalmol* 2009, 147(2):189–97.e2.

2. Nagy ZZ: New technology update: femtosecond laser in cataract surgery. *Clin Ophthalmol* 2014, 8:1157–67.

3. Proust H, Baeteman C, Matonti F, Conrath J, Ridings B, Hoffart L: Femtosecond laser-assisted decagonal penetrating keratoplasty. *Am J Ophthalmol* 2011, 151(1):29–34.

4. Shehadeh-Mashor R, Chan C, Yeung SN, Lichtinger A, Amiran M, Rootman DS: Long-term outcomes of femtosecond laser-assisted mushroom configuration deep anterior lamellar keratoplasty. *Cornea* 2013, 32(4):390–5.

5. Deshmukh R, Stevenson LJ, Vajpayee RB: Laser-assisted corneal transplantation surgery. *Surv Ophthalmol* 2021, 66(5):826–37.

6. Chan CC, Ritenour RJ, Kumar NL, Sansanayudh W, Rootman DS: Femtosecond laser-assisted mushroom configuration deep anterior lamellar keratoplasty. *Cornea* 2010, 29(3):290–5.

7. Vogel A, Noack J, Hüttmann G, Paltauf G: Mechanisms of femtosecond laser nanosurgery of cells and tissues. *Applied Physics B* 2005, 81:1015–47.

8. Ratkay-Traub I, Ferincz IE, Juhasz T, Kurtz RM, Krueger RR: First clinical results with the femtosecond neodynium-glass laser in refractive surgery. *J Refract Surg* 2003, 19(2):94–103.

9. Farid M, Steinert RF: Femtosecond laser-assisted corneal surgery. *Curr Opin Ophthalmol* 2010, 21(4):288–92.

10. Hovhannisyan V, Lo W, Hu C, Chen S-J, Dong CY: Dynamics of femtosecond laser photo-modification of collagen fibers. *Optics Express* 2008, 16(11):7958–68.

11. Fung SS, Aiello F, Maurino V: Outcomes of femtosecond laser-assisted mushroom-configuration keratoplasty in advanced keratoconus. *Eye (Lond)* 2016, 30(4):553–61.

12. Monterosso C, Antonini M, Di Zazzo A, Gaudenzi D, Caretti L, Coassin M, Rapizzi E: Femtosecond laser-assisted deep anterior lamellar keratoplasty: a safer option in keratoconus surgery. *Eur J Ophthalmol* 2022, 32(1):59–65.

13. Price FW, Jr., Price MO: Femtosecond laser shaped penetrating keratoplasty: one-year results utilizing a top-hat configuration. *Am J Ophthalmol* 2008, 145(2):210–4.

14. Menabuoni L, Canovetti A, Rossi F, Malandrini A, Lenzetti I, Pini R: The 'anvil' profile in femtosecond laser-assisted penetrating keratoplasty. *Acta Ophthalmol* 2013, 91(6):e494–5.

15. Price FW, Jr., Price MO, Jordan CS: Safety of incomplete incision patterns in femtosecond laser-assisted penetrating keratoplasty. *J Cataract Refract Surg* 2008, 34(12):2099–103.

16. Daniel MC, Böhringer D, Maier P, Eberwein P, Birnbaum F, Reinhard T: Comparison of long-term outcomes of femtosecond laser-assisted keratoplasty with conventional keratoplasty. *Cornea* 2016, 35(3):293–8.

17. Thompson MJ: Femtosecond laser-assisted half-top-hat keratoplasty. *Cornea* 2012, 31(3):291–2.

18. Maier P, Böhringer D, Birnbaum F, Reinhard T: Improved wound stability of top-hat profiled femtosecond laser-assisted penetrating keratoplasty in vitro. *Cornea* 2012, 31(8):963–6.

19. Choi M, Lee YE, Whang WJ, Yoo YS, Na KS, Joo CK: Correlation between corneal button size and intraocular pressure during femtosecond laser-assisted keratoplasty. *Cornea* 2016, 35(3):383–7.

20. Pedrotti E, Bonacci E, De Rossi A, Bonetto J, Chierego C, Fasolo A, De Gregorio A, Marchini G: Femtosecond laser-assisted big-bubble deep anterior lamellar keratoplasty. *Clin Ophthalmol* 2021, 15:645–50.

21. Salouti R, Zamani M, Ghoreyshi M, Dapena I, Melles GRJ, Nowroozzadeh MH: Comparison between manual trephination versus femtosecond laser-assisted deep anterior lamellar keratoplasty for keratoconus. *Br J Ophthalmol* 2019, 103(12):1716–23.

22. Lu Y, Chen X, Yang L, Xue C, Huang Z: Femtosecond laser-assisted deep anterior lamellar keratoplasty with big-bubble technique for keratoconus. *Indian J Ophthalmol* 2016, 64(9):639–42.

23. Liu YC, Wittwer VV, Yusoff NZM, Lwin CN, Seah XY, Mehta JS, Seiler T: Intraoperative optical coherence tomography-guided femtosecond laser-assisted deep anterior lamellar keratoplasty. *Cornea* 2019, 38(5):648–53.

24. Buzzonetti L, Petrocelli G, Valente P, Iarossi G, Ardia R, Petroni S, Parrilla R: The big-bubble full femtosecond laser-assisted technique in deep anterior lamellar keratoplasty. *J Refract Surg* 2015, 31(12):830–4.

25. Gogri PY, Bore MC, Rips AGT, Reddy JC, Rostov AT, Vaddavalli PK: Femtosecond laser-assisted big bubble for deep anterior lamellar keratoplasty. *J Cataract Refract Surg* 2021, 47(1):106–10.

26. Niknam S, Rajabi MT: Fixed dilated pupil (urrets-zavalia syndrome) after deep anterior lamellar keratoplasty. *Cornea* 2009, 28(10):1187–90.

27. Goweida MB, Mahmoud S, Sobhy M, Liu C: Deep anterior lamellar keratoplasty with large descemet's membrane perforation: should we stop conversion to penetrating keratoplasty? *J Curr Ophthalmol* 2021, 33(2):171–6.

28. Bozkurt KT, Acar BT, Acar S: Fixed dilated pupilla as a common complication of deep anterior lamellar keratoplasty complicated with Descemet membrane perforation. *Eur J Ophthalmol* 2013, 23(2):164–70.

29. Tran TM, Farid M: Update on femtosecond laser-enabled keratoplasty. *Cornea* 2023, 42(4):395–403.

30. Khodaparast M, Shahraki K, Jabbarvand M, Shahraki K, Rafat M, Moravvej Z: Sutureless femtosecond laser-assisted anterior lamellar keratoplasty using a bioengineered cornea as a viable alternative to human donor transplantation for superficial corneal opacities. *Cornea* 2020, 39(9):1184–9.

31. Lin A, Gaster RN: Suction loss during femtosecond laser incision for penetrating kerato-plasty. *Cornea* 2009, 28(3):362–4.

32. Angunawela RI, Riau A, Chaurasia SS, Tan DT, Mehta JS: Manual suction versus femtosec-ond laser trephination for penetrating keratoplasty: intraocular pressure, endothelial cell damage, incision geometry, and wound healing responses. *Invest Ophthalmol Vis Sci* 2012, 53(6):2571–9.

33. Feizi S, Daryabari SH, Najdi D, Javadi MA, Karimian F: Big-bubble deep anterior lamellar keratoplasty using central vs peripheral air injection: a clinical trial. *Eur J Ophthalmol* 2016, 26(4):297–302.

34. Jhanji V, Sharma N, Vajpayee RB: Intraoperative perforation of Descemet's membrane during "big bubble" deep anterior lamellar keratoplasty. *Int Ophthalmol* 2010, 30(3):291–5.

35. Ziaei M, Ormonde SE: Descemet's membrane macroperforation during interface irrigation in big bubble deep anterior lamellar keratoplasty. *Oman J Ophthalmol* 2017, 10(3):241–3.

36. Anwar M, Teichmann KD: Big-bubble technique to bare Descemet's membrane in anterior lamellar keratoplasty. *J Cataract Refract Surg* 2002, 28(3):398–403.

37. Roberts HW, Maycock NJ, O'Brart DP: Late stromal rejection in deep anterior lamellar kerato-plasty: a case series. *Cornea* 2016, 35(9):1179–81.

38. Hosseini H, Nowroozzadeh MH, Salouti R, Nejabat M: Anti-VEGF therapy with bevaci-zumab for anterior segment eye disease. *Cornea* 2012, 31(3):322–34.

39. Dua HS, Said DG, Messmer EM, Rolando M, Benitez-Del-Castillo JM, Hossain PN, Shortt AJ, Geerling G, Nubile M, Figueiredo FC, Rauz S, Mastropasqua L, Rama P, Baudouin C: Neurotrophic keratopathy. *Prog Retin Eye Res* 2018, 66:107–31.

40. Kezic JM, Wiffen S, Degli-Esposti M: Keeping an 'eye' on ocular GVHD. *Clin Exp Optom* 2022, 105(2):135–42.

41. Alio JL, Rodriguez AE, WróbelDudzińska D: Eye platelet-rich plasma in the treatment of ocular surface disorders. *Curr Opin Ophthalmol* 2015, 26(4):325–32.

42. Tong L, Sun CC, Yoon KC, Lim Bon Siong R, Puangsricharern V, Baudouin C: Cyclosporine anionic and cationic ophthalmic emulsions in dry eye disease: a literature review. *Ocul Immunol Inflamm* 2021, 29(7–8):1606–15.

43. St Clair RM, Sharma A, Huang D, Yu F, Goldich Y, Rootman D, Yoo S, Cabot F, Jun J, Zhang L, Aldave AJ: Development of a nomogram for femtosecond laser astigmatic keratotomy for astigmatism after keratoplasty. *J Cataract Refract Surg* 2016, 42(4):556–62.

44. Nubile M, Carpineto P, Lanzini M, Calienno R, Agnifili L, Ciancaglini M, Mastropasqua L: Femtosecond laser arcuate keratotomy for the correction of high astigmatism after kerato-plasty. *Ophthalmology* 2009, 116(6):1083–92.

45. Wetterstrand O, Holopainen JM, Krootila K: Treatment of postoperative keratoplasty astig-matism using femtosecond laser-assisted intrastromal relaxing incisions. *J Refract Surg* 2013, 29(6):378–82.

46. Shehadeh-Mashor R, Chan CC, Bahar I, Lichtinger A, Yeung SN, Rootman DS: Comparison between femtosecond laser mushroom configuration and manual trephine straight-edge configuration deep anterior lamellar keratoplasty. *Br J Ophthalmol* 2014, 98(1):35–9.

47. Li X, Zhao Y, Chen H, Li Y, Hong J, Xu J: Clinical properties and risk factors for descemet membrane folds after deep anterior lamellar keratoplasty in patients with keratoconus. *Cornea* 2019, 38(10):1222–7.

48. Fontana L, Parente G, Sincich A, Tassinari G: Influence of graft-host interface on the quality of vision after deep anterior lamellar keratoplasty in patients with keratoconus. *Cornea* 2011, 30(5):497–502.

49. Prazeres TM, Muller RT, Rayes T, Hirai FE, de Sousa LB: Comparison of descemet-on versus descemet-off deep anterior lamellar keratoplasty in keratoconus patients: a randomized trial. *Cornea* 2015, 34(7):797–801.

50. Salouti R, Masoumpour M, Nowroozzadeh MH, Zamani M, Ghoreyshi M, Melles GR: Changes in corneal endothelial cell profile measurements after deep anterior lamellar kerato-plasty for keratoconus. *Cornea* 2013, 32(6):751–6.

51. Janiszewska-Bil D, Czarnota-Nowakowska B, Krysik K, Lyssek-Boroń A, Dobrowolski D, Grabarek BO, Wylęgała E: Comparison of long-term outcomes of the lamellar and penetrating keratoplasty approaches in patients with keratoconus. *J Clin Med* 2021, 10(11).

52. Yüksel B, Kandemir B, Uzunel UD, Çelik O, Ceylan S, Küsbeci T: Comparison of visual and topographic outcomes of deep-anterior lamellar keratoplasty and penetrating keratoplasty in keratoconus. *Int J Ophthalmol* 2017, 10(3):385–90.

53. Han DCY, Mehta JS, Por YM, Htoon HM, Tan DTH: Comparison of outcomes of lamellar keratoplasty and penetrating keratoplasty in keratoconus. *Am J Ophthalmol* 2009, 148(5):744–51.e1.

54. Chen Y, Hu D-N, Xia Y, Yang L, Xue C, Huang Z: Comparison of femtosecond laser-assisted deep anterior lamellar keratoplasty and penetrating keratoplasty for keratoconus. *BMC Ophthalmology* 2015, 15(1):144.

55. Kubaloglu A, Coskun E, Sari ES, Guneş AS, Cinar Y, Piñero DP, Kutluturk I, Ozerturk Y: Comparison of astigmatic keratotomy results in deep anterior lamellar keratoplasty and penetrating keratoplasty in keratoconus. *Am J Ophthalmol* 2011, 151(4):637–43.e1.

56. Lu Y, Grisolia AB, Ge YR, Xue CY, Cao Q, Yang LP, Huang ZP: Comparison of femtosecond laser-assisted descemetic and predescemetic lamellar keratoplasty for keratoconus. *Indian J Ophthalmol* 2017, 65(1):19–23.

57. Li H, Chen M, Dong YL, Zhang J, Du XL, Cheng J, Gao H, Xie LX: Comparison of long-term results after manual and femtosecond assisted corneal trephination in deep anterior lamellar keratoplasty for keratoconus. *Int J Ophthalmol* 2020, 13(4):567–73.

58. Janiszewska-Bil D, Czarnota-Nowakowska B, Krysik K, Mistarz M, Dobrowolski D, Grabarek BO, Lyssek-Boroń A: Prospective safety evaluation of the femtosecond laser-assisted keratomileusis procedure in correcting residual ametropia in patients after deep anterior lamellar keratoplasty. *Med Sci Monit* 2023, 29:e939691.

59. Bahar I, Kaiserman I, Lange AP, Levinger E, Sansanayudh W, Singal N, Slomovic AR, Rootman DS: Femtosecond laser versus manual dissection for top hat penetrating keratoplasty. *Br J Ophthalmol* 2009, 93(1):73–8.

23 Keratoconus: Optical and Surgical Management
Management of Post-Keratoplasty Astigmatism

Saeed Raeisi, Zahra Bibak Bejandi, and Seyed Farzad Mohammadi

INTRODUCTION

Keratoplasty is a staged procedure. At stage one, you remove a diseased cornea and replace it with a healthy one. Then, you have to handle the refractive aspect, and this, in fact, has remained as the bigger challenge. Advances in donor cornea punch and recipient bed trephination have excluded gross mismatches from happening. However, suturing is still manual, and its symmetry and strength are adjusted grossly and visually. Considering our current state-of-the-art refractive precision, these are primitive and underdeveloped techniques, and, despite the initial enthusiasm for the advent of the femtosecond laser for keratoplasty, laser cuts did not resolve the astigmatism challenge. Additionally, we do not know the refractive translation of the inherent features of the donor cornea.

Despite having normal biomechanics and thickness, grafted corneas have high refractive mismatches with the recipient biometry and generally severe shape distortions. Every refractive correction which we use for virgin eyes have been used for grafted eyes as well, and we review them in the following sections.

CONTACT LENSES (CLS)

CLs are used to correct high degrees of irregular astigmatism and aberrations that are not fully correctable and/or tolerable by spectacles.[1]

CLs include rigid gas-permeable (RGP), scleral, miniscleral, hybrid, and piggy-back CLs.[1,2] A fitting success rate of 80%,[3] 88%,[4] and 83.3%[5] were reported for RGP, scleral lenses, and hybrid lenses, respectively. It should be noted that corneal neovascularization and the presence of corneal sutures are not a contraindication for CL use.[1,6] In general, larger-diameter CLs are preferred as they avoid pressure on the graft host junction (GHJ). Smaller-diameter CLs decenter, dislocate, or spontaneously eject more frequently.[7]

ASTIGMATIC KERATOTOMY

Astigmatic keratotomy (AK) involves one or two corneal incisions on the steepest meridian of astigmatism and is used to correct high astigmatism which is not corrected by spectacles or contact lenses.[8] The incisions may be asymmetric.

Using manual techniques must be conducted according to standardized nomograms; for example, one study described a standardized approach of paired incisions of 60-degree arc lengths, 600 μm in depth at a 6-mm optical zone (rule of 6);[6] manual procedures can cause complications, such as corneal perforation, overcorrection, wound dehiscence, and graft failure or rejection.[9]

Two factors make AKs inherently unpredictable: keratotomy exists in the context of asymmetrically distributed tissue which, in addition to limbus, has an additional irregular donor–recipient anchor. Advanced dynamic biomechanical maps, combined with intra-operative aberrometry and titratable interventions, are needed.

COMPRESSION SUTURES

Placing tight sutures on the flat axis may help to reduce astigmatism after keratoplasty (Figures 23.1–23.3). They are reversible and easy choices. Nylon 10-0 sutures are usually used for such procedures.

A combination of AK on the steep axis and placing compression sutures on the axis 90° away from it has proved useful[10] and induced more diopter shift, but the risk of perforation and a very high astigmatic shift must be evaluated. The problem is that one should remove the suture, or it will decay anyway. Reversibility and longer-term unpredictability are the pitfalls.[3]

A 45-year-old man with a history of keratoplasty (DALK) for KCN six years ago was referred to our clinic for correction of high astigmatism, so he was planned for compression sutures in the flat axis.

Cyclo refraction before compression sutures: +5.5 −10.00 × 177 BCVA: 7/10

Cyclo refraction three months after compression sutures: +2.00 −5.75 × 110 BCVA: 10/10

LASER REFRACTIVE SURGERY

Surface Ablation

Indications for excimer laser refractive surgery are anisometropia and contact lens intolerance,[11] and it is considered three to six months after complete suture removal, a minimum pachymetry of more than 500 μm, and simulated keratometry values between 38 D and 55 D.[12]

For mild to moderate spherocylindrical errors, laser refractive surgery is the procedure of choice. Despite the older teaching of recommending LASIK for a grafted cornea to avoid the PRK risk of haze, three factors have now changed this:

- mitomycin C (MMC) very effectively reduces the haze risk

- despite advances achieved with the femto-laser, it frequently ends up with an uneven bed and/or disordered flaps

- finally, yet importantly, in surface ablation, we can perform a topo-guided procedure more effectively, now in its most refined approach, which is a trans-epithelial topo-guided surface ablation.

If the eye has a sizable combination of irregular astigmatism and spherocylindrical error, the senior author [SFM] suggests a staged procedure of lenticule extraction to address the spherocylindrical error to be followed by a trans-epithelial topo-guided ablation for irregular astigmatism, taking into account the cap thickness.

Corneal grafts are more prone to haze and regression after PRK; MMC treatment for longer than usual and up to two minutes has been shown to reduce corneal haze by up to 20%.[13] Patients with irregular astigmatism (–7.5 D to –2.0 D) underwent TG-PRK with MMC, after which astigmatism decreased significantly ($P = 0.003$) from 5.10 ± 0.4 D to 3.37 ± 0.06 D after 12 months.[14]

Lenticule Extraction

Lenticule extraction within the graft button has a potential advantage over the LASIK flap because the flap is more likely to breach and weaken the GHJ scar.

The study shows significant improvement in UCVA and BCVA after lenticule extraction. GHJ dehiscence during lenticule separation was a complication which was reported.[15]

One study included patients having up to 6 D of astigmatism and a donor button size of >8 mm with a minimum of 500 μm thickness at the thinnest location. The authors reported 67 ± 25.5% as a mean percentage astigmatism reduction.[16]

Lenticule extraction and toric implantable collamer lens (TICL) implantation effectively correct myopic astigmatism, but lenticule extraction showed better correction accuracy in the magnitude and axis of astigmatism.[17]

INTRASTROMAL CORNEAL RING SEGMENTS (ICRS)

Studies recommend that ICRS implantation after PKP must be performed a minimum of one year after PKP and a minimum of three months after complete suture removal.[18]

Almost all of the studies have suggested using small-diameter rings, such as Keraring or Ferrara rings to reduce the risk of GHJ dehiscence or stromal vascularization.[19]

Patients intolerant of CL wear and astigmatism higher than 6 diopters underwent ICRS followed by PRK. Mean refractive astigmatism decreased from 7.10 ± 1.13 D in the pre-operative condition to 4.61 ± 1.61 D after ICRS ($P < 0.0001$) and to 2.58 ± 1.49 D after PRK ($P < 0.0001$).[20]

TORIC INTRAOCULAR LENS

We can use toric IOL during cataract surgery or clear lens extraction after keratoplasty following suture removal with regular astigmatism and minimal HOA.[21] The advantage is that any degree of spherical error can be targeted to be corrected, but it should be kept in mind that IOL producers do not manage all spherocylindrical errors. Most studies suggested toric IOLs to treat astigmatism of 1.5–4.25 D; for high astigmatism, one can use combined toric IOL implantation with a corneal procedure, such as LASIK, PRK, or FSAK.[21,22]

For pseudophakic and aphakic eyes with high post-PKP astigmatism, we can use iris-fixated toric IOLs[23] and transscleral-fixation toric IOLs,[24] respectively. Also, posterior chamber phakic toric IOLs have been used in younger ages with clear lenses.

There are some challenges for toric IOL in grafted eyes, such as unpredictable IOL power calculation, rotation of toric IOL, and endothelial cell loss (ECL).

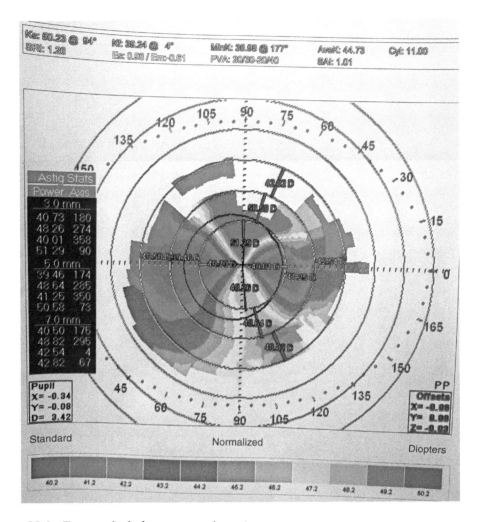

Figure 23.1   Topography before compression suture.

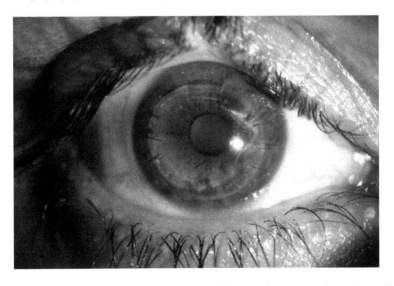

Figure 23.2   Six Nylon 10-0 compression sutures in flat axis (suture tension adjusted with intra-operative keratoscopy).

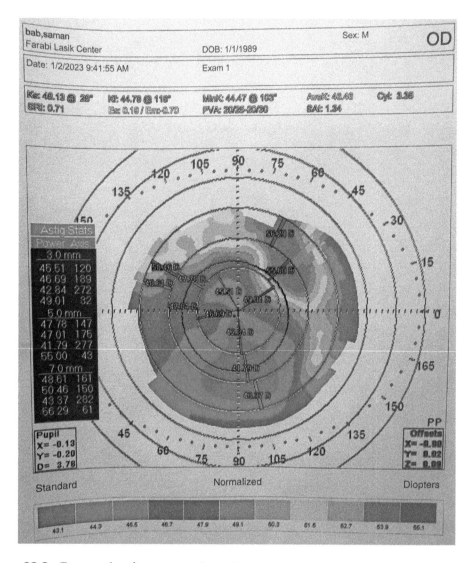

Figure 23.3 Topography after compression suture.

To improve the accuracy of IOL power calculation, we can use multimodal approaches, such as topography, tomography, biometry data, and refraction.[22]

High-power toric IOL (in the range of 9.0–15.5 D cylinders) effectively reduced high-value astigmatism over the one-year follow-up.[25]

One study with three years follow-up reported an ECL of 34.8 ± 26.3%. Also, a few cases have reported graft rejection and failure.[26]

REPEAT KERATOPLASTY

Repeat grafts are recommended when all other interventions have failed to treat high or irregular astigmatism.[8]

Excellent outcomes were reported for repeat PKP for management of high irregular astigmatism with excimer laser trephination larger than the previous GHJ.[27]

CONCLUSION

Following keratoplasty, the cornea surgeon must handle resultant regular spherocylindrical errors and inevitable irregular astigmatism. Asymmetric donor tissue distribution brings about the most challenging refractive errors, sometimes necessitating a re-graft. Despite this, the surgeon can nowadays carry out astigmatic keratotomy (preferably with a femto-laser), implant a toric intraocular lens, and/or perform a topo-guided excimer ablation to reach the precious emmetropia. In general, if there is poor tissue distribution, corneoplasty procedures of compression suture, AK, intracorneal ring segments, and regrafts are employed to be followed by laser refractive procedures or toric intraocular lenses.

REFERENCES

1. Asena L, Altınörs DD. Visual rehabilitation after penetrating keratoplasty. *Experimental and Clinical Transplantation: Official Journal of the Middle East Society for Organ Transplantation.* 2016;14(Suppl 3):130–4.

2. Altay Y, Balta O, Burcu A, Ornek F. Hybrid contact lenses for visual management of patients after keratoplasty. *Nigerian Journal of Clinical Practice.* 2018;21(4):451.

3. Moramarco A, Gardini L, Iannetta D, Versura P, Fontana L. Post penetrating keratoplasty ectasia: incidence, risk factors, clinical features, and treatment options. *Journal of Clinical Medicine.* 2022;11(10):2678.

4. Lee JC, Chiu GB, Bach D, Bababeygy SR, Irvine J, Heur M. Functional and visual improvement with prosthetic replacement of the ocular surface ecosystem scleral lenses for irregular corneas. *Cornea.* 2013;32(12):1540–3.

5. Abdalla YF, Elsahn AF, Hammersmith KM, Cohen EJ. SynergEyes lenses for keratoconus. *Cornea.* 2010;29(1):5–8.

6. Barnett M, Lien V, Li JY, Durbin-Johnson B, Mannis MJ. Use of scleral lenses and miniscleral lenses after penetrating keratoplasty. *Eye & Contact Lens.* 2016;42(3):185–9.

7. Severinsky B, Behrman S, Frucht-Pery J, Solomon A. Scleral contact lenses for visual rehabilitation after penetrating keratoplasty: long term outcomes. *Contact Lens & Anterior Eye: The Journal of the British Contact Lens Association.* 2014;37(3):196–202.

8. Feizi S, Zare M. Current approaches for management of postpenetrating keratoplasty astigmatism. *Journal of Ophthalmology.* 2011;2011:1–8.

9. Wilkins MR, Mehta JS, Larkin DFP. Standardized arcuate keratotomy for postkeratoplasty astigmatism. *Journal of Cataract & Refractive Surgery.* 2005;31(2):297–301.

10. Fares U, Sarhan ARS, Dua HS. Management of post-keratoplasty astigmatism. *Journal of Cataract & Refractive Surgery.* 2012;38(11):2029–39.

11. Vajpayee RB, Sharma N, Sinha R, Bhartiya P, Titiyal JS, Tandon R. Laser in-situ keratomileusis after penetrating keratoplasty. *Survey of Ophthalmology.* 2003;48(5):503–14.

12. Koay PY, McGhee CN, Weed KH, Craig JP. Laser in situ keratomileusis for ametropia after penetrating keratoplasty. *Journal of Refractive Surgery (Thorofare, NJ: 1995).* 2000;16(2):140–7.

13. Laíns I, Rosa AM, Guerra M, Tavares C, Lobo C, Silva MF, et al. Irregular astigmatism after corneal transplantation—efficacy and safety of topography-guided treatment. *Cornea.* 2016;35(1):30–6.

14. e Silva FB, Hazarbassanov RM, Martines E, Güell JL, Hofling-Lima AL. Visual outcomes and aberrometric changes with topography-guided photorefractive keratectomy treatment of irregular astigmatism after penetrating keratoplasty. *Cornea.* 2018;37(3):283–9.

15. Kim BK, Mun SJ, Lee DG, Chung YT. Bilateral small incision lenticule extraction (SMILE) after penetrating keratoplasty. *Journal of Refractive Surgery.* 2016;32(9):644–7.

16. Massoud TH, Ibrahim O, Shehata K, Abdalla MF. Small incision lenticule extraction for post-keratoplasty myopia and astigmatism. *Journal of Ophthalmology.* 2016;2016:1–9.

17. Wan T, Yin H, Wu Z, Yang Y. Vector analysis of small incision lenticule extraction and toric implantable collamer lens implantation for astigmatism correction. *European Journal of Ophthalmology.* 2021;31(3):994–1001.

18. Chang DH, Hardten DR. Refractive surgery after corneal transplantation. *Current Opinion in Ophthalmology.* 2005;16(4):251–5.

19. Coscarelli S, Ferrara G, Alfonso JF, Ferrara P, Merayo-Lloves J, Araújo LP, et al. Intrastromal corneal ring segment implantation to correct astigmatism after penetrating keratoplasty. *Journal of Cataract & Refractive Surgery.* 2012;38(6):1006–13.

20. Bertino P, Magalhães RS, de Souza Jr CJ, Rocha G, Santhiago MR. Intrastromal corneal ring segments followed by PRK for postkeratoplasty high astigmatism: prospective study. *Journal of Cataract & Refractive Surgery.* 2022;48(8):912–23.

21. Müftüoglu IK, Akova YA, Egrilmez S, Yilmaz SG. The results of toric intraocular lens implantation in patients with cataract and high astigmatism after penetrating keratoplasty. *Eye & Contact Lens.* 2016;42(2):e8–e11.

22. Sorkin N, Kreimei M, Einan-Lifshitz A, Mednick Z, Telli A, Trinh T, et al. Stepwise combination of femtosecond astigmatic keratotomy with phacoemulsification and toric intraocular lens implantation in treatment of very high postkeratoplasty astigmatism. *Cornea.* 2020;39(1):71–6.

23. Tehrani M, Schwenn O, Dick HB. [Toric intraocular lens to correct high astigmatism after penetrating keratoplasty in a pseudophakic eye - a case report]. *Klinische Monatsblatter fur Augenheilkunde.* 2001;218(12):795–9.

24. Borkenstein AF, Reuland A, Limberger IJ, Rabsilber TM, Auffarth GU. Transscleral fixation of a toric intraocular lens to correct aphakic keratoplasty with high astigmatism. *Journal of Cataract and Refractive Surgery.* 2009;35(5):934–8.

25. Reddy J, Pooja C, Prabhakar G. High power custom toric intraocular lens for correcting high corneal astigmatism in post-keratoplasty and keratoconus patients with cataract. *Indian Journal of Ophthalmology.* 2021;69(7):1766.

26. Tahzib NG, Cheng YY, Nuijts RM. Three-year follow-up analysis of Artisan toric lens implantation for correction of postkeratoplasty ametropia in phakic and pseudophakic eyes. *Ophthalmology.* 2006;113(6):976–84.

27. Alfaro Rangel R, Szentmáry N, Lepper S, Daas L, Langenbucher A, Seitz B. 8.5/8.6-mm excimer laser-assisted penetrating keratoplasties in a tertiary corneal subspecialty referral center: indications and outcomes in 107 eyes. *Cornea.* 2020;39(7):806–11.

24 Post-Keratoplasty Astigmatism Management by Relaxing Incisions

Mohammad Naser Hashemian and Sadegh Ghafarian

KERATOPLASTY AND ETIOLOGY OF ASTIGMATISM

Corneal transplantation is the most common and successful transplantation worldwide. Penetrating keratoplasty, a procedure with a long history exceeding a century, has been the main treatment for corneal diseases causing vision loss. Nowadays, anterior lamellar keratoplasty and endothelial keratoplasty are increasingly favored over penetrating keratoplasty (PK) in the management of corneal diseases because of fewer complications and faster visual recovery.[1,2]

Astigmatism is the most common cause of visual impairment after corneal transplantation, despite the clarity of the corneal graft. Up to one-third of patients undergoing PK may develop post-operative astigmatism greater than 5 diopters (D). Mild to moderate levels of regular astigmatism can be corrected with spectacles or contact lenses, although irregular astigmatism is associated with higher-order aberrations which ultimately limit the vision, even with optical correction. This explains why, in 10–20% of PK cases, vision is not satisfactorily corrected by spectacles or contact lenses.[2,3]

A variety of factors are involved in causing excessive astigmatism after keratoplasty, and these can be classified as pre-operative, intra-operative, or post-operative. Pre-existing corneal thinning and vascularization or eccentric trephination of the donor or host tissue are a few examples. Quality of wound healing, astigmatism of the donor cornea, and the tension, length, depth, and configuration of corneal suture placement have been implicated (Table 24.1).[4]

GENERAL CONSIDERATIONS AND AVAILABLE APPROACHES FOR MANAGEMENT OF POST-PKP ASTIGMATISM

The corneal graft–host junction generally heals one year after transplantation, and the corneal surface stabilizes 3–4 months after complete suture removal. However, this duration may vary considerably depending on the patient's age, general health conditions, and use of topical and systemic immunosuppressants. Therefore, surgical procedures for post-keratoplasty astigmatism correction should be postponed for at least three to four months after complete suture removal.

Before any surgical procedure, a complete ophthalmic examination incorporating uncorrected (UCVA) and best-corrected distance visual acuity (BCDVA) should be performed. Slit-lamp biomicroscopy is the best tool for evaluation of graft size, graft centration, graft clarity, and detection of any areas of opacity or neovascularization. The graft–host interface should be investigated with extra attention being paid to the quality of apposition (override or underride) and stability of the surgical wound.

A comprehensive ophthalmological assessment should be performed prior to any surgical procedure. Through examination, this must include uncorrected (UCVA) and best-corrected distance visual acuity (BCDVA), intraocular pressure measurement, slit-lamp biomicroscopy, and dilated fundus examination. Meticulous slit-lamp biomicroscopy is crucial to assessing graft centralization, transparency, and areas of opacification or neovascularization. Attention should be paid to the quality of the apposition (over-ride or under-ride) and the stability of the surgical wound at the graft–host interface.

Astigmatism should be evaluated through a combination of manifest refraction, keratometry, corneal topography, and occasionally wavefront analysis. Central and peripheral pachymetry are required if laser or incisional refractive surgery is planned. Anterior segment OCT is a very useful device for evaluation of corneal thickness in different optical zones and evaluation of the graft–host junction.

Commonly practiced techniques to reduce astigmatism after keratoplasty include post-operative suture manipulation (running suture tension adjustment and selective interrupted suture removal), optical correction (spectacles and contact lenses), relaxing incisions, compression sutures, a combination of relaxing incisions and compression sutures (augmented relaxing incisions), laser refractive surgery (PRK and LASIK), insertion of intrastromal corneal ring segments, wedge resection, toric phakic intraocular lenses, and, finally, regrafting. Relaxing incision may be the primary surgical procedure used by many surgeons to minimize astigmatism after keratoplasty. Advantages of relaxing incisions include the ease of performing the technique, a short stabilization time (3–6 weeks), and the correction of a wide range of astigmatic errors compared

DOI: 10.1201/9781003371601-24

Table 24.1 Factors Contributing to Post-Keratoplasty Astigmatism

Pre-Operative Factors	Intra-Operative Factors	Post-Operative Factors
Severity of the underlying disorder (e.g., keratoconus or PMD)	Infant donor cornea	Time of suture adjustment
	oval or eccentric trephination	Time of suture removal
Pre-existing corneal thinning or vascularization	graft size	Post-operative medications
	Donor–recipient disparity	Post-operative inflammation
Systemic comorbidities (e.g., diabetes mellitus, Down syndrome)	Corneal thickness mismatch	Graft vascularization
	Poor suturing technique	Graft rejection
		Wound dehiscence

with other methods. Disadvantages of relaxing incisions include less predictable results with potential overcorrection, wound destabilization, and inadvertent corneal perforations requiring wound re-suture.[5]

PRINCIPLE OF RELAXING INCISIONS AND SURGICAL TECHNIQUE

Relaxing incision is the first method of choice for many surgeons to reduce astigmatism after keratoplasty. A relaxing incision placed in the graft is termed "astigmatic keratotomy" (AK). The term "arcuate keratotomy" describes the arc shape of relaxing incisions. Incisions can be placed either at the graft–host junction or on the graft itself. Incisions in the recipient corneas are not recommended because scarring at the graft–host junction alters the corneal biomechanics. In addition, the graft–host junction is believed to form a new limbus, that blocks the effect of relaxing incisions in the recipient cornea.[6]

In patients with significant astigmatism after keratoplasty, relaxing incisions can be performed three to four months after complete suture removal. The main principle of relaxing incision is to flatten the steep corneal meridian by making one or two incisions perpendicular to it. This simultaneous flattening of the steep meridian in which the incision is placed and the steepening of the flat meridian 90 degrees away from the incision is known as a "coupling effect". The "coupling ratio" is defined as the amount of flattening at the meridian of the incision divided by the induced steepening in the opposite meridian. A coupling ratio of 1.0 implies equal changes in both steep and flat meridians and no subsequent change in spherical equivalent. A positive coupling ratio (>1.0) causes a hyperopic shift. On the other hand, a negative coupling ratio (<1.0) results in a myopic shift. AK incisions that are straighter than the graft curve yield a myopic shift in the spherical equivalent, and incisions that are more curved than the graft–host wound will induce a hyperopic shift in the spherical equivalent.[7,8]

Corneal thickness should be carefully measured in the optical zone and the steep meridian using ultrasound pachymetry, Scheimpflug corneal topography, or the anterior segment OCT. The outline of the area of the planned incision should be marked prior to surgery. The location of the relaxing incisions is based on the steep axis of astigmatism. Corneal topography is preferred for guidance over keratometry and refraction alone. Relaxing incisions are usually located at a 6- or 7-mm optical zone with an arc length of 45° to 90°. Relaxing incisions should be centered on the visual axis, even in cases of graft decentration. If it is not possible to make a 7-mm optical zone incision within the graft due to the graft eccentricity, the incisions are placed at 0.5–1.0 mm inside the graft–host junction. Incisions in the optical zone smaller than 5 mm are associated with a high level of irregular astigmatism and should be avoided. The optical zone, arc length, and depth are set according to nomograms. The effect of astigmatic correction increases with greater incision depth, smaller optical zone, increasing patient age, and longer incision length.

Relaxing incisions can be performed manually (freehand with a diamond knife or mechanized with a Hanna arcitome) or with femtosecond laser technology. The femtosecond laser is currently being used in these circumstances and results are encouraging. Femtosecond laser AK can be an effective alternative to manual AK, allowing more controlled and more precise incision of corneal tissue in terms of depth, length, and curvature.[9,10]

Combining incisional surgery with compression sutures can achieve greater astigmatic correction. Compression sutures can be placed at the graft–host interface 90 degrees away from the steep meridian. The goal is to overcorrect the astigmatism to allow for selective suture removal post-operatively to titrate the desired astigmatic effect.[5]

NOMOGRAMS

The optical zone, arc length, and depth of relaxing incisions are determined using nomograms. The Hanna nomogram and the Lindstrom nomogram are available for planning manual AK

Table 24.2   Hanna Nomogram for AK in Native Corneas

Refractive Astigmatism (D)	Optical Zone Diameter (mm)	Incision Depth (% of Corneal Thickness)	Angular Length of Incision (Degrees)
2.50 to 3.75	6.75	75	60
4.00 to 5.00	6.50	75	60
5.00 to 6.25	6.50	75	70
6.50 to 7.50	6.25	75	70
7.75 to 8.75	6.25	75	80
9.00 to 15.00	6.00	75	80

incisions in native corneas. The Hanna nomogram is based on refractive astigmatism, from 2.50 D to 15 D. The optical zone diameter for AK in the range 6.00–6.75 mm, with an incision depth of 75% of corneal pachymetry and an angular length from 60 to 80° (Table 24.2).[7,11]

Based on a modified Lindstrom nomogram, Abbey et al.[12] introduced a femtosecond laser AK nomogram for the correction of astigmatism in native corneas based on a modified Lindstrom nomogram. Nomograms developed for native corneas cannot be used for corneas after keratoplasty because they do not react the same way as native corneas to incisional surgery. The effect of relaxing incisions in post-keratoplasty eyes was proportional to the degree of astigmatism, which is not the case in native corneas. Saint-Clair has developed a new modified nomogram for femtosecond laser astigmatic keratotomy after keratoplasty, taking into account multiple factors associated with the incision and the amount of pre-existing astigmatism (Table 24.3).[13]

MANUAL VS FSAK

Astigmatic keratotomy can be done manually with a handheld diamond knife, or mechanized like the Hanna arcitome. The advent of the femtosecond laser has promised improved accuracy, safety, and reproducibility in the treatment of high levels of astigmatism after keratoplasty compared with manual and mechanized incision. Intra-operative OCT on a femtosecond laser platform allows surgeon to precisely adjust location, depth, and centration of the incision. FSAK is also associated with a reduced risk of wound dehiscence, epithelial down growth, infection, and corneal incisions perforation.

Studies have shown that both manual AK and FSAK are safe and effective in reducing astigmatism after keratoplasty. However, FSAK had better visual and keratometric results compared with manual AK.[10,14,15]

IRREGULAR ASTIGMATISM

The goal of relaxing incisions in post keratoplasty is to treat astigmatism that cannot be corrected with spectacles or contact lenses. This includes high levels of regular astigmatism and variable degrees of irregular astigmatism. Certain levels of nonorthogonal astigmatism could be observed after uneventful keratoplasty due to unpredictable course of wound healing in such cases. Irregular astigmatism could reduce both corrected and uncorrected distance visual acuity.[4]

Table 24.3   Nomogram for Femtosecond Laser AK after Keratoplasty

Pre-Op DK	Incision Magnitude	Correction (%)	Incision Depth (% Corneal Thickness)	Arc Length (Degrees)	Optical Zone Diameter (mm)
2	1.311	0.87	85	60	7.0
3	1.784	0.82	85	75	6.8
4	2.176	0.78	85	85	6.7
5	2.508	0.72	85	90	6.6
6	2.791	0.98	90	90	6.6
7	3.036	0.91	90	90	6.5
8	3.249	0.87	90	90	6.4
9	3.438	0.83	90	90	6.3
10	3.605	0.81	90	90	6.2

Most studies have evaluated the effect of relaxing incisions in regular astigmatism. Studies of irregular astigmatism are limited, and there is no modified nomogram in such cases. However, available studies concluded that femtosecond laser-assisted AK is also effective in reducing irregular astigmatism after PKP. It should be noticed that relaxing incisions should be performed using single or paired asymmetric (same or different length) incisions centered on the topographic location of the steep meridian. Paired incisions needed to be centered on the steep axis of each meridian, even if the meridians were not aligned. Unsuccessful correction and overcorrection occur more in cases with irregular astigmatism because of irregular nature of such cases and instability of asymmetric incisions over time. Refinement of the treatment nomogram for femtosecond laser-assisted AK for high astigmatism after PKP remains a major issue.[16]

OTHER TECHNIQUES

Beveled Astigmatic Keratotomy

Femtosecond laser astigmatic keratotomy (FLAK) demonstrates accuracy, safety, and reproducibility in the treatment of high post-keratoplasty astigmatism compared with conventional manual relaxing incisions. Most of the studies applied incisions at 90 degrees to the corneal surface. This technique has a lower incidence of complications, such as full thickness perforation. However, a 90-degree incision orientation is still associated with the same problem of wound gaping that occurs with manual astigmatic keratotomy incisions. The wound healing process after astigmatic keratotomy can take from six months to five years; at first, the wound gape becomes filled with an epithelial plug, and then replaced with hypercellular scar tissue. This complex process could explain late changes in corneal curvature, which occur due to increased separation of the edges of the wound. A wound gape is also a potential site for infection and causes foreign body sensation and discomfort for the patient.[14,17]

Some authors hypothesized that oblique incisions made at a 135° angle to the corneal surface could decrease wound gaping by allowing for the anterior cornea to slide forward. Moreover, these beveled incisions can be made at a 65–75% depth, rather than 90%, with a reported comparable reduction in astigmatism versus the traditional 90 degrees femtosecond laser-assisted arcuate keratotomy (FSAK) incisions.[18]

ISAK (Intrastromal Astigmatic Keratotomy)

Relaxing incisions extend from the anterior corneal surface to the posterior stroma at 90% depth in order to flatten the steep corneal meridian. Recently, nonpenetrating or intrastromal astigmatic keratotomy (ISAK) was introduced to minimize both early and late anterior wound complications. The absence of an open wound in such incisions can avoid wound gape, infections or epithelial disruption. ISAK was successful for treatment of mild to moderate astigmatism such as naturally occurring and post-cataract surgery astigmatism and residual astigmatism after refractive surgery.[19,20]

Some authors have tried ISAK for treatment of high amount of astigmatism after keratoplasty. Wetterstrand et al. reported the results of ISAK after penetrating keratoplasty of 16 patients. Intrastromal incisions were made with a depth of 90% of corneal thickness, optical zone of 6.0–7.0 mm, and a safe area of 90 µm anteriorly. Desired intact posterior corneal border also kept close to 90 µm for protection of the endothelium. At 3 months follow-up, refractive cylinders decreased from 6.8 ± 2.2 D to 3.7 ± 1.7 D, with no severe adverse effect. Post-keratoplasty astigmatism reduced up to 53% by ISAK.[21] This technique seems to be relatively safe and effective. However further studies are needed for introduction of reliable nomograms.

DIAKIK (Deep Intrastromal Arcuate Keratotomy with In Situ Keratomileusis)

To eliminate early and late complications of relaxing incisions because of anteriorly opened wound, the idea of nonpenetrating incisions had formed. Loriaut et al. described a novel technique, deep intrastromal arcuate keratotomy with in situ keratomileusis (DIAKIK) for treatment of high natural occurring and post-keratoplasty astigmatism. In this technique deep ISAK performed under a LASIK flap:

The first step is ISAK. This is performed at 75% depth of corneal stroma. A 100 µm LASIK flap was then made, lifted to open the ISAK, and the flap replaced. Excimer laser ablation can be performed one month later to correct any residual refractive error under the flap.

DIAKIK technique allows a greater astigmatism correction and can reduce the astigmatism by over 80%, however there are still potential complications of the LASIK itself like epithelial ingrowth and microperforations.[22,23]

COMPLICATIONS AND SOLUTIONS

Astigmatic keratotomy can be very effective in reducing post-keratoplasty astigmatism, however like other ophthalmic procedure inadvertent complications could be observed such as overcorrection, undercorrection, corneal perforation, wound gape, corneal ectasia, infectious keratitis, allograft rejection, and even endophthalmitis. The technology of femtosecond laser brings more safety and predictability to astigmatic keratotomy but complications still exist.[15]

Predictability

Poor predictability is the major concern in post-keratoplasty astigmatic keratotomy. The rate of overcorrection has been reported up to 43.5% of patients who underwent FSAK after PKP or DALK.[14] The unpredictability seems to be correlated with many variables such as the value of the initial cylinder, pattern of astigmatism, individual variability and misalignment in correction. Individual variability may be due to compression force distribution in corneal graft and variability in biomechanical constraints. Misalignment could be prevented by precise limbal marking just before procedure and control of cyclotorsion intraoperatively. The pattern of irregular astigmatism (where the flat and the steep meridians are not orthogonal) could also lead to unpredictable results. Some authors suggested using topography-guided placement of relaxing incision in such cases.[24]

Long-term instability in refraction is another challenge which can be explained by the inherent dynamic instability and effect of epithelial remodeling in such incisions over time. Nonpenetrating relaxing incisions may eliminate epithelial induced complications and long-term instability.[21,22]

Corneal Perforation

The risk of deep incision and inadvertent corneal perforation is higher in manual procedures, because pre-operative visualization of the corneal thickness is not possible. In manual astigmatic keratotomy, depth is routinely set at 75–85% of central corneal thickness (CCT) without *in-vivo* visualization. Deep incisions are also associated with late wound dehiscence. Femtosecond laser technology, combined with anterior OCT, provides more depth accuracy as we have a clear intraoperative view of the cornea thickness. Microperforations are usually self-sealing but sometimes may requiring sutures. Overcorrection or late wound dehiscence can also be managed with compressive sutures.[9]

Infections

Infections are rare but possible, typically occurring between six to 12 months post-operatively. Infectious keratitis frequency has been reported as being from 0% to 4.8% with FSAK after PKP and all cases were resolved with topical antibiotics.[9,16] Topical post-operative antimicrobial prophylaxis should be administered and it should be sufficient. Rarely, fibrosis at the incision site may not properly form and epithelial disruption would be a trigger for infection that can occur as late as 15 years after the procedure.[25]

Only one case of endophthalmitis has been reported after FSAK. Endophthalmitis occurred five days after procedure, with no clinical evidence of wound leakage intra-operatively. The patient was treated for 9 D of cylinder. The endophthalmitis resolved with intravitreal antibiotic therapy but with a loss of two lines of BCVA.[16]

Graft Rejection

Allograft rejections have also been reported after astigmatic keratotomy; however, all have been resolved with topical steroids. Administration of prophylactic topical steroids may prevent such rejections.[13,26]

CONCLUSION

Astigmatic keratotomy is the first surgical procedure used by many cornea surgeons to reduce high levels of astigmatism after keratoplasty. Advantages of relaxing incisions over other methods include the ease of technique, minimal surface disturbance, rapid visual recovery, and the correction of a wide range of both orthogonal and nonorthogonal astigmatisms.

With either manual or femtosecond laser-assisted techniques, overall astigmatic reduction ranged from 30 to 72%. Most of the patients with astigmatism higher than 6 D had residual cylinder less or equal to 3 D after the procedure, which can then be considered for other corrective methods.[6,9,15,27]

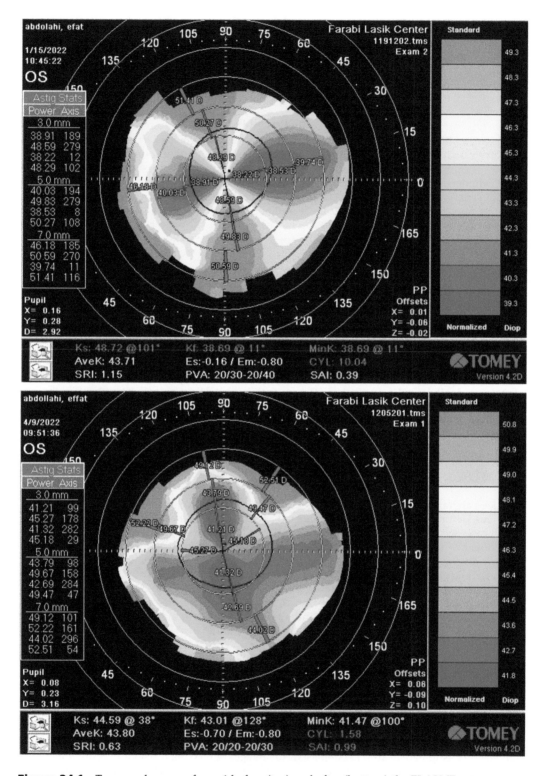

Figure 24.1 Topography map of case 1 before (top) and after (bottom) the FLAK (Femto-Assisted Astigmatic Keratotomy) procedure, illustrating a marked reduction in the topographic astigmatism from 10.04 D pre-operatively to 1.58 D three months after the procedure. D, diopter.

In the reported comparative studies, FSAK appears to be safer (especially with less wound dehiscence) and more predictable than manual keratotomy. However, all studies showed great variability in results, despite using the same surgical method. There is no standard surgical procedure nor well-predicted nomogram for post-keratoplasty astigmatic correction due to its unpredictable nature. A recently introduced nomogram for surgical planning of FSAK for post-keratoplasty astigmatism, which was created using regression analysis, has the co-efficient of determination of about 0.67, meaning that 33% of the variation in Surgically Induced Astigmatism (SIA) correction amount cannot be attributed to known pre-operative parameters.[13]

Further prospective studies should be conducted to introduce new nomograms by considering more variables with higher predictability. We may never reach a predictable and ideal nomogram in post-keratoplasty astigmatism due to the unpredictable nature of the healing process in corneal grafts. Surgeons should use available nomograms as a guide, and constantly monitor and adjust them based on their own experience and surgical outcomes. However, the ultimate goal of AK is to reduce advanced astigmatism, which can be corrected with optical correction or more predictable surgery, such as excimer laser ablation or toric IOL implantation.

CASE PRESENTATION

A 51-year-old keratoconic woman with a history of Big Bubble DALK, performed for keratoconus, had high astigmatism 12 months after complete suture removal. Before the procedure, UCVA was 20/400, which improved to 20/100 with +7.5 −8.50 × 10. Keratometry readings were 38.69 × 11/48.72 × 101 Figure 24.1, top). Two arcuate incisions with 75 degrees length were made by a femtosecond laser at a 7.00-mm optical zone with 70% depth. Arc center position was located at 105° and 185° at the steepest meridians. At the last follow-up examination, which was performed three months after the FLAK, UCVA was 20/100 which improved to 20/50 with +3.00 −2.0 × 10 and keratometry reading were 43.01 × 128/44.59 × 38, respectively, indicating a reduction of 8.00 D in keratometric astigmatism (Figure 24.1, bottom).

REFERENCES

1. Shimmura S, Tsubota K. Deep anterior lamellar keratoplasty. *Curr Opin Ophthalmol.* 2006;17(4):349–355. doi:10.1097/01.ICU.0000233953.09595.91

2. Olson RJ, Pingree M, Ridges R, Lundergan ML, Alldredge C, Clinch TE. Penetrating keratoplasty for keratoconus: a long-term review of results and complications. *J Cataract Refract Surg.* 2000;26(7):987–991. doi:10.1016/S0886-3350(00)00430-2

3. Coster DJ, Lowe MT, Keane MC, Williams KA. A comparison of lamellar and penetrating keratoplasty outcomes: a registry study. *Ophthalmology.* 2014;121(5):979–987. doi:10.1016/J.OPHTHA.2013.12.017

4. Deshmukh R, Nair S, Vaddavalli PK, et al. Post-penetrating keratoplasty astigmatism. *Surv Ophthalmol.* 2022;67(4):1200–1228. doi:10.1016/J.SURVOPHTHAL.2021.11.005

5. Feizi S, Zare M. Current approaches for management of postpenetrating keratoplasty astigmatism. *J Ophthalmol.* 2011;2011:1–8. doi:10.1155/2011/708736

6. Ho Wang Yin G, Hoffart L. Post-keratoplasty astigmatism management by relaxing incisions: a systematic review. *Eye Vis (Lond).* 2017;4(1). doi:10.1186/S40662-017-0093-7

7. Hardten DR, Lindstrom RL. Surgical correction of refractive errors after penetrating keratoplasty. *Int Ophthalmol Clin.* 1997;37(1):1–35. doi:10.1097/00004397-199703710-00003

8. Rowsey JJ, Fouraker BD. Corneal coupling principles. *Int Ophthalmol Clin.* 1996;36(4):29–38. doi:10.1097/00004397-199603640-00006

9. al Sabaani N, al Malki S, al Jindan M, al Assiri A, al Swailem S. Femtosecond astigmatic keratotomy for postkeratoplasty astigmatism. *Saudi J Ophthalmol.* 2016;30(3):163–168. doi:10.1016/j.sjopt.2016.04.003

10. Chang JSM. Femtosecond laser-assisted astigmatic keratotomy: a review. *Eye and Vision.* 2018;5(1). doi:10.1186/s40662-018-0099-9

11. Hoffart L, Touzeau O, Borderie V, Laroche L. Mechanized astigmatic arcuate keratotomy with the Hanna arcitome for astigmatism after keratoplasty. *J Cataract Refract Surg.* 2007;33(5):862–868. doi:10.1016/J.JCRS.2007.01.031

12. Abbey A, Ide T, Kymionis GD, Yoo SH. Femtosecond laser-assisted astigmatic keratotomy in naturally occurring high astigmatism. *Br J Ophthalmol.* 2009;93:1566–1569.

13. st. Clair RM, Sharma A, Huang D, et al. Development of a nomogram for femtosecond laser astigmatic keratotomy for astigmatism after keratoplasty. *J Cataract Refract Surg.* 2016;42(4):556–562. doi:10.1016/J.JCRS.2015.12.053

14. Hashemian MN, Ojaghi H, Mohammadpour M, et al. Femtosecond laser arcuate keratotomy for the correction of postkeratoplasty high astigmatism in keratoconus. *J Res Medi Sci.* 2017;22(1). doi:10.4103/1735-1995.200267

15. Al-Qurashi M, al Sabaani N, al Malki S. Comparison of manual and femtosecond laser arcuate keratotomy procedures for the correction of post-keratoplasty astigmatism. *Saudi J Ophthalmol.* 2019;33(1):12–17. doi:10.1016/j.sjopt.2018.11.001

16. Fadlallah A, Mehanna C, Saragoussi JJ, Chelala E, Amari B, Legeais JM. Safety and efficacy of femtosecond laser-assisted arcuate keratotomy to treat irregular astigmatism after penetrating keratoplasty. *J Cataract Refract Surg.* 2015;41(6):1168–1175. doi:10.1016/J.JCRS.2014.08.046

17. Donnenfeld E, Rosenberg E, Boozan H, Davis Z, Nattis A. Randomized prospective evaluation of the wound integrity of primary clear corneal incisions made with a femtosecond laser versus a manual keratome. *J Cataract Refract Surg.* 2018;44(3):329–335. doi:10.1016/J.JCRS.2017.12.026

18. Cleary C, Tang M, Ahmed H, Fox M, Huang D. Beveled femtosecond laser astigmatic keratotomy for the treatment of high astigmatism post-penetrating keratoplasty. *Cornea.* 2013;32(1):54–62. doi:10.1097/ICO.0B013E31825EA2E6

19. Byun YS, Kim S, Lazo MZ, et al. Astigmatic correction by intrastromal astigmatic keratotomy during femtosecond laser-assisted cataract surgery: factors in outcomes. *J Cataract Refract Surg.* 2018;44(2):202–208. doi:10.1016/J.JCRS.2017.11.018

20. Day AC, Lau NM, Stevens JD. Nonpenetrating femtosecond laser intrastromal astigmatic keratotomy in eyes having cataract surgery. *J Cataract Refract Surg.* 2016;42(1):102–109. doi:10.1016/J.JCRS.2015.07.045

21. Wetterstrand O, Holopainen JM, Krootila K. Treatment of postoperative keratoplasty astigmatism using femtosecond laser-assisted intrastromal relaxing incisions. *J Refract Surg.* 2013;29(6):378–382. doi:10.3928/1081597X-20130515-01

22. Loriaut P, Sandali O, el Sanharawi M, Goemaere I, Borderie V, Laroche L. New combined technique of deep intrastromal arcuate keratotomy overlayed by LASIK flap for treatment of high astigmatism. *Cornea.* 2014;33(10):1123–1128. doi:10.1097/ICO.0000000000000236

23. Shalash RB, Elshazly MI, Salama MM. Combined intrastromal astigmatic keratotomy and laser in situ keratomileusis flap followed by photoablation to correct post-penetrating keratoplasty ametropia and high astigmatism: one-year follow-up. *J Cataract Refract Surg.* 2015;41(10):2251–2257. doi:10.1016/J.JCRS.2015.10.028

24. Geggel HS. Arcuate relaxing incisions guided by corneal topography for postkeratoplasty astigmatism: vector and topographic analysis. *Cornea*. 2006;25(5):545–557. doi:10.1097/01. ICO.0000214222.13615.B6

25. Heidemann DG, Dunn SP, Chow CYC. Early- versus late-onset infectious keratitis after radial and astigmatic keratotomy: clinical spectrum in a referral practice. *J Cataract Refract Surg*. 1999;25(12):1615–1619. doi:10.1016/S0886-3350(99)00285-0

26. Javadi M, Feizi S, Mirbabaee F, Fekri Y. Office-based relaxing incision procedure for correction of astigmatism after deep anterior lamellar keratoplasty. *J Ophthalmic Vis Res*. 2017;12(2):156–164. doi:10.4103/jovr.jovr_24_16

27. Ho Wang Yin G, Hoffart L. Post-keratoplasty astigmatism management by relaxing incisions: a systematic review. *Eye and Vision*. 2017;4(1). doi:10.1186/s40662-017-0093-7

25 Intra-Operative and Post-Operative Suture-Related Considerations and Complications of Corneal Graft for Keratoconus

Alireza Peyman, Asieh Aslani, and Mohsen Pourazizi

INTRODUCTION

Keratoconus is a progressive corneal disease that results in thinning and protrusion of the cornea, leading to visual impairment. In cases where conservative treatments are no longer effective, corneal transplantation is the standard of treatment. Corneal grafting, specifically penetrating keratoplasty (PK) and deep anterior lamellar keratoplasty (DALK), are commonly used surgical interventions for advanced keratoconus.[1,2]

Advances in surgical techniques and suture materials have aimed to reduce the risk of suture-related complications and improve the outcomes of corneal transplantation for keratoconus. This chapter will review prerequisite, intra-operative, and post-operative suture-related considerations and complications of corneal graft for keratoconus.[1,3] We will discuss the factors that influence suture-related complications, the different types of suture materials and techniques used, and the management of suture-related complications. By providing a comprehensive overview of these issues, this chapter aims to improve the understanding of suture-related complications and inform best practices for the successful management of corneal transplantation for keratoconus.

PREREQUISITES

Learning Curve and Teaching Methods

Successful management of suture-related complications during corneal transplantation for keratoconus requires a high level of skill and expertise. However, achieving proficiency in this area is not an easy task and requires a significant learning curve. During this period, surgeons may encounter different types of suture-related complications and develop techniques to avoid or manage them.

Therefore, a structured training program is necessary to ensure that ophthalmology residents and corneal fellows acquire the necessary skills to perform corneal suturing and manage suture-related complications. Such programs should include didactic lectures, supervised surgical training, and surgical simulation.

Didactic lectures should cover the principles of suture placement, suture tension, and suture material selection. Additionally, the anatomy of the cornea, wound healing, and different suturing techniques should be discussed in detail. These lectures should be supplemented with instructional videos and surgical demonstrations.

Supervised surgical training should involve hands-on experience under the direct supervision of an experienced corneal surgeon. Surgical simulation is another valuable tool for training. Simulation training allows the practice of suturing techniques in a controlled environment without risking patient safety. There are various models available for corneal suturing simulation, such as the use of corneal buttons or synthetic models.

Instrumentation

Corneal suturing is an integral part of keratoplasty, and selecting the appropriate instrumentation is essential for achieving optimal outcomes. The choice of instruments should be based on their ability to provide accurate, precise, and consistent suturing while minimizing tissue trauma.[4]

Forceps Forceps are essential for manipulating the corneal tissue during suturing. Fine, delicate forceps are preferred to minimize tissue trauma. The tips of the forceps should be flat to avoid creating pressure points on the corneal tissue. Ideally, forceps should be lightweight and ergonomic, allowing for comfortable and precise manipulation of the tissue. Forceps with angled tips can be useful for suturing in difficult-to-reach areas.

Needles Needles are used to pass the suture through the cornea. Tapered needles are preferred due to their ability to penetrate the cornea more easily and create smaller suture tracks. Cutting needles can be used where a more aggressive approach is required, but they can also increase tissue trauma. Spatulated needles can be useful for creating smoother suture tracks or when passing sutures through thick tissue.

Needle Holders Needle holders are necessary for holding the needle during suturing. They should be lightweight and ergonomic, allowing for comfortable and precise manipulation of the

DOI: 10.1201/9781003371601-25

needle. They might have a locking mechanism to prevent the needle from slipping or rotating during suturing, although some surgeons prefer a non-locking needle holder. The jaws of the needle holder should be smooth to avoid damaging the suture.

Scissors Scissors are used to cut the suture. Fine, delicate scissors are preferred to minimize tissue trauma. Curved scissors can be useful for suturing in difficult-to-reach areas. The scissors should be held perpendicular to the suture to ensure a clean and precise cut.

Surgical Blades Surgical blades are used to create the initial incision in the cornea. They should be sharp and precise, with a small profile to minimize tissue trauma. The blade should be held perpendicular to the corneal surface to create a clean and precise incision. Ideally, the blade should be disposable to minimize the risk of infection.

Sutures Different types of sutures are available for suturing, including sutures composed of absorbable or non-absorbable materials. The choice of suture material depends on the surgeon's preference and the specific needs of the patient. Non-absorbable sutures are preferred for long-term stability, while absorbable sutures are useful for temporary fixation or when long-term suturing is not required. The size of the suture should be chosen based on the thickness of the corneal tissue, and the suture material should be selected based on its biocompatibility and tensile strength.

Suture Material and Needle Types

Suture material is an important consideration in corneal graft and keratoplasty procedures, as it plays a crucial role in the success of the surgery. The choice of suture material depends on several factors, including the duration of the post-operative period, the tension on the wound, and the surgeon's preference.[4,5]

Non-Absorbable Suture Materials Non-absorbable suture materials are commonly used in corneal graft and keratoplasty procedures. These sutures are made of materials that are not broken down by the body's enzymes and remain in place for extended periods. Nylon, polyester, and polypropylene are the most used non-absorbable suture materials in corneal surgery. Nylon is preferred due to its strength, flexibility, and excellent knot-tying ability. Polyester and polypropylene are used in cases where higher tensile strength is required for a longer time.

Absorbable Suture Materials Absorbable suture materials are less frequently used alternatives to non-absorbable sutures and are useful when the suture is needed for only a short period while the removal is expected to be bothersome, such as in the pediatric age group. These sutures are made of materials that are degraded by the body's enzymes and eliminated within a few weeks. Polyglactin and poliglecaprone are the absorbable suture materials used in corneal surgery but are not suitable for corneal grafts when long-term strength of the suture is necessary.

Suture Thickness The choice of suture thickness depends on the tensile strength necessary and the surgeon's preference. In general, 11-0 to 8-0 sutures are used in corneal surgery. 10-0 sutures are preferred by most surgeons. However, thicker sutures may be required in cases of thicker corneas or to provide additional tensile strength, such as 11-0 sutures.

Needle Types The choice of needle type also plays a role in the success of corneal repair and keratoplasty procedures. The two most commonly used needle types in corneal surgery are tapered and cutting needles.

Tapered Needles Tapered needles are used in corneal surgery due to their ability to penetrate the cornea more easily and create smaller suture tracks. These needles have a sharp, pointed tip, tapering to a smaller diameter toward the end of the needle. Tapered needles are ideal for use on thin corneas or when a smaller suture track is required.

Cutting Needles: Cutting needles have a sharp, triangular tip that cuts through tissue more easily than tapered needles. These needles are useful in cases where a more aggressive approach is required, such as for use on thicker or more fibrotic corneas. However, the use of cutting needles can increase tissue trauma and may result in a larger suture track.

Spatulated Needles Spatulated needles are useful for creating smoother suture tracks. These needles easily pass through thick or fibrotic tissue.

INTRA-OPERATIVE TECHNIQUE

Suturing Technique

The suture material and needle type are chosen based on the surgeon's preference and the surgical procedure. Typically, interrupted and running sutures are used in cornea suturing. Interrupted sutures are more reliable and robust and preferred in cases with a diseased recipient bed. Running sutures are usually used in combination with interrupted sutures; they are quicker to place, and some surgeons feel better astigmatic control with running sutures.[5,6] Torque, anti-torque, and no-torque running suturing methods were devised to improve the outcome in different surgical situations. The first suture is usually placed at the 12 o'clock position, and subsequent sutures are placed at 6 o'clock, 3 o'clock, and 9 o'clock positions. The sutures are placed deep in the stroma and reach 90–95% depth, approximately 0.5 to 1 mm from the edge of the cornea wound. The suture is then passed through the donor cornea, starting from the opposite side of the recipient cornea. The suture is then tied with a square knot, and the excess suture is trimmed away.[4]

Suture Knots

Suture knots are an important aspect of keratoplasty surgery, as they are used to secure the suture material in place and maintain proper tension on the cornea. Several different knot-tying techniques and suture materials are used in keratoplasty surgery, each with its own advantages and disadvantages.

One common knot-tying technique used in keratoplasty surgery is the square knot. This knot is created by making two opposing loops and then interlocking them to secure the suture material in place. The square knot is a strong knot and is easy to tie, making it a popular choice in keratoplasty surgery.

Another knot-tying technique used in keratoplasty surgery is the slip knot. This knot is created by making a loop in the suture material and then passing the free end of the suture through the loop. The slip knot is a versatile knot and can be adjusted to achieve the desired tension on the cornea.

The type of suture material used in keratoplasty surgery can also affect the knot-tying technique used. Non-absorbable sutures, such as nylon and polyester, are commonly used in keratoplasty surgery due to their strength and durability.

Several studies have compared different knot-tying techniques and suture materials in keratoplasty surgery. One study found that the use of a modified slip knot technique with non-absorbable sutures resulted in better outcomes compared with other knot-tying techniques, including the square knot and the surgeon's knot.

Suture Tension

Suture tension is a critical factor in achieving optimal outcomes in keratoplasty. The tension of the sutures can affect the curvature of the cornea and, therefore, the degree of astigmatism that develops post-operatively.

Sutures are typically placed in a specific pattern during keratoplasty, with each suture contributing to the overall tension on the cornea. If the tension of the sutures is too high, it can cause the cornea to become steep, resulting in a high degree of astigmatism. Conversely, if the tension is too low, it can cause the cornea to become flat, resulting in a low degree of astigmatism.

The tension of the sutures is typically adjusted during the surgery to achieve the desired curvature of the cornea. This is done by manipulating the tension of each suture individually, either by tightening or loosening the suture as necessary. The surgeon must use their judgment and experience to determine the appropriate tension for each suture to achieve the desired outcome.

Various techniques can be used to measure and adjust suture tension during keratoplasty. One common technique is to use a hand-held surgical keratoscope to visualize the mires indicating curvature of the cornea and the distribution of tension on the sutures. The surgeon can use this information to adjust the tension of each suture as needed. Grossly, a perfectly circular donor might have an even curvature while an oval donor is a sign of high astigmatism. Studies have shown that the tension of the sutures is a significant factor in determining the degree of post-operative astigmatism in keratoplasty.[3,7]

Tissue Position

Correct tissue position is a critical factor in achieving optimal long-term astigmatic outcome in cornea grafts. The alignment of the donor cornea with the recipient bed is crucial for reducing astigmatism and achieving good visual acuity.

During the surgery, the donor cornea is sutured onto the recipient bed using interrupted sutures. The sutures are placed in a specific pattern, usually at the 12 o'clock, 6 o'clock, 3 o'clock, and 9 o'clock positions. The tension of the sutures is adjusted to ensure that the donor cornea is aligned with the recipient bed. If the donor cornea is not positioned correctly, it can result in a high degree of astigmatism, which can significantly affect visual acuity. In addition, if the sutures are not placed at the correct depth, it can cause an uneven wound, which can also contribute to astigmatism.

A common technique to ensure correct tissue position during a cornea graft is to use a surgical marker to mark the center of the recipient cornea and the center of the donor cornea, and mark the donor and recipient cardinal points. The surgeon can use these marks as a guide to ensure that the donor cornea is aligned correctly with the recipient bed. A corneal radial marker can be invaluable in complicated cases; some surgeons use dye on the trephine appendages as a marker.[3,7]

POST-OPERATIVE CONSIDERATIONS

Despite proper technique and materials, sutures in keratoplasty can still result in post-operative complications. These complications can include suture-related infections, suture loosening, suture breakage, suture abscess formation, and suture infiltrations. These complications can lead to wound leaks, astigmatic changes, and graft rejection.[7-9]

Leakage

Suture leakage occurs when the cornea wound is not properly sealed by the sutures, leading to fluid outflow from the cornea wound. This can occur as a result of loose sutures, broken sutures, or wound dehiscence due to cheese wiring of sutures, and can lead to ocular hypotonia, infectious endophthalmitis, and subsequent complications. Treatment may involve repositioning or replacing the sutures and, in some cases, the use of tissue adhesives.

Loose Sutures

Loose sutures can result in inadequate wound closure and increased risk of infection. Loose sutures can lead to wound dehiscence and exposure of the graft, which can result in infection and graft failure. A loose suture could also trigger cornea neovascularization and graft rejection. Treatment may involve removing or replacing the loose sutures. A running loose suture should be removed at once, but some surgeons try to anchor a loose running suture to limbus or sclera using a single suture which usually works for a short time and the sutures could be removed with or without replacement.

Suture Infiltration

Suture infiltration occurs when the suture tract becomes surrounded by inflammatory cells due to incited inflammation or infection, leading to tissue loss or neovascularization. Treatment may involve removal of the affected sutures, use of topical, subconjunctival, or intra-corneal antibiotics, and replacement with new sutures, when necessary.[9]

Suture Abscess Formation

Suture abscess formation can occur when bacteria or other microorganisms gain entry to the wound site along the suture tract. This can result in infection and inflammation, leading to corneal opacity and astigmatism. Treatment may involve removal of the affected sutures and administration of antibiotics. Some extreme uncontrolled cases might result in cornea melting which necessitates a repeat graft or a patch cornea graft.[9]

Suture Breakage

Suture breakage can occur due to material fatigue or trauma to the suture. This can result in incomplete wound closure and exposure of the graft, leading to infection and graft failure. Treatment involves removal of the affected sutures and re-suturing the wound.

Astigmatism

Astigmatism is a common complication following keratoplasty and can result from misplaced tissue, suture tension, erroneous suture placement, or uneven wound healing. To manage astigmatism, a variety of techniques can be employed, including selective suture removal or adjustment, relaxing incisions, and laser-assisted techniques. A relaxing keratotomy on the steep meridian, usually performed at least three months after removal of the sutures, could be done as an incision or induced dehiscence at the surgical wound guided by keratoscopy or a nomogram. Femto-laser assisted incisions at the junction or inside the donor tissue is another option, aiming to decrease astigmatism. A compression suture at the flat meridian will augment the effect of the astigmatic incisions; a wedge cornea tissue incision at the flat meridian might help to treat the most extreme cases. A smaller degree of astigmatism might be addressed using a cornea laser vision correction procedure in an appropriate subject (usually femto-LASIK), Toric phakic IOLs are another alternative. For irregular or extremely high astigmatism, the physician may discuss the possibility of a repeat keratoplasty. Proper management of astigmatism can improve visual outcomes following keratoplasty.[7]

Suture Removal

All non-absorbable sutures must be removed. For a regular cornea incision, many surgeons remove the sutures at about six weeks after surgery, although, for a large vertical wound of a keratoplasty, removing any suture before three months might increase the risk of wound dehiscence. Some interrupted sutures at the steep meridian might be removed to control the astigmatism about three months after surgery. Any loose or infiltrated sutures should be removed immediately to decrease the risk of infection or neovascularization. All sutures must be covered by cornea epithelium; visible shining of the suture plastic material is a sign of suture baring and risk of imminent loosening of the suture.[7,10] Many surgeons use a topical antiseptic (usually a 5% povidone-iodine drop) just before suture removal and a few days of topical antibiotic drops to decrease the risk of cornea infection or even infectious endophthalmitis for a full thickness suture. After a year of keratoplasty, the surgeon decides to remove the sutures. For patients with some astigmatism, removal of all sutures could be helpful for addressing the astigmatism with other procedures, although, in patients with small degrees of astigmatism, the surgeon may decide to leave the sutures in place for a longer time. Gradual degradation of the nylon suture material, especially under the upper eyelid will cause spontaneous breakage of the suture which, on some occasions, makes it bothersome to the patients and it is sometimes not easy to remove a degraded thin suture using regular forceps.[10]

REFERENCES

1. Keane M, Coster D, Ziaei M, Williams K. Deep anterior lamellar keratoplasty versus penetrating keratoplasty for treating keratoconus. *The Cochrane Database of Systematic Reviews.* 2014(7):Cd009700. https://doi.org/10.1002/14651858.cd009700.pub2

2. Henein C, Nanavaty MA. Systematic review comparing penetrating keratoplasty and deep anterior lamellar keratoplasty for management of keratoconus. *Contact Lens & Anterior Eye: The Journal of the British Contact Lens Association.* 2017;40(1):3–14.

3. Feizi S, Javadi MA, Karimian F, Bayat K, Bineshfar N, Esfandiari H. Penetrating keratoplasty versus deep anterior lamellar keratoplasty for advanced stage of keratoconus. *American Journal of Ophthalmology.* 2023;248:107–115.

4. Pagano L, Shah H, Al Ibrahim O, et al. Update on suture techniques in corneal transplantation: a systematic review. *Journal of Clinical Medicine.* 2022;11(4):1078.

5. Acar BT, Vural ET, Acar S. Does the type of suturing technique used affect astigmatism after deep anterior lamellar keratoplasty in keratoconus patients? *Clinical Ophthalmology (Auckland, NZ).* 2011;5:425–428.

6. Javadi MA, Naderi M, Zare M, Jenaban A, Rabei HM, Anissian A. Comparison of the effect of three suturing techniques on postkeratoplasty astigmatism in keratoconus. *Cornea.* 2006;25(9):1029–1033.

7. Deshmukh R, Nair S, Vaddavalli PK, et al. Post-penetrating keratoplasty astigmatism. *Survey of Ophthalmology.* 2022;67(4):1200–1228.

8. Moramarco A, Gardini L, Iannetta D, Versura P, Fontana L. Post penetrating keratoplasty ectasia: incidence, risk factors, clinical features, and treatment options. *Journal of Clinical Medicine.* 2022;11(10):2678.

9. Song A, Deshmukh R, Lin H, et al. Post-keratoplasty infectious keratitis: epidemiology, risk factors, management, and outcomes. *Frontiers in Medicine.* 2021;8:707242.

10. Fares U, Sarhan AR, Dua HS. Management of post-keratoplasty astigmatism. *Journal of Cataract and Refractive Surgery.* 2012;38(11):2029–2039.

26 Corneal Graft Rejection: Pathophysiology, Clinical Presentations, Prevention, and Management

Mohammad-ali Javadi, Kiana Hassanpour, and Hossein Mohammad-Rabei

INTRODUCTION

The corneal graft is the most successful solid-tissue transplantation.[1] Despite containing corneal antigens in donor tissue, the high success rate of corneal transplantation mainly relates to the immune privilege (IP) of the cornea and one of the IP components, anterior chamber-associated immune deviation (ACAID). IP and ACAID alter the classical recognition of corneal antigens by the immune system.[2,3] Since these processes are relative, immunologic graft rejection is one of the most frequent complications after corneal transplantation, both penetrating and lamellar, and remains the most common cause of graft failure.[4,5] Corneal graft rejection refers to the process in which a graft, which has been clear for at least two weeks, becomes edematous because of an immunologic reaction.[6] Like other transplant rejections, corneal graft rejection is immunologically mediated, although this type of transplantation enjoys the advantage of immunotolerance which is rarely seen in other organ transplantations.[7] Up to one-third of eyes with penetrating keratoplasty experience at least one episode of immunologic reaction and about 5–7% result in subsequent graft failure.[8] It has been reported that approximately 12% of graft rejection episodes in low-risk settings and 40% in high-risk settings lead to subsequent graft failure.[9,10] Our experience, however, indicates that timely diagnosis and appropriate treatment of rejection episodes can reduce its rate significantly. The graft survival rate has significantly improved using topical preventive measures.

PATHOPHYSIOLOGY

Immune Privilege of the Cornea

■ Corneal graft, a solid tissue transplantation, has a higher success rate than other transplants. The normal cornea is an immune-privileged site, and multiple mechanisms lead to the immune privilege of the cornea.[11] These include the absence of blood vessels and lymphatic channels in the cornea, the presence of Major Histocompatibility Complex II (MHC II) antigen-presenting cells in limbus far from the corneal center, lower expression of MHC-containing alloantigen on epithelial donor cells, expression of CD-95 ligand or Fas ligand on the different corneal layer (epithelium, stromal layer, and endothelium), the immunomodulatory environment in aqueous humor including transforming growth factor B2, alpha-melanocytic stimulating hormone, vasoactive intestinal peptide, calcitonin gene-related peptide, and finally anterior chamber-associated immune deviation (ACAID).[12,13] Inflammation and neovascularization can lower the immune privilege of the cornea. Corneal graft rejection is mainly a cell-mediated response coordinated by the CD4+ T cell.[14,15] Vessels and lymphatics grow into the cornea as a result of inflammation or trauma.[16–18] APCs normally residing in the limbus are attracted into the central corneal stroma in response to inflammatory stimuli. Of note, major histocompatibility complex antigen expression on corneal cells is also upregulated due to pro-inflammatory cytokines.[19] Foreign antigens on the cells of the corneal allografts are recognized by the host immune system and an immune cascade is started (afferent immune response arm). Following host sensitization, a particular immune response is developed (efferent immune response arm).[20] The mechanisms involved in the allograft rejection reaction are compared with the neural arc consisting of an afferent (or sensory) nerve, central nervous system, and efferent (or motor) nerve.[21]

Anterior Chamber-Associated Immune Deviation (ACAID)

ACAID is another active regulatory process that requires time (six to eight weeks, on average) to develop and may be insufficient to prevent active sensitization to foreign alloantigens.[22–24]

Various studies demonstrated that the introduction of antigens in AC causes a deviation in the immune response, leading to inhibition of delayed-type hypersensitivity (DTH) and complement-associated antibodies.[25–28] Antigen entrance through the ocular veins is captured by APC and will reach the spleen rather than lymphatic nodes. The immune response caused in the spleen activates regulatory T-cells rather than cytotoxic T-cells. Therefore, the suppressed immune response, as a result of ACAID, will not eliminate the antigen. Of note, the ACAID is a dynamic process rather than a static phenomenon.[27]

DOI: 10.1201/9781003371601-26

Immunohistochemical studies using markers of lymphatic endothelium along with ultra-structural and drainage studies support the existence of corneal lymphangiogenesis.[29] Corneal lymphangiogenesis is always less extensive than hemangiogenesis although they develop concurrently.[30] Corneal blood vessels allow the influx of immune effector cells, and corneal lymphangiogenesis provides an exit route for antigenic material and APCs from the graft to the regional lymph nodes.[30] The presence of corneal lymphangiogenesis with APC uptake into lymphatic vessels compromises ACAID and enhances the chance of graft rejection.[31]

Corneal Alloantigen

Major histocompatibility complex (MHC) or Human Leukocyte Antigens (HLA), which are cell surface glycoproteins, are encoded by four genes on chromosome 6. All nucleated cells, including corneal epithelium, keratocytes, and the endothelial cells, express HLA-A, B, and C antigens known as Class I whereas Class II (HLA-DR, DQ, DP) antigens are placed on immune cells like Langerhans cells, B-lymphocytes, and macrophages.[32] Minor Histocompatibility Complex (mHC) is a group of antigens not included in the two aforementioned groups. It is believed that mHC has a more important role in corneal graft rejection (Table 26.1).[33,34]

The expression of Class II antigens is upregulated by inflammatory reaction and interferon-gamma (IFN-gamma), leading to the start of an inflammatory response.[35] Host sensitization occurs by the processing of donor antigens by APCs of the host or the donor cornea. The processed antigens are then presented to the host immune system by APC and peptides.[35] Animal studies have demonstrated that T CD4+-knocked-out rats do not develop allogenic rejection against transplanted tissue.[36] Once sensitized, the host develops an immune response against the antigens in the graft.[37] The activated Th-1 cells release IL-2, IFN-gamma, macrophage activation factor (MAF), migration inhibition factor (MIF), and several other lymphokines and cytokines. IL-2 further stimulates the activation and proliferation of other T and B lymphocytes.[38] IFN-gamma induces the expression of Class II antigens, which are effective stimulators of the rejection response. Cytotoxic T lymphocytes serve as effector cells, attacking the cells with the foreign antigen. B cells secrete antibodies against the foreign antigen, attracting innate immunity inflammatory cells such as macrophages, antibody-dependent cell-mediated cytotoxic cells (ADCC), natural killer cells, and complement activation.[5,38,39]

Mechanisms Involved in Corneal Graft Rejection

The exact mechanism of corneal graft rejection is yet to be discovered.

Generally, cells involved in an immune rejection are divided into B and T cells. T cells are divided into T-helper (CD4+) and cytotoxic lymphocytes (CD8+). It is believed that delayed-type hypersensitivity is caused by cells expressing CD4. These cells are divided into T-helpers 1, 2, and 17. Th1 causes the secretion of IL2, IFN-γ, and TNF and is responsible for DTH. The role of Th1 is regulated by Th2 which secretes IL 4, 6, 9, 10, and 13.

It has been shown that the deletion of CD4+ cells by antibodies against these cells leads to a severe reduction in rejection reactions, whereas antibodies against CD8+ cells may not prevent immune rejection response.[40]

Immune rejection response is divided into three components.[41]

Table 26.1 Effect of Major and Minor Histocompatibility Complex on Corneal Graft Rejection

Donor/Host Disparity	Rejection Rate	Animal Model
MHC + minors	38–100%	Mouse
	55–100%	Rat
MHC only	27%	Mouse
Minors only	30–90%	Mouse
	26%	Rat
MHC Class I only	30%	Mouse
	18%	Rat
MHC Class II only	17%	Mouse
	0%	Rat

- The **afferent limb** collects and transfers them to lymphatic organs.

- **Central processing** that orchestrates immune responses against antigens.

- The **efferent limb** consists of blood vessels and conveys effector cells into the site of transplanted tissue.

To better understand immune regulation, immunologists propose a similarity between immune response and nerve reflex. Any disorder in the immune reflex arc causes an altered or deleted response. Regional immunity and IP are examples of immune reactions in the immune reflex arc that are altered by inhibitory agents.

Afferent Limb

The afferent limb involves the distance between antigen entrance into the body and antigen presentation to B and T lymphocytes. Macrophage and dendritic cells are named APCs. APCs capture the entered antigens and reach the lymphatic organs through lymphatic channels. APCs migrating from peripheral tissues express ligands which act as auxiliary ligands for B and T cells. These ligands are recognized as co-stimulatory molecules because activation of resting lymphocytes depends on both antigen recognition and co-stimulation by APCs.

Activation of B and T lymphocytes occurs when the responsible cells receive two separate signals.

Signal I is the interaction of lymphocyte receptors with antigen-presenting cells.

Signal II, perceived by naïve T-lymphocyte in the lymph nodes, occurs when the co-stimulatory stimuli are delivered by APC through the expression of surface molecules like CD 80, CD 86, ICAM-1, LFA-3, CD 40, and the secretion of cytokines like IL 12 and IL 1β.[42,43]

Central Processing Mechanism

The central processing mechanism is a complicated process in which received signals from the lymph node or spleen convert to the effector cells like CD4+, CD8+, and B cells secreting various types of immunoglobulins.

Efferent Limb

Blood vessels enable immune agents, activated and released in the central processing stage, to reach targeted tissue and organs. These mediators and cells are aimed at eliminating the offending antigens. Despite the interaction between antigen and APCs resulting in the adaptive immune response, the majority of antigen elimination takes place by innate immunity cells.

CD4+ are minimally capable of removal of antigens. However, these cells secrete lymphokines like IFN-γ and IFN-α that potentiate innate immune response.[44]

Based on the type of antigen presentation to the immune system, the time interval between transplantation and graft rejection can vary. In acute graft rejection, or the direct pathway, the immune system of the recipient is stimulated by the donor's APC antigen complex presented to the immune system.[45] The indirect pathway results in subacute or chronic rejection, and the APC of the recipient recognizes the donor antigen and introduces the antigen to the immune system through the afferent limb. After central processing, the efferent limb will induce an immune response.[46]

Despite the traditional belief that the indirect pathway is dominant in graft rejection, a direct pathway also plays a role, especially in the high-risk setting of the graft.[47–50]

The exact role of antibodies in corneal transplantation is controversial. Corneal graft rejection can occur in the absence of donor-specific IgG alloantibody. Both complement-dependent or complement-independent factors can result in the antibody-mediated killing of the corneal endothelium.[51,52]

RISK FACTORS

The risk factors for corneal graft rejection are divided into two groups:[53] Factors related to donor cornea like antigen incompatibility (ABO and HLA), and the presence of APC on the donor cornea.[54–56] Other donor factors influencing graft rejection include the method and the nature of donor button cutting. Pretreatment of donor tissue with ultraviolet radiation may reduce the chances of the development of rejection.[57,58]

■ Factors related to the host cornea with a more significant role include:

- Stromal tissue vascularization. The Collaborative on Corneal Transplant Study (CCTS) demonstrated that two or more quadrants of vascularization put the graft at high risk of corneal graft rejection. The depth and size of vascularization predict the time and intensity of graft rejection. Moreover, in patients with immune rejection episodes, the recovery rate depends on the amount of corneal vascularization.[10,59,60]

- Previous PKP. Especially when the graft failed due to immune rejection. CCTS also demonstrated that the risk of graft rejection increases up to 50% with each previous PKP.[61–63]

- Peripheral anterior synechiae (PAS) cause direct contact between the donor cornea and the host's vascular system. PAS in three or four quadrants greatly increase the rejection risk. Moreover, PAS cause tension on the endothelial cells and increases the risk of glaucoma, both increasing the risk of EC loss and subsequent graft failure.[62,63]

- Another factor includes previous intraocular surgeries, like lensectomy, vitrectomy, glaucoma surgeries, and concomitant surgeries, like combined transplant and vitrectomy. The larger diameter of the donor especially more than 8.25 mm or decentered grafts approximates the donor to the limbal area and host immune system.[62,63]

- Age of recipient. It is observed that corneal transplantation under the age of 40 could increase the risk of graft rejection two fold.[62,63]

- Ocular inflammatory diseases like uveitis and ocular surface inflammatory diseases like atopic keratoconjunctivitis (AKC), mucous membrane pemphigoid (MMP), and Stevens–Johnson syndrome (SJS) cause chronic inflammation and severe inflammatory responses. The inflammation causes the activation of both efferent and afferent arms of the immune system. On the other hand, AKC could cause permanent damage to limbal stem cells.

- Limbal stem cell deficiency (LSCD) in patients with chemical burns, AKC, and SJS is a risk factor for graft failure. In patients with LSCD, limbal stem cell transplantation should be considered before a corneal transplant.

- Herpes simplex or Varicella–Zoster keratopathy increases the risk of graft rejection. Furthermore, graft rejection more frequently leads to graft failure in patients undergoing PKP due to HSK scar compared with PKP due to keratoconus.[62–64]

- Post-immunized patients and patients with high T4/T8 ratios also run a high risk of graft rejection.[65]

Recently, there has been a growing concern regarding acute corneal allograft rejection after vaccination for COVID-19. Various studies, mostly case reports and case series, reported rejection episodes after vaccination with BNT162b2 (Pfizer), mRNA-1273 (Moderna), ChAdOx1 (AstraZeneca), and CoronaVac (Sinovac). The causality relationship between vaccination and graft rejection is yet to be understood. However, the temporality between rejection episodes and COVID-19 vaccination (ranging between one day and six weeks) and also previous reports of rejection after other vaccines like hepatitis B and influenza necessitate attention being paid to this possible risk factor. Various theories are proposed to explain the role of vaccination in acute graft rejection, including the activation of T cell-related immune responses and the release of IFN-gamma and IL-2 after vaccination.[66]

CLINICAL MANIFESTATIONS OF CORNEAL GRAFT REJECTION

Symptoms of acute graft rejection include eye redness, photophobia, ocular discomfort, and blurred vision. However, graft rejection episodes could be symptomless in nearly 30% of patients. These episodes are discovered in a regular follow-up examination.

It is believed that graft rejection is due to immunologic reactions that occur in three main types: **Acute rejection** in the first seven to 14 days

Subacute rejection occurs after 14 to 56 days.

Chronic rejection occurs after 56 days.

Acute rejection mostly occurs in the high-risk setting while subacute and chronic rejection could happen in normal eyes.

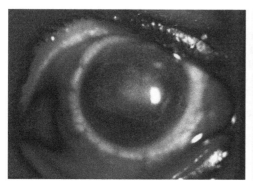 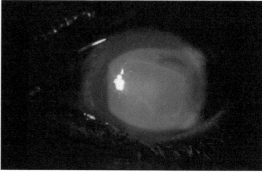

Figure 26.1 Epithelial rejection line in a patient with penetrating keratoplasty. Right-hand image demonstrates the line with fluorescein staining.

Corneal graft rejection clinically presents in four typical categories in combination or separately:

- **Epithelial rejection**, comprising 10–15% of total rejection cases, is a direct immune response against the donor's epithelial cells. It is believed that the donor epithelium is not completely replaced by the host's epithelium. Epithelial rejection occurs within 1–13 months after transplantation and usually occurs earlier than other rejection types. Infiltration of lymphocytes forms an epithelial ridge, usually starting from the periphery and moving toward the center after multiple days to weeks. The epithelial ridge stains with fluorescein or Rose Bengal. Patients might lack any symptoms. Since epithelial rejection could harbor other rejection types, it should be considered significant and should promptly be treated (Figure 26.1).

- **Subepithelial rejection**, first described by Krachmer and Allderge,[67] is another rejection type, presenting with white subepithelial opacities formed by lymphocytic infiltration just beneath the Bowman's layer. The deposits resemble Adenovirus-associated keratoconjunctivitis and could be differentiated with the following criteria:

  - Subepithelial rejection usually accompanies other rejection types.

  - The opacities in subepithelial rejection occur only in the donor tissue.

  - There is no history of conjunctivitis on prior days.

Patients' symptoms could vary from a lack of symptoms to seeing halos around the objects. Whether the lymphocytic infiltration is in response to epithelial cells or the donor's keratocytes is yet to be investigated.[67] In slit-lamp biomicroscopy, the subepithelial opacities are better observed with oblique illumination (Figure 26.2).

Subepithelial rejection usually improves with timely treatment. However, the risk of recurrence or harboring other rejection types should be strongly considered. To avoid subsequent endothelial rejection, aggressive treatment is necessary.

- **Stromal rejection** rarely occurs in the absence of rejection in other corneal layers after PKP. In lamellar keratoplasty, stromal rejection is more common and presents with local stromal opacities adjacent to corneal vascularization and might progress toward the corneal center within 24–48 hours. The stromal opacity consists of lymphocytes, plasma cells, and PMNs. Stromal keratolysis may occur at the border of the host and donor cornea and could resemble a corneal abscess in severe and prolonged rejections. Descemetocele formation, stromal necrosis, and corneal perforation may occur as a result of stromal rejection (Figure 26.3).

- **Endothelial rejection** remains the most common and severe form of rejection. This rejection type may seriously damage the endothelial cells and subsequently lead to graft failure. The patients generally present with eye redness, pain, photophobia, blepharospasm, and vision loss. Keratic precipitates (KPs), deposits of inflammatory cells on the endothelium, are variably present from a few to many deposits. KPs could linearly deposit, forming an endothelial rejection line (ERL) or in a diffuse form. The ERL, known as Khodadoust's line, generally appears in the inferior part or near corneal vascularization. Corneal edema usually coexists at the location of the Khodadoust line. A mild reaction in the anterior chamber could also be observed.

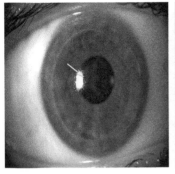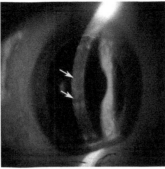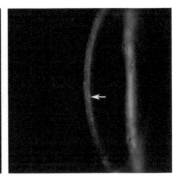

Figure 26.2 White round subepithelial opacities in a patient with history of penetrating keratoplasty. Oblique illumination to reveal the opacities in the middle image. The right-hand image demonstrates the level of opacities in the anterior stroma.

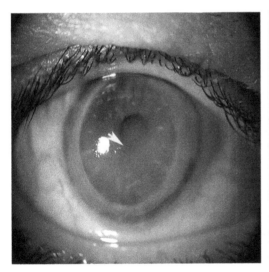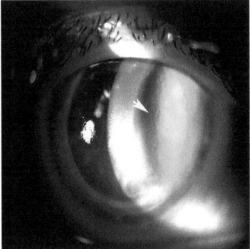

Figure 26.3 Stromal rejection presenting as stromal edema and Descemet folding in a patient with a history of penetrating keratoplasty.

Functional impairment of endothelial pumps leads to folding in Descemet's membrane, stromal thickening, and microcystic corneal edema. Stromal edema could be limited to the ERL and graft borders while diffuse edema may occasionally occur leading to the invisibility of KPs. Other clinical findings include conjunctival hyperemia, iris vessel congestion, especially in presence of iridocorneal adhesions (ICA), and miosis.

In endothelial keratoplasties (DSAEK and DMEK), an endothelial rejection line is not usually present and KPs are diffusely scattered on the endothelial cells (Figure 26.4).

In the pediatric population, graft rejection may atypically present with corneal epithelial defect and ocular inflammation.

In repeated transplantations, immune rejection episodes may present differently. The rejection episode may occur as soon as the first two weeks. There is an increased risk of progressing toward graft failure. Khodadoust's line may be absent and KPs are usually diffuse.[5,53,67–70]

Immunologic rejection reactions can be divided into mild, moderate, and severe forms based on the number of KPs and AC inflammation degree. The presence of fewer than 5 KPs is considered mild rejection, while between 5 and 25 KPs is considered moderate, and more than 25 KPs indicates a severe rejection episode.[70]

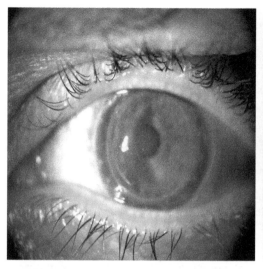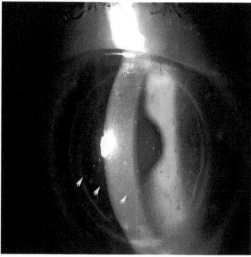

Figure 26.4   Endothelial rejection presenting with moderate KP. The right-hand image demonstrates the endothelial rejection line.

DIFFERENTIAL DIAGNOSIS

Episodes of graft rejection should be differentiated from differential diagnoses, including Herpes simplex keratopathy, Cytomegalovirus (CMV)-associated keratopathy, epithelial downgrowth, corneal fungal infection, or infection with *Streptococcus* hemolytic species. The most important differential diagnosis remains HSK. Dendritic corneal epithelial lesions favor the diagnosis of HSK. Stromal and endothelial HSK presents with iritis, stromal edema, and KPs. The simultaneous presence of KP on the donor's and host's endothelium favors the diagnosis of HSK rather than graft rejection.[70]

PREVENTIVE MEASURES

There exists no standard protocol to prevent allograft rejection in high-risk grafts.

There are conflicting results in the literature regarding the role of HLA and ABO matching in the prevention of graft rejection.[71-74] There is an ongoing systematic review of the literature to investigate the evidence against or for HLA matching.[75]

Recent studies revealed that the density of immune cells investigated by *in-vivo* confocal microscopy could identify graft rejection earlier than the patients' signs and symptoms. However, the clinical use of immune cells in the early diagnosis of graft rejection is yet to be understood.[76]

The main goals in the follow-up of high-risk grafts remain prevention, early diagnosis, and timely and prompt treatment of rejection episodes. Preventive measures focus on the following approaches:

- Immunosuppressive drugs including steroids[60]

- Inhibition of LC migration (IL-1Ra and TNF-α)[77]

- Blockade of costimulatory pathways (CD 28 with B7 molecules found on APCs)[78]

- Overexpression of immunomodulatory cytokines[79]

- Inhibition of adhesion molecules (suppression of efferent limb)[79]

- Reduction of corneal neovascularization[80]

- Induction of ACAID[81,82]

- Gene therapy[83]

Preoperative Measures to Reduce the Risk of Rejection

Providing a healthy non-inflamed ocular surface through optimization of the ocular surface is mandatory to guaranteeing graft survival. In inflammatory corneal diseases like AKC, VKC, SJS, and MMP, the inflammation should be maximally controlled.[84]

In patients with extensive corneal neovascularization, cauterization of blood vessels or use of anti-vascular endothelial growth factor (anti-VEGF) injections are recommended before the surgery.[84]

Post-Operative Management of Corneal Graft

The immunologic outcome of corneal graft rejection depends heavily on the post-operative regimen. The main goals are prevention of rejection, prompt diagnosis, and timely treatment. Patients must be educated about rejection symptoms like ocular discomfort, and photophobia. They also must be recommended to refer quickly when symptoms occur, and the importance of regular follow-up should be emphasized.

Loose sutures and sutures along the corneal vascular tracts should be removed upon diagnosis. Topical antibiotics and steroids should be administered after suture removal.

Immunosuppressive Regimen

Topical and systemic immunosuppressive regimens are prescribed to prevent immune rejection. To date, corticosteroids are the mainstay of the postoperative regimen.[60,84] In high-risk grafts, the addition of specific immunosuppressive agents might be needed.

Corticosteroids

Topical corticosteroids, like betamethasone and prednisolone acetate 1%, are the most frequently prescribed drugs. While less potent steroids have a better safety profile, more potent steroids are required in the early post-operative period (Table 26.2).[60]

Bioavailability of Topical Steroids

Bioavailability means the proportion of the unchanged part of the drug entering into the systemic blood vessels and depends on the corneal penetration. Ideal steroids are biphasic, meaning being lipid soluble (hydrophobic) to pass from epithelium and endothelium and being water soluble (hydrophilic) to cross the stroma. Acetate and alcohol derivatives are lipophiles and sodium phosphate is hydrophile. In intact corneal epithelium, penetration of the acetate form is higher while phosphate forms enter easier when the corneal epithelial defect is present. Presumably, acetate and alcohol derivatives are more potent in the control of inflammation rather than phosphates.[85–87]

Corticosteroid Role in Corneal Graft Rejection

Based on a survey in 2011, prednisolone acetate (PA) is the most commonly prescribed steroid by members of The Cornea Society.[60] In lower-risk PKP, the prophylactic regimen includes topical corticosteroid (betamethasone or PA) four times a day for three months (time of ACAID formation) tapered within 4–6 months.

To taper the steroids, attention to cataracts and IOP is essential. Steroids could be continued for a longer period in pseudophakic patients with a normal optic nerve. In patients with IOP rise, potent steroids should be replaced with loteprednol or fluorometholone.

In high-risk PKP, the prophylactic regimen includes betamethasone or PA 1% four to six times in regards to inflammation up to four to six months. Although it is recommended by some cornea surgeons to taper the steroid within six to 12 months, we believe that the period of application of steroid should be decided on an individual basis and, in most patients, steroid use for six months will be sufficient.

In patients undergoing PKP due to complications of HSK, an oral prophylactic regimen with acyclovir or valacyclovir should be continued for a long duration.

In DSAEK, despite the lower risk of endothelial graft rejection, prophylactic measures are highly recommended.[88,89] It is emphasized again that the time for ACAID development is six to eight weeks. The use of steroids in this period is mandatory.

Table 26.2 Comparison of Ophthalmic Corticosteroids Commonly Prescribed in Prevention and Treatment of Corneal Graft Rejection

Type of Drug	Available Formulation	Form	Anti-Inflammatory Activity	Intraocular Penetrance	IOP Rise	Consideration
Difloprednate		Drop — Emulsion	Very high	High	Very High	
Prednisolone	Acetate, Sodium Phosphate	Drop 1% — Suspension; Drop 0.125% — Solution; Drop 0.5% — Solution	High	High	High	Effective in intraocular and ocular surface inflammations. The presence of epithelial defect increases the intraocular penetration of prednisolone, sodium phosphate.
Dexamethasone	Alcohol Derivatives, Sodium Phosphate	Drop 0.1%, Ointment	High	Moderate	High	Dexamethasone is resistant to metabolism after entrance into AC and is very effective in controlling intraocular inflammation. Dexamethasone ointment could be prescribed at night in high-risk grafts.
Betamethasone	Acetate, Sodium Phosphate	Drop 0.1%, Ointment — Suspension, Solution	Moderate	Moderate	Moderate	Betamethasone sodium phosphate 1% is the most commonly prescribed drop with significant anti-inflammatory effects.
Hydrocortisone		Drop 1%, Ointment 0.5, 1, 3%	Moderate	Low	Low	
Fluorometholone	Alcohol Derivatives Sodium Phosphate	Drop 1%	High	Low	Low	In steroid responders who need to use steroids, Fluorometholone is the drug of choice.
Medrysone	Structurally similar to progesterone	Drop 1% — Suspension	Low	Low	Low	A low-potency steroid used in ocular surface inflammation, not in intraocular inflammation
Loteprednol	Ester with Etabonate	Drop 0.1%, 0.5%	High	Low	Low	It is commonly prescribed to treat allergic or vernal keratoconjunctivitis

Immunosuppressive Drugs

Based on the study of Holland et al.,[90] a steroid-sparing regimen could be added to steroids in high-risk grafts. These regimens include calcineurin inhibitors and anti-proliferative drugs, blocking the activation and action of T-cells.

Calcineurin inhibitors include cyclosporine A and tacrolimus.

Cyclosporine A is a non-myelotoxic immunosuppressive drug with anti-inflammatory effects. It adheres to the cytoplasmic proteins named cyclophilin A and D that are important in the function of T-lymphocytes.[60,68,84,89,90]

Effects of cyclosporine A on the ocular surface include

- Reduction of T-cell migration toward the donor

- Reduction of blood growth in the donor cornea

- Prevention of lymphocyte infiltration in the conjunctiva and lacrimal gland.[60,68,84,89,90]

Topical cyclosporine A is used in dry eye disease; however, the efficacy in corneal graft rejection is in doubt.[60]

Regarding the low effect and high adverse effects of systemic cyclosporine A, it has a minimal role to play in the immunosuppressive regimen after corneal transplantation.

Tacrolimus is a macrolide antibiotic with potent immunosuppressive effects. Tacrolimus inhibits lymphocyte signals and subsequent IL 2 secretion through adhesion to calcineurin. Topical tacrolimus (FK506) can penetrate the intact cornea and is effective to prevent corneal rejection at a dose of 0.05%. However, tacrolimus does not affect the treatment of corneal rejection.[60,68,84,89,90] Oral tacrolimus, with the generic name Prograf®, is effective in the prevention of corneal graft rejection. Compared to oral cyclosporine A, tacrolimus lowers the number of rejection episodes and increases graft survival.[60,68,84,89,90]

Antiproliferative drugs include mycophenolate mofetil (MMF), rapamycin, and azathioprine.

MMF, with the generic name of Cellcept®, inhibits the proliferation of B and T lymphocytes. MMF is used in the treatment of posterior uveitis and the prevention of corneal graft rejection in high-risk grafts. MMF has higher efficacy and lower side effects compared to cyclosporine. Cellcept is available in 500-mg tablets and is prescribed 2 g daily. Due to its favorable tolerability, MMF is the first-line prophylactic regimen in high-risk grafts.[60,68,84,89,90]

Novel and Future Immunosuppressive Agents

In experimental models, monoclonal antibodies against IL12, CD8, CD4, and CD3 have been investigated. daclizumab (Zanapax) and basiliximab (Simulect) attach to the alpha subunit of IL 2 and inhibit T cell activity. It has been shown that basiliximab has lower efficacy than cyclosporine A and also adverse events.[91,92]

An antibody against CD 52 with the generic name of alemtuzumab is another novel monoclonal antibody. CD 52 is a receptor on T cells, B cells, NK cells, and monocytes. Alemtuzumab is widely used after liver, kidney, and lung transplantation. There are studies investigating alemtuzumab after corneal transplantation which demonstrated longer graft survival.[93]

Tocilizumab, another monoclonal antibody, binds to the IL-6 receptor on T cells and inhibits the attachment of IL6 to T cells. IL 6 plays a pivotal role in the growth and differentiation of T cells. It is believed that the use of tocilizumab decreases T-helper 17 population and increases T-reg cells. In an experimental model, tocilizumab reduced graft neovascularization as well as immunologic rejection.[94]

Gene Therapy

Gene therapy in corneal transplantation is an ongoing field of research. Regarding the pathophysiology of corneal graft rejection, anti-angiogenesis, regulation of immune response, and anti-apoptosis are the main targets used in gene therapy. Viral vectors, including adenovirus and lentivirus, and non-viral vectors have been used in these approaches. The targeted genes in anti-angiogenesis approaches are neuropilin 2, Flt23k, and VEGFR1. CTLA1, 4, IL 10, 4, 12, TNF-R, and DC have been targeted in studies using immunomodulator approaches. P35, BclxL, and PD-L1 comprise targets of anti-apoptosis approaches. To the best of our knowledge, no clinical trial has reported the successful outcome of these strategies yet; therefore, further research is needed to use gene therapy as a clinical measure in the prevention of corneal graft rejection.[95,96]

TREATMENT OF ACUTE GRAFT REJECTION

The most effective strategy in the management of corneal graft rejection remains early diagnosis and prompt treatment with frequent doses.

The mainstay treatment of corneal graft rejection is topical corticosteroid; betamethasone 0.1%, prednisolone acetate 0.1%, or dexamethasone 0.1% should be prescribed every one to three hours in the first days based on the severity, then tapered off, based on the clinical outcome. Topical corticosteroids should be continued until the resolution of the last KP.[97]

In patients with recurrent corneal graft rejection, long-term treatment with steroid eye drop every or every other night is recommended. Betamethasone eye ointment could be added in patients with a history of rejection. However, the bioavailability of ointments is lower than eye drops.

Patients should be regularly visited in short intervals and steroids should be prescribed with caution in patients with high IOPs and HSK.

Subtenon injection of 20 mg triamcinolone acetonide or 2 mg dexamethasone can be used in patients with severe rejection episodes or low response to frequent drops.[98]

The use of oral corticosteroids (1 mg/kg) is controversial and there is a lack of evidence supporting the role of systemic steroids. Intravenous methylprednisolone (125–500 mg) has also been studied.[99]

It seems that oral prednisolone is controversial. In one study, the addition of subtenon injection of triamcinolone acetonide (TA) 20 mg in addition to topical PA 1% compared with IV methylprednisolone 500 mg was added to PA 1%. Several studies showed that cyclosporine 0.05% has no additional benefit on acute corneal graft rejection.[100–102] Topical tacrolimus 0.05% has also been investigated in the treatment of acute graft rejection in endothelial transplantation but decreases the incidence of future rejection episodes.[103]

REFERENCES

1. Dana MR, Qian Y, Hamrah P. Twenty-five–year panorama of corneal immunology: emerging concepts in the immunopathogenesis of microbial keratitis, peripheral ulcerative keratitis, and corneal transplant rejection. *Cornea*. 2000 Sep 1;19(5):625–43.

2. Niederkorn JY. Corneal transplantation and immune privilege. *International Reviews of Immunology*. 2013 Jan 13;32(1):57–67.

3. Javadi MA, Motlagh BF, Jafarinasab MR, Rabbanikhah Z, Anissian A, Souri H, Yazdani S. Outcomes of penetrating keratoplasty in keratoconus. *Cornea*. 2005 Nov;24(8):941–6.

4. Coster DJ, Williams KA. The impact of corneal allograft rejection on the long-term outcome of corneal transplantation. *American Journal of Ophthalmology*. 2005 Dec 1;140(6):1112–22.

5. Panda A, Vanathi M, Kumar A, Dash Y, Priya S. Corneal graft rejection. *Survey of Ophthalmology*. 2007 Jul 1;52(4):375–96.

6. Williams KA, Esterman AJ, Bartlett C, Holland H, Hornsby NB, Coster DJ. How effective is penetrating corneal transplantation? Factors influencing long-term outcome in multivariate analysis. *Transplantation*. 2006 Mar 27;81(6):896–901.

7. Streilein JW. New thoughts on the immunology of corneal transplantation. *Eye*. 2003 Nov;17(8):943–8.

8. Rahman I, Carley F, Hillarby C, Brahma A, Tullo AB. Penetrating keratoplasty: indications, outcomes, and complications. *Eye*. 2009 Jun;23(6):1288–94.

9. Chong EM, Dana MR. Graft failure IV. Immunologic mechanisms of corneal transplant rejection. *International Ophthalmology*. 2008 Jun;28(3):209–22.

10. Maguire MG, Stark WJ, Gottsch JD, Stulting RD, Sugar A, Fink NE, Schwartz A, Collaborative Corneal Transplantation Studies Research Group. Risk factors for corneal graft failure and rejection in the collaborative corneal transplantation studies. *Ophthalmology*. 1994 Sep 1;101(9):1536–47.

11. Hori J. Mechanisms of immune privilege in the anterior segment of the eye: what we learn from corneal transplantation. *Journal of Ocular Biology, Diseases, and Informatics*. 2008 Dec;1(2):94–100.

12. Cursiefen C. Immune privilege and angiogenic privilege of the cornea. *Immune Response Eye*. 2007;92:50–57.

13. Taylor AW. Ocular immune privilege. *Eye*. 2009 Oct;23(10):1885–9.

14. Larkin DF, Alexander RA, Cree IA. Infiltrating inflammatory cell phenotypes and apoptosis in rejected human corneal allografts. *Eye*. 1997 Jan;11(1):68–74.

15. Yamada J, Kurimoto I, Streilein JW. Role of CD4+ T cells in immunobiology of orthotopic corneal transplants in mice. *Investigative Ophthalmology & Visual Science*. 1999 Oct 1;40(11):2614–21.

16. Chauhan SK, Dohlman TH, Dana R. Corneal lymphatics: role in ocular inflammation as inducer and responder of adaptive immunity. *Journal of Clinical & Cellular Immunology*. 2014;5:256.

17. Clements JL, Dana R. *Inflammatory corneal neovascularization: etiopathogenesis. In Seminars in Ophthalmology* 2011 Sep 1 (Vol. 26, No. 4–5, pp. 235–45). Taylor & Francis.

18. Feizi S, Azari AA, Safapour S. Therapeutic approaches for corneal neovascularization. *Eye and Vision*. 2017 Dec;4(1):1.

19. Hamrah P, Huq SO, Liu Y, Zhang Q, Dana MR. Corneal immunity is mediated by heterogeneous population of antigen-presenting cells. *Journal of Leukocyte Biology*. 2003 Aug;74(2):172–8.

20. Niederkorn JY. The immune privilege of corneal allografts1. *Transplantation*. 1999 Jun 27;67(12):1503–8.

21. Niederkorn JY. Immune privilege of corneal allografts. *Cornea and External Eye Disease*. 2010;128:1–2.

22. Streilein JW. Anterior chamber associated immune deviation: the privilege of immunity in the eye. *Survey of Ophthalmology*. 1990 Jul 1;35(1):67–73.

23. Kaplan HJ, Niederkorn JY. Regional immunity and immune privilege. *Immune Response and The Eye*. 2007;92:11–26.

24. Stein-Streilein J, Streilein JW. Anterior chamber associated immune deviation (ACAID): regulation, biological relevance, and implications for therapy. *International Reviews of Immunology*. 2002 Jan 1;21(2–3):123–52.

25. Wilbanks GA, Streilein JW. Distinctive humoral immune responses following anterior chamber and intravenous administration of soluble antigen. Evidence for active suppression of IgG2-secreting B lymphocytes. *Immunology*. 1990 Dec;71(4):566.

26. Wilbanks GA, Wayne Streilein J. Fluids from immune privileged sites endow macrophages with the capacity to induce antigen-specific immune deviation via a mechanism involving transforming growth factor- β. *European Journal of Immunology*. 1992 Apr;22(4):1031–6.

27. Wilbanks GA, Streilein JW. Characterization of suppressor cells in anterior chamber-associated immune deviation (ACAID) induced by soluble antigen. Evidence of two functionally and phenotypically distinct T-suppressor cell populations. *Immunology*. 1990 Nov;71(3):383.

28. Li XY, D'orazio T, Niederkorn JY. Role of Th1 and Th2 cells in anterior chamber-associated immune deviation. *Immunology*. 1996 Sep;89(1):34–40.

29. Cursiefen C, Schlötzer-Schrehardt U, Küchle M, Sorokin L, Breiteneder-Geleff S, Alitalo K, Jackson D. Lymphatic vessels in vascularized human corneas: immunohistochemical investigation using LYVE-1 and podoplanin. *Investigative Ophthalmology & Visual Science*. 2002 Jul 1;43(7):2127–35.

30. Cursiefen C, Chen L, Dana MR, Streilein JW. Corneal lymphangiogenesis: evidence, mechanisms, and implications for corneal transplant immunology. *Cornea*. 2003 Apr 1;22(3):273–81.

31. Hou Y, Bock F, Hos D, Cursiefen C. Lymphatic trafficking in the eye: modulation of lymphatic trafficking to promote corneal transplant survival. *Cells*. 2021 Jul 2;10(7):1661.

32. Anaya JM, Shoenfeld Y, Rojas-Villarraga A, Levy RA, Cervera R, editors. *Autoimmunity: From Bench to Bedside* [Internet]. Bogota (Colombia): El Rosario University Press; 2013 Jul 18. PMID: 29087650.

33. Qazi Y, Hamrah P. Corneal allograft rejection: immunopathogenesis to therapeutics. *Journal of Clinical & Cellular Immunology*. 2013 Nov 20;2013(Suppl 9):6.

34. Sano Y, Ksander BR, Wayne SJ. Minor H, rather than MHC, alloantigens offer the greater barrier to successful orthotopic corneal transplantation in mice. *Transplant Immunology*. 1996 Mar 1;4(1):53–6.

35. Qazi Y, Turhan A, Hamrah P. Trafficking of immune cells in the cornea and ocular surface. *Advances in Ophthalmology*. 2012 Mar 7: 79–104.

36. Hu J, Zhang W, Xu L, Hu L. JAK2 gene knockout inhibits corneal allograft rejection in mice by regulating dendritic cell-induced T cell immune tolerance. *Cell Death Discovery*. 2022 Jun 16;8(1):1–9.

37. Niederkorn JY. Immune mechanisms of corneal allograft rejection. *Current Eye Research*. 2007 Dec;32(12):1005–16. https://doi.org/10.1080/02713680701767884. PMID: 18085464.

38. Niederkorn JY. Mechanisms of corneal graft rejection: the sixth annual Thygeson Lecture, presented at the Ocular Microbiology and Immunology Group meeting, October 21, 2000. *Cornea*. 2001 Oct 1;20(7):675–9.

39. Lam H, Dana MR. Corneal graft rejection. *International Ophthalmology Clinics*. 2009 Jan 1;49(1):31–41.

40. Joo CK, Pepose JS, Stuart PM. T-cell mediated responses in a murine model of orthotopic corneal transplantation. *Investigative Ophthalmology & Visual Science*. 1995 Jul 1;36(8):1530–40.

41. Pleyer U, Schlickeiser S. The taming of the shrew? The immunology of corneal transplantation. *Acta Ophthalmologica*. 2009 Aug;87(5):488–97.

42. Streilein JW. Regional immunity and ocular immune privilege. *Chemical Immunology*. 1999 Jan 1;73:11–38.

43. Hamrah P, Dana MR. Corneal antigen-presenting cells. *Immune Response and The Eye*. 2007;92:58–70.

44. Streilein JW. Immunological non-responsiveness and acquisition of tolerance in relation to immune privilege in the eye. *Eye.* 1995 Mar;9(2):236–40.

45. Huq S, Liu Y, Benichou G, Dana MR. Relevance of the direct pathway of sensitization in corneal transplantation is dictated by the graft bed microenvironment. *The Journal of Immunology.* 2004 Oct 1;173(7):4464–9.

46. Sano Y, Streilein JW, Ksander BR. Detection of minor alloantigen-specific cytotoxic T cells after rejection of murine orthotopic corneal allografts: evidence that graft antigens are recognized exclusively via the" indirect pathway" 1. *Transplantation.* 1999 Oct 15;68(7):963–70.

47. Amouzegar A, Chauhan SK, Dana R. Alloimmunity and tolerance in corneal transplantation. *The Journal of Immunology.* 2016 May 15;196(10):3983–91.

48. Hegde S, Beauregard C, Mayhew E, Niederkorn JY. CD4+ T-cell–mediated mechanisms of corneal allograft rejection: role of fas-induced apoptosis. *Transplantation.* 2005 Jan 15;79(1):23–31.

49. Niederkorn JY, Stevens C, Mellon J, Mayhew E. CD4+ T-cell–independent rejection of corneal allografts. *Transplantation.* 2006 Apr 27;81(8):1171–8.

50. Niederkorn JY, Mayhew E, Mellon J, Hegde S. Role of tumor necrosis factor receptor expression in anterior chamber-associated immune deviation (ACAID) and corneal allograft survival. *Investigative Ophthalmology & Visual Science.* 2004 Aug 1;45(8):2674–81.

51. Hargrave SL, Mayhew E, Hegde S, Niederkorn J. Are corneal cells susceptible to antibody-mediated killing in corneal allograft rejection? *Transplant Immunology.* 2003 Jan 1;11(1):79–89.

52. He YG, Niederkorn JY. Depletion of donor-derived Langerhans cells promotes corneal allograft survival. *Cornea.* 1996 Jan 1;15(1):82–9.

53. Dua HS, Azuara-Blanco A. Corneal allograft rejection: risk factors, diagnosis, prevention, and treatment. *Indian Journal of Ophthalmology.* 1999 Jan 1;47(1):3.

54. Armitage WJ, Goodchild C, Griffin MD, Gunn DJ, Hjortdal J, Lohan P, Murphy CC, Pleyer U, Ritter T, Tole DM, Vabres B. High-risk corneal transplantation: recent developments and future possibilities. *Transplantation.* 2019 Dec;103(12):2468.

55. Batchelor JR, Casey TA, Gibbs DC, Lloyd DF, Werb A, Prasad SS, James A. HLA matching and corneal grafting. *The Lancet.* 1976 Mar 13;307(7959):551–4.

56. Roy R, Des Marchais B, Bazin R, Boisjoly HM, Dubé I, Laughrea PA. Role of ABO and Lewis blood group antigens in donor-recipient compatibility of corneal transplantation rejection. *Ophthalmology.* 1997 Mar 1;104(3):508–12.

57. Dana R, Olkowski S, Ahmadian H, Stark WJ, Young EM. Low-dose ultraviolet-B irradiation of donor corneal endothelium and graft survival. *Investigative Ophthalmology & Visual Science.* 1990.

58. Singh RB, Marmalidou A, Amouzegar A, Chen Y, Dana R. Animal models of high-risk corneal transplantation: a comprehensive review. *Experimental Eye Research.* 2020 Sep 1;198:108152.

59. Di Zazzo A, Kheirkhah A, Abud TB, Goyal S, Dana R. Management of high-risk corneal transplantation. *Survey of Ophthalmology.* 2017 Nov 1;62(6):816–27.

60. Azevedo Magalhaes O, Shalaby Bardan A, Zarei-Ghanavati M, Liu C. Literature review and suggested protocol for prevention and treatment of corneal graft rejection. *Eye.* 2020 Mar;34(3):442–50.

61. Fasolo A, Capuzzo C, Fornea M, Franch A, Birattari F, Carito G, Cucco F, Prosdocimo G, Sala M, Delle Noci N, Primavera V. Risk factors for graft failure after penetrating keratoplasty: 5-year follow-up from the corneal transplant epidemiological study. *Cornea.* 2011 Dec 1;30(12):1328–35.

62. Weisbrod DJ, Sit M, Naor J, Slomovic AR. Outcomes of repeat penetrating keratoplasty and risk factors for graft failure. *Cornea.* 2003 Jul 1;22(5):429–34.

63. Dunn SP, Gal RL, Kollman C, Raghinaru D, Dontchev M, Blanton CL, Holland EJ, Lass JH, Kenyon KR, Mannis MJ, Mian SI. Corneal graft rejection ten years after penetrating keratoplasty in the cornea donor study. *Cornea.* 2014 Oct;33(10):1003.

64. Kuffova L, Knickelbein JE, Yu T, Medina C, Amescua G, Rowe AM, Hendricks RL, Forrester JV. High-risk corneal graft rejection in the setting of previous corneal herpes simplex virus (HSV)-1 infection. *Investigative Ophthalmology & Visual Science.* 2016;57(4):1578–87.

65. Steinemann TL, Koffler BH, Jennings CD. Corneal allograft rejection following immunization. *American Journal of Ophthalmology.* 1988 Nov 1;106(5):575–8.

66. Fujio K, Sung J, Nakatani S, Yamamoto K, Iwagami M, Fujimoto K, Shokirova H, Okumura Y, Akasaki Y, Nagino K, et al. Characteristics and clinical ocular manifestations in patients with acute corneal graft rejection after receiving the covid-19 vaccine: a systematic review. *Journal of Clinical Medicine.* 2022;11:4500. https://doi.org/10.3390/jcm11154500

67. Alldredge OC, Krachmer JH. Clinical types of corneal transplant rejection. Their manifestations, frequency, preoperative correlates, and treatment. *Archives Ophthalmology.* 1981 Apr;99(4):599–604.

68. Kharod-Dholakia B, Randleman JB, Bromley JG, Stulting RD. Prevention and treatment of corneal graft rejection: current practice patterns of the Cornea Society, 2011. *Cornea.* 2015 Jun 1;34(6):609–14.

69. Vanathi M, Panda A, Vengayil S, Chaudhuri Z, Dada T. Pediatric keratoplasty. *Survey of Ophthalmology.* 2009 Mar-Apr;54(2):245–71.

70. Brightbill FS, McDonnell PJ, McGhee CN, Farjo AA, Serdarevic O. *Corneal Surgery E-Book: Theory Technique and Tissue.* Elsevier Health Sciences; 2008 Nov 28.

71. Armitage WJ. HLA matching and corneal transplantation. *Eye.* 2004 Mar;18(3):231–2.

72. Van Essen TH, Roelen DL, Williams KA, Jager MJ. Matching for human leukocyte antigens (HLA) in corneal transplantation–To do or not to do. *Progress in Retinal and Eye Research.* 2015 May 1;46:84–110.

73. Völker-Dieben HJ, Claas FH, Schreuder GM, Schipper RF, Pels E, Persijn GG, Smits J, D'Amaro J. Beneficial effect of HLA-DR matching on the survival of corneal allografts1. *Transplantation.* 2000 Aug 27;70(4):640–8.

74. Armitage WJ, Winton HL, Jones MN, Crewe JM, Rogers CA, Tole DM, Dick AD. Corneal transplant follow-up study II (CTFS II): a prospective clinical trial to determine the influence of HLA class II matching on corneal transplant rejection: baseline donor and recipient characteristics. *British Journal of Ophthalmology.* 2019 Jan 1;103(1):132–6.

75. Sachdeva GS, Cabada JP, Karim SS, Kahandawa DL, Thomas KA, Kumar A, Barry RJ, Butt GF. Effectiveness of matching human leukocyte antigens (HLA) in corneal transplantation: a systematic review protocol. *Systematic Reviews*. 2021 Dec;10(1):1–6.

76. Chirapapaisan C, Abbouda A, Jamali A, Müller RT, Cavalcanti BM, Colon C, Witkin D, Sahin A, Dana R, Cruzat A, Hamrah P. In vivo confocal microscopy demonstrates increased immune cell densities in corneal graft rejection correlating with signs and symptoms. *American Journal of Ophthalmology*. 2019 Jul;203:26–36.

77. Yamada J, Dana MR, Zhu SN, Alard P, Streilein JW. Interleukin 1 receptor antagonist suppresses allosensitization in corneal transplantation. *Archives of Ophthalmology*. 1998 Oct 1;116(10):1351–7.

78. Poirier N, Blancho G, Vanhove B. A more selective costimulatory blockade of the CD28-B7 pathway. *Transplant International*. 2011 Jan;24(1):2–11.

79. Di Zazzo A, Lee SM, Sung J, Niutta M, Coassin M, Mashaghi A, Inomata T. Variable responses to corneal grafts: insights from immunology and systems biology. *Journal of Clinical Medicine*. 2020 Feb 21;9(2):586.

80. Cursiefen C, Hos D. Cutting edge: novel treatment options targeting corneal neovascularization to improve high-risk corneal graft survival. *Cornea*. 2021 Dec 31;40(12):1512–8.

81. Sano Y, Okamoto S, Streilein JW. Induction of donor-specific ACAID can prolong orthotopic corneal allograft survival in" high-risk" eyes. *Current Eye Research*. 1997 Jan 1;16(11):1171–4.

82. Sonoda A, Sonoda Y, Muramatu R, Streilein JW, Usui M. ACAID induced by allogeneic corneal tissue promotes subsequent survival of orthotopic corneal grafts. *Investigative Ophthalmology & Visual Science*. 2000 Mar 1;41(3):790–8.

83. Qazi Y, Hamrah P. Gene therapy in corneal transplantation. In *Seminars in Ophthalmology* 2013 Sep 1 (Vol. 28, No. 5–6, pp. 287–300). Taylor & Francis.

84. Jabbehdari S, Baradaran-Rafii A, Yazdanpanah G, Hamrah P, Holland EJ, Djalilian AR. Update on the management of high-risk penetrating keratoplasty. *Current Ophthalmology Reports*. 2017 Mar;5(1):38–48.

85. McGhee CN. Pharmacokinetics of ophthalmic corticosteroids. *British Journal of Ophthalmology*. 1992 Nov;76(11):681–4.

86. Abud TB, Di Zazzo A, Kheirkhah A, Dana R. Systemic immunomodulatory strategies in high-risk corneal transplantation. *Journal of Ophthalmic and Vision Research*. 2017 Jan-Mar;12(1):81–92.

87. Shimazaki J, Iseda A, Satake Y, Shimazaki-Den S. Efficacy and safety of long-term corticosteroid eye drops after penetrating keratoplasty: a prospective, randomized, clinical trial. *Ophthalmology*. 2012 Apr;119(4):668–73.

88. Ang M, Soh Y, Htoon HM, Mehta JS, Tan D. Five-year graft survival comparing descemet stripping automated endothelial keratoplasty and penetrating keratoplasty. *Ophthalmology*. 2016 Aug;123(8):1646–52.

89. Jordan CS, Price MO, Trespalacios R, Price FW Jr. Graft rejection episodes after Descemet stripping with endothelial keratoplasty: part one: clinical signs and symptoms. *British Journal of Ophthalmology*. 2009 Mar;93(3):387–90.

90. Holland EJ, Mogilishetty G, Skeens HM, Hair DB, Neff KD, Biber JM, Chan CC. Systemic immunosuppression in ocular surface stem cell transplantation: results of a 10-year experience. *Cornea*. 2012 Jun;31(6):655–61.

91. Williams KA, Coster DJ. Monoclonal antibodies in corneal transplantation. *British Journal of Ophthalmology*. 1992 Oct;76(10):577

92. Fu H, Larkin DF, George AJ. Immune modulation in corneal transplantation. *Transplantation Reviews (Orlando)*. 2008 Apr;22(2):105–15.

93. Thiel MA, Kaufmann C, Coster DJ, Williams KA. Antibody-based immunosuppressive agents for corneal transplantation. *Eye (London)*. 2009 Oct;23(10):1962–5.

94. Wu XS, Lu XL, Wu J, Ma M, Yu J, Zhang ZY. Tocilizumab promotes corneal allograft survival in rats by modulating Treg-Th17 balance. *International Journal of Ophthalmology*. 2019 Dec 18;12(12):1823–1831.

95. Ritter T, Wilk M, Nosov M. Gene therapy approaches to prevent corneal graft rejection: where do we stand? *Ophthalmic Research*. 2013;50(3):135–40.

96. Williams KA, Jessup CF, Coster DJ. Gene therapy approaches to prolonging corneal allograft survival. *Expert Opinion on Biological Therapy*. 2004 Jul 1;4(7):1059–71.

97. Randleman JB, Stulting RD. Prevention and treatment of corneal graft rejection: current practice patterns (2004). *Cornea*. 2006 Apr;25(3):286–90.

98. Athanasiadis I, de Wit D, Tsatsos M, Patel AK, Sharma A. Subconjunctival injection of triamcinolone acetonide in the management of corneal graft rejection and new vessels. *The Journal of Clinical Pharmacology*. 2012 Apr;52(4):607–12.

99. Hill JC, Maske R, Watson P. Corticosteroids in corneal graft rejection. Oral versus single pulse therapy. *Ophthalmology*. 1991 Mar;98(3):329–33.

100. Poon A, Constantinou M, Lamoureux E, Taylor HR. Topical Cyclosporin A in the treatment of acute graft rejection: a randomized controlled trial. *Clinical & Experimental Ophthalmology*. 2008 Jul;36(5):415–2.

101. Poon AC, Forbes JE, Dart JK, Subramaniam S, Bunce C, Madison P, Ficker LA, Tuft SJ, Gartry DS, Buckley RJ. Systemic cyclosporin A in high risk penetrating keratoplasties: a case-control study. *British Journal of Ophthalmology*. 2001 Dec;85(12):1464–9.

102. Javadi MA, Feizi S, Karbasian A, *et al*. Efficacy of topical ciclosporin A for treatment and prevention of graft rejection in corneal grafts with previous rejection episodes. *British Journal of Ophthalmology* 2010;94:1464–1467.

103. Hashemian MN, Latifi G, Ghaffari R, Ghassemi H, Zarei-Ghanavati M, Mohammadi SF, Yasseri M, Fallah Tafti MR, Tafti ZF. Topical tacrolimus as adjuvant therapy to corticosteroids in acute endothelial graft rejection after penetrating keratoplasty: a randomized controlled trial. *Cornea*. 2018 Mar;37(3):307–312.

27 Ocular Surface Considerations in Corneal Transplantation in Keratoconus

Siamak Zarei-Ghanavati and Mehrdad Motamed Shariati

INTRODUCTION

Keratoconus (KC) is an asymmetric bilateral ocular disease, characterized by progressive corneal thinning and steepening.[1] Changes in the curvature and thickness of the cornea cause irregular astigmatism and visual impairment, necessitating corneal transplantation in severe stages of the disease.[2] Recent studies have reported changes in the inflammatory cytokine profile of the ocular surface in KC patients.[3] In addition, the level of oxidative stress biomarkers is higher in the tear film and cornea of these patients, while the level of antioxidants is lower in the tear film and aqueous humor of KC eyes.[4] It can be claimed that KC is associated with an abnormal ocular surface. From a clinical point of view, this issue becomes more important when a patient is planned for corneal transplantation or any other intervention.

In this chapter, we aim to review the ocular surface considerations in corneal transplantation of patients with KC.

OCULAR SURFACE: DEFINITION AND EVALUATION

The ocular surface is an integrated exposed part of the eye, which plays a significant role in the quality of vision. It consists of the cornea, conjunctiva, and tear film secretion system, including goblet cells, meibomian glands, main and accessory lacrimal glands, and eyelids. These anatomical structures, along with the sensory and motor nervous systems integrating them, comprise the lacrimal function unit (LFU).[5] The main task of LFU is to maintain the tear film osmolarity within a physiological range and create an optimal microenvironment for the corneal and conjunctival epithelia.[6] However, dysfunction of this system can lead to dry eye disease (DED).[7]

Ocular surface disorders are multifactorial conditions with multiple mechanisms. Diseases involving the eyelids, such as orbicularis muscle dysfunction, eyelid retraction, entropion or ectropion (through disruption of the spread of the tear layer and intensification of inflammation), seborrheic or staphylococcal blepharitis, and allergic conjunctivitis, may result in ocular surface disorders. Any disturbance in each of the LFU components causes changes in the volume, composition, and distribution of tears, resulting in DED.[8] Tear hyperosmolarity and tear film instability are two main mechanisms with synergic interactions. Evidence suggests that there is a bidirectional relationship between ocular surface inflammation and tear osmolarity. By increasing the tear osmolarity, epithelial cells release inflammatory cytokines due to cellular osmotic stress. Inflammation can also cause tear film instability owing to the destruction of goblet cells, as well as the reduction of mucin production.[9,10]

Ocular surface health assessments comprise subjective and objective evaluations. Various types of questionnaires, such as ocular surface disease index (OSDI) and dry eye questionnaire-5, have been designed for the subjective evaluation of DED, considering the symptoms of this disease, including foreign body sensation, pain, burning sensation, photophobia, eyestrain, transient visual disturbances, red eye, and tearing.[11] In addition, the evaluation of tear film instability, using the tear breakup time (TBUT) test, examination of epithelial cells using fluorescein, and evaluation of the staining pattern, Schirmer's test, meibomian gland assessments via infrared imaging, and corneal topography, are all available options for the objective evaluation of the ocular surface.[12]

ROLE OF INFLAMMATION IN KERATOCONUS (KC)

Although KC has been regarded as a non-inflammatory condition with dysregulated extracellular matrix (ECM) remodeling, evidence shows that subclinical inflammatory processes contribute to this disorder.[13] The greater prevalence of this disease in atopic individuals can be explained by the mechanical stress on the cornea, caused by eye rubbing and inflammatory processes.[14] According to recent studies, the cytokine and inflammatory profiles of the ocular surface differ in patients with KC.[3] The levels of pro-inflammatory molecules, including interleukin-1β (IL-1β), interleukin-6 (IL-6), tumor necrosis factor-α (TNF-α), matrix metalloproteinase-2 (MMP-2), and perforin, are significantly higher in the tear film of patients with KC compared with healthy individuals.[3,4] Furthermore, it has been shown that rubbing the eyes for a minute increases the tear levels of MMP-13, IL-6, and TNF-α in normal individuals.[15]

DOI: 10.1201/9781003371601-27

Regarding the critical role of the dynamic interaction between structural tissue cells and immune cells in establishing tissue homeostasis, the hypothesis of abnormal ECM remodeling and corneal biomechanical decompensation due to local immune system disturbances can be proposed. In brief, according to the immuno-inflammatory hypothesis of KC pathogenesis, external stimuli (e.g., eye rubbing, oxidative stress, and atopy) cause changes in structural and immune cells, leading to alterations in the inflammatory cytokine secretion; these changes disrupt the homeostasis of core ECM proteins and arrangements, resulting in aberrant ECM remodeling of the cornea and biomechanical weakness.[3,13,16]

OCULAR SURFACE IN KERATOCONUS

Considering the interactions between epithelial cells and the basement membrane, which mainly consists of type IV collagen and laminin isoforms, changes in ECM arrangements and increased levels of inflammatory cytokines can disturb the ocular surface homeostasis.[17] Multiple studies suggest that the keratoconus proteome is an atypical finding. It is important to consider that changes affect the epithelium and tear film, as well as the corneal stroma. Although the available methods vary significantly, some protein groups are expressed differently in KC (Table 27.1).[4,13,18,19] The difference in the expression of structural proteins, catabolic enzymes, and inflammatory cytokines in KC patients can potentially lead to ocular surface disturbances.

Table 27.1   The Corneal Proteome in Keratoconus (KC) Patients

	Changes in KC Patients	Potential Effects on the Ocular Surface
Structural proteins	Downregulation of the expression of collagen I, II, and IV and structural proteins, including lumican, keratocan, and decorin.	Proteoglycans and glycoproteins are essential to normal corneal function for maintaining not only stromal transparency, but also the air–tear interface. In addition, the interaction of corneal epithelial cells with type IV collagen and laminin isoforms, located at the basement membrane, is vital to maintenance of the ocular surface integrity.[17]
Catabolic enzymes	The tear fluid contains higher levels of degenerative enzymes, such as cathepsins and matrix metalloproteases (MMPs), as well as phosphatases, lipases, and esterases. The expression of protease inhibitors is reduced. The increased total proteinase activity is regarded as a crucial component of KC, as it is assumed to drive the significant reorganization of the corneal architecture.	The increased expression of degenerative enzymes in tears can lead to corneal epithelial barrier weakening and disturb the ocular surface homeostasis.[20]
Oxidative stress and inflammation proteins	The upregulation of classic proinflammatory proteins, including interleukin-1 (IL-1), IL-6, MMP-9, transforming growth factor-beta (TGF-β), and tumor necrosis factor-alpha (TNF-α), occurs. The inducible nitric oxide synthase (iNOS) expression is also increased. Decreased superoxide dismutase activity impairs the ability of the KC cornea to respond to oxidative stress appropriately. Augmented lipid peroxidation is attributed to changes in Class 3 aldehyde dehydrogenase (ALDH-3) enzymes.	Increased inflammation can affect the ocular surface in various ways. Dysfunction of goblet cells and decreased mucin production, dysfunction of meibomian glands, increased tear evaporation, and decreased tear production are some of these mechanisms that ultimately increase the tear osmolarity and stress on epithelial cells.[20]

From a clinical point of view, understanding different aspects of the pathogenesis of KC is crucial for treatment planning. Overall, breaking the vicious immuno-inflammatory cycle and establishing homeostasis at the ocular surface can help prevent disease progression and stabilize the cornea. Ocular surface optimization is also essential for patients who are candidates for corneal transplantation. In addition, ocular surface diseases affect the patient's graft rejection rate and optical quality.[21]

Table 27.2   Ocular Surface Complications Associated with the Use of Contact Lenses (CLs) in Keratoconus (KC) Patients

Hypoxic or hypercapnic stress

Immunologic reactions against deposits on the lens

Infection

Mechanical trauma

Giant papillary conjunctivitis

Squamous metaplasia of bulbar conjunctiva

Increased levels of proinflammatory cytokines in tears

Increased size of corneal epithelial cells

Decreased keratocyte density on the corneal surface

Increased polymegathism and pleomorphism in the endothelial cells of the cornea

EFFECTS OF PREVIOUS INTERVENTIONS (E.G., CONTACT LENSES AND COLLAGEN CROSS-LINKING) ON THE OCULAR SURFACE

It is common for KC patients to use contact lenses (CLs) due to irregular astigmatism.[22] Although complications of CLs are uncommon, they might be very serious. Metabolic damage to corneal epithelial cells due to hypoxia, stimulation of corneal neovascularization, and toxic and mechanical stress are some complications disturbing the homeostasis of the ocular surface.[23] KC patients are known to be prone to ocular surface complications induced by CLs (Table 27.2).[24]

With respect to the progressive nature of KC, some patients were previously treated with corneal collagen cross-linking (CXL). However, various short-term and long-term ocular surface complications have been documented in patients undergoing CXL. Undiagnosed ocular surface diseases, such as dry eye and blepharitis, may increase the risk of these complications post-operatively. Microbial keratitis is one of these potentially vision-threatening complications that can be anticipated in patients due to the epithelial defect, caused by intra-operative debridement, bondage CL application, and topical corticosteroid application in the post-operative period. Other complications that may occur following CXL include corneal haze formation, endothelial damage, peripheral sterile infiltration, and herpes reactivation.[25] Nevertheless, the exact impact of this procedure on the inflammatory profile of the ocular surface is yet to be fully determined.

Based on the results of a study by Uysal et al.,[26] improvement of TBUT test results, conjunctival squamous metaplasia, and goblet cell density suggest that CXL has a positive impact on the ocular surface and tear film of KC patients in the long term (18-month follow-up) owing to a relative improvement in corneal irregularity. In another study, the levels of tear cytokines, including IL-4, IL-5, IL-6, IL-7, IL-8, and TNF-α, decreased significantly three months after CXL.[27] Nonetheless, ultraviolet-A (UV-A) radiation utilized in CXL can potentially cause oxidative nuclear DNA damage to long-lived stem cells in the limbal region, which can be easily prevented by covering the limbus during the procedure.[28] Limbal stem cells (LSCs) are pivotal to maintaining the corneal epithelial integrity and regeneration. Damage to these cells results in conjunctival epithelial invasion and corneal neovascularization.[29]

OCULAR SURFACE DISORDERS ASSOCIATED WITH ALLERGIC CONJUNCTIVAL DISORDERS (ACDS) IN KERATOCONUS (KC) PATIENTS

Allergic conjunctival disorders (ACDs) include allergic conjunctivitis, vernal keratoconjunctivitis (VKC), atopic keratoconjunctivitis (AKC), and giant papillary conjunctivitis (GPC).[30] Generally, VKC is a T-helper-2 (Th2) lymphocyte-driven disease, characterized by the infiltration of inflammatory cell types, such as eosinophils, mast cells, and T lymphocytes, into the conjunctiva.[31,32] Atopic keratoconjunctivitis (AKC), which may involve both Th1 and Th2 inflammatory cascades, differs from VKC.[33] In the pathological examination of tears, higher levels of TNF-α, histamine, tryptase, immunoglobulin E (IgE), and immunoglobulin G (IgG) antibodies are found.[32]

The association of DED with ACD, both ocular surface inflammatory disorders, is an important clinical finding. The incidence rate of DED in patients with ACD is nearly 50%. Furthermore, MGD is more prevalent in patients with AKC and VKC. In a study by Osama et al., meibomian gland expressibility and meibomian gland dropout scores were significantly worse in AKC than in

Table 27.3   Ocular Surface Complications Associated with Allergic Conjunctival Disorders (ACDs)

Corneal punctate epithelial erosions and epithelial defects	Conjunctival hyperemia
Giant papilla	Corneal ulcers-shield ulcers
Limbal stem cell deficiencies (VKC and AKC)	Higher levels of inflammatory cytokines in tears
Meibomian gland dysfunction	

obstructive MGD patients.[34] Factors that lead to the development and exacerbation of DED in ACD patients include tear-film lipid layer instability, tear protein changes in ACD, increased inflammatory cytokines, prolonged use of antihistamines, squamous metaplasia of the conjunctival epithelium, and decreased goblet cell density.[35] Previous studies have reported a significantly higher prevalence of KC in ACD. According to a popular etiological hypothesis, the release of inflammatory mediators through ocular allergy and eye rubbing may change the biomechanical properties of the cornea and cause corneal ectasias.[14] Ocular surface findings of ACDs are described in Table 27.3 and should be considered before any surgical interventions, such as corneal transplantation.[36] The immunological and optical outcomes of corneal transplantation are significantly influenced by some ocular surface defects in ACDs, such as corneal stem cell deficiencies (CSCDs) in VKC and AKC through corneal vascularization.[37,38]

CORNEAL TRANSPLANTATION IN KERATOCONUS (KC)

Generally, KC is a progressive disease, and corneal transplantation remains the traditional treatment option for advanced cases that cannot be managed successfully with CLs. This disease is recognized as the underlying cause of nearly 18% of penetrating keratoplasty (PK) cases and 40% of deep anterior lamellar keratoplasty (DALK) interventions.[39] Generally, PK is one of the most widely used corneal surgical procedures, which involves the removal of full corneal thickness and replacement with a donor tissue.[40] Another surgical procedure is DALK, in which the damaged recipient stroma is replaced with the donor corneal stroma, while maintaining the recipient corneal endothelium and posterior limiting lamina.[41,42] Corneal transplantation is a plausible and highly successful treatment option for KC patients. Five-year graft survival rates of up to 97% have been reported for this procedure.[43] It has been proposed that the visual and refractive outcomes of DALK are comparable with those of PK. Ocular surface homeostasis is one of the most critical factors determining the long-term success of keratoplasty. The presence of active inflammation on the ocular surface, as reported in ACDs, may significantly increase the graft failure rate.[38]

NECESSITY OF OCULAR SURFACE OPTIMIZATION IN CANDIDATES FOR CORNEAL TRANSPLANTATION DUE TO KERATOCONUS (KC)

As discussed in previous sections of this chapter, a wide range of changes occur on the ocular surface of patients with KC. Dysregulation of the ocular surface immune system is a major finding in KC corneas. Furthermore, ophthalmic surgeries, including corneal transplantation, by damaging the epithelium and sensory nerves, compromising the tear film, and increasing inflammation, may have further adverse effects on the cornea.[44–47] A preexisting ocular surface disease can potentially jeopardize the success of corneal transplantation through chronic inflammation.[47] In addition to other possible adverse effects, surgical operations of eyes with a preexisting ocular surface disease may aggravate the disease and impede optimal vision.

The post-operative success of keratoplasty is related to the preservation of the corneal epithelium, tear film, and meibomian gland activity to promote ocular surface homeostasis.[44,47] Optimization of the ocular surface before surgery may enhance the surgical outcomes, improve post-operative patient satisfaction, and reduce post-operative complications.[48] It is essential to consider different factors that affect graft survival, visual function, and subjective symptoms when seeking satisfactory keratoplasty outcomes. Allograft rejection, endothelial decompensation, and ocular surface disorders (e.g., infectious or sterile keratitis and corneal scarring) are common causes of graft failure.[46] A history of ocular surface disorders or inflammation should be considered as an important factor, influencing the graft survival, visual function, and subjective symptoms following corneal transplantation. After keratoplasty, delayed epithelial healing or persistent epithelial defects may limit the graft viability by aggravating infection, melting, scarring, and neovascularization.[49,50]

Table 27.4 Important Ocular Surface Disorders in Candidates for Keratoplasty Due to Keratoconus (KC)

Blepharitis	Anterior blepharitis is a chronic inflammation of the eyelid that affects the lid edge and eyelash follicles and causes irritation and redness of the eyelids. Atypical tear film and ocular surface inflammation, leading to keratitis, conjunctivitis, or DED, are frequent sequelae. It also potentially increases the risk of post-operative infectious corneal ulcers if ignored during the peri-operative period.[51] Punctate epithelial erosions, marginal infiltration, peripheral neovascularization, and pannus are complications of blepharitis, compromising graft survival.[52]
Meibomian gland dysfunction (MGD)	A chronic condition, called MGD, results in diminished or abnormal meibum secretion because of terminal duct occlusion and/or impaired glandular activity. With increased tear evaporation, the risk of tear film hyperosmolarity, blepharitis, DED, and ocular surface injury is increased. The symptoms of this disease include ocular irritation and visual disturbances. Before corneal transplantation, it is crucial to identify and treat MGD to improve surgical outcomes.[53]
Allergic conjunctival disorders (ACDs)	A common feature of these disorders is the increased inflammation of the ocular surface, including the infiltration of immune cells and the release of inflammatory mediators. MGD, DED, and structural or functional alterations of the ocular surface arise from this inflammation.[30] Corneal limbal stem cell deficiency, persistent epithelial defects, peripheral vascularization, and increased susceptibility to infectious keratitis are the complications of ACDs, with significant effects on graft survival.[54]
Dry eye disease (DED)	Loss of tear film homeostasis is a hallmark of a chronic, multifactorial condition, known as DED. Conventional categories of DED involve aqueous tear deficiency and evaporative subtypes. However, current research indicates that these conditions typically coexist or manifest as a spectrum.[55–57] The vicious cycle of ocular surface inflammation and damage arises from the tear film abnormality, which can impair vision and produce uncomfortable ocular symptoms. According to the immuno-inflammatory hypothesis for the pathogenesis of KC,[3] inflammation can be proposed as an intermediate link between KC and DED. DED can represent a higher risk of surgical complications and post-operative infections after keratoplasty.[44]

Following corneal transplantation, ocular surface abnormalities with positive corneal staining are frequent, and post-operative tear film instability has been linked to visual function. Common preexisting ocular surface disorders in patients with KC who are candidates for keratoplasty are summarized in Table 27.4.

To effectively manage ocular surface diseases, each condition must be treated according to standard protocols. Numerous therapeutic options include topical and systemic medications, interventional therapies, and dietary modification. Ocular surface diseases are mainly multifactorial. Accordingly, multifaceted therapeutic approaches are frequently required to treat specific symptoms. Moreover, ocular surface diseases frequently manifest as a spectrum, requiring thorough treatments that address each manifestation.[12,58]

OCULAR SURFACE ASSESSMENT BEFORE SURGERY

A thorough inspection of any ocular surface abnormalities is essential before scheduling a patient for corneal transplantation (Table 27.5).

The rest of this chapter reviews the available treatment options, including medical treatment and relatively invasive interventions, to optimize the ocular surface of KC eyes before corneal transplantation.

MEDICAL AND PROCEDURAL MANAGEMENT OPTIONS TARGETING THE OCULAR SURFACE BEFORE CORNEAL TRANSPLANTATION

Various medicines are available to treat ocular surface abnormalities. Treatment approaches are customized according to preexisting disorders. In other words, a patient receives one or more treatments, depending on the identified problems. The main topical and systemic agents are described below.

ARTIFICIAL TEARS

Different types of topical lubricants are available, including preservative-free or preserved artificial tears, gels, and ointments. The main use of lubricants is to improve the quality and quantity of tears in patients. Viscosity-enhancing agents, electrolytes, osmoprotectants, lipid-based agents and surfactants, antioxidants, and preservatives are the main components used in the composition of

Table 27.5   Ocular Surface Evaluations of Patients with Keratoconus (KC) Scheduled for Corneal Transplantation

Subjective evaluations	• Assessment of the patient's symptoms via history-taking, using the Dry Eye Questionnaire-5 (DEQ-5) and Ocular Surface Disease Index (OSDI) • History of ocular conditions, including allergic conjunctivitis and dry eye syndrome • History of using contact lenses (CLs) • History of ocular surgeries, including collagen cross-linking (CXL) and corneal laser ablation
Objective evaluations	• Eyelid examination (attention to texture and morphology, indicating floppy eyelid syndrome) • Tarsal and bulbar conjunctival examinations (papilla and hyperemia) • Ocular surface staining pattern (fluorescein, Rose Bengal, and lissamine green stains) • Meibomian gland expressibility: Meibum quality and volume, and meibography • Tear film lipid layer, thickness, spread time, and rate. • Tear osmolarity test • TBUT • Meniscus height • Schirmer's test

artificial tears.[59] The most frequently used components, which comprise the main bulk of artificial tears, are viscosity-enhancing agents, including cellulose derivatives, carbomer, hyaluronic acid, polyvinyl alcohol, povidone, and dextran; these agents have a branched structure similar to mucin 1 and are known as mucomimetic agents.[59]

Regarding the high levels of inflammatory biomarkers at the ocular surface of KC corneas, artificial tears, by diluting these factors, can play an influential role in restoring homeostasis on the ocular surface. When a patient has allergic conjunctivitis or DED, these medicines become more important. The inflammation caused by an increase in tear osmolarity is the primary pathophysiology of DED. Artificial tears decrease the inflammation by reducing the tear osmolarity.[60] In ACD, which is quite prevalent among patients with KC, artificial tears reduce inflammation by diluting antigens and cytokines on the ocular surface.[61] Considering the irritating effects of preservatives used in eye drops for the prevention of microbial growth inside bottles, it seems logical to select preservative-free agents when their use exceeds four to six times per day.[62] Benzalkonium chloride is the most common preservative agent used in eye drop solutions, which has recognized toxicity. Although other soft preservatives, such as polyquaternium-1, sodium chlorite, and edetate disodium, exhibit much lower levels of cytotoxicity, the absence of preservatives improves ocular surface health.[59] Artificial tears only have transitory effects and are often inadequate for long-term management, as they do not affect the underlying etiology of ocular surface abnormalities.

ANTIHISTAMINES

The H_1 receptor antagonists are the mainstay of treatment for patients with allergic conjunctivitis. Regarding the high prevalence of VKC and allergic conjunctivitis in patients with KC, surgeons should consider antihistamines in the management of ocular surface inflammation, especially when the patient is a candidate for corneal transplantation. Patients with allergic conjunctivitis, especially VKC, can benefit from antihistamines, because they can prevent conjunctival epithelial cells from secreting proinflammatory cytokines. Although first-generation antihistamines are well-tolerated and exhibit long-term safety, they have disadvantages, such as painful instillation, brief duration of action, and low potency. Although more recent antihistamines, such as antazoline, emedastine, and levocabastine, are also H_1 antagonists, their duration of action is longer (4–6 hours), and they are tolerated better than older antihistamines.[63–65]

Prescription of oral antihistamines for ACD patients is increasingly popular, since preservatives in the eye drops exacerbate the ocular surface inflammation. Obviously, these side effects do not occur with the use of systemic agents. Moreover, regarding the anticholinergic effects, antihistamines (via topical or systemic routes of administration) may have adverse effects on the exacerbation of dry eye in patients.[66] In addition, these agents have short-term effects in reducing the ocular surface inflammation and relieving the patient's symptoms, as they do not target the underlying etiopathogenesis of the disease.

MAST CELL STABILIZERS

Eosinophils, neutrophils, macrophages, mast cells, and other cells involved in allergic inflammation all respond to mast cell stabilizers. Mast cell stabilizers (used two to four times daily) are excellent first-line treatments, used alongside antihistamines and dual-acting medications for lowering inflammation in ACDs.[31,67] Traditional mast cell stabilizers, such as cromolyn sodium, lodoxamide, and pemirolast, show full efficacy after several days to weeks. On the contrary, dual-acting agents, with both antihistamine and mast cell stabilizing effects, can alleviate allergic manifestations much more rapidly. Numerous generic dual-acting agents are commercially available, including alcaftadine, azelastine, bepotastine besilate, epinastine hydrochloride (HCl), ketotifen fumarate, and olopatadine HCl. The latter is currently available as a 0.2% formulation for once-daily dosing.[68] The most common side effects of mast cell stabilizers include burning sensation and discomfort after administration.[68]

NON-STEROIDAL ANTI-INFLAMMATORY DRUGS (NSAIDS)

Cyclooxygenase inhibitors reduce inflammation by lowering prostaglandin synthesis. Topical NSAIDs, such as diclofenac sodium 0.1% and diclofenac tromethamine, are mainly used to prevent and treat cystoid macular edema and reduce post-operative inflammation and pain. However, epithelial toxicity is a serious concern that prevents the routine use of these agents for patients with ocular surface diseases. Furthermore, corneal melting associated with the use of these agents has been reported.[69]

CORTICOSTEROIDS

Corticosteroids help control inflammation by inhibiting the metabolism of arachidonic acids. Due to the decreased production of many inflammatory mediators, these agents are frequently used to treat various ocular surface conditions, including DED, ACD, blepharitis, and MGD.[70] Regarding the anti-inflammatory potency of corticosteroids, a range of topical steroids are available. The patient's condition, including intraocular pressure (IOP), and the severity of ocular surface inflammation are major determinants of drug selection. Fluorometholone 0.1%, with a high relative potency and low to moderate adverse effects on IOP, is a reasonable choice for most conditions. Loteprednol, durezol, and rimexolone are other newer topical steroids that are claimed to have minimal effects on IOP.[71]

In patients with more severe ocular surface inflammation, such as acute VKC, increased use of more potent agents, such as prednisolone acetate 1% or dexamethasone 0.1%, is recommended.[32] Preservative-free corticosteroid eye drops should be considered in some cases of allergic conjunctivitis or DED, especially in association with corneal epithelial defects. Regarding the ocular side effects of topical and systemic corticosteroids, such as cataract and glaucoma, prescription of immunomodulatory agents should be considered in patients who require prolonged anti-inflammatory treatments.

IMMUNOMODULATORS

Cyclosporine A is a calcineurin inhibitor, which alleviates inflammation by inhibiting T lymphocytes. Lower concentrations of this drug (0.05%) are widely used against DED, as it has been proven to increase the production of tears.[72] Eye drops with higher concentrations of cyclosporine (1% and 5%) are applicable against ACDs (32). In recent years, the use of topical tacrolimus has increased in patients with ACDs. Tacrolimus (0.02–0.1%) is a T cell inhibitor, which reduces inflammation and prevents serious ocular complications, such as shield ulcers and limbal stem cell deficiency.[73] However, the increased susceptibility of patients to infectious keratitis has limited its application in severe refractory cases of ACD.[74]

The use of oral cyclosporine A (2.5–5 mg/kg) is limited to patients with severe refractory AKC, who show poor response to topical agents. This therapeutic approach is extremely rare in VKC and other forms of ACDs. Oral tacrolimus, which is assumed to be 25–100 times more immunosuppressive than cyclosporine A, is mainly used against severe ocular surface inflammations and high-risk cases of corneal graft rejection (inflamed and vascular host beds).[75] The use of immunomodulators in patients who are candidates for corneal transplantation can help improve the surgical outcomes by reducing inflammation in the ocular surface microenvironment and establishing homeostasis.

ANTIBIOTICS

Antimicrobials are primarily used for patients with MGD and blepharitis. Reduction of bacterial load, especially staphylococci, on the ocular surface helps control inflammation before surgery. Since azithromycin is a macrolide antibiotic with anti-inflammatory and lipid-regulating effects, it can be widely used against MGD and posterior blepharitis. Azithromycin ophthalmic solution (1%) is one of the commercially available options.[76] The bacteriostatic characteristics of tetracyclines, their ability to inhibit bacterial lipase, and their ability to reduce the formation of inflammatory mediators make them effective in the treatment of DED and MGD, as well as tear film stabilization.[77] Moreover, oral azithromycin is an effective treatment alternative, with no ocular topical surface side effects attributed to eye drops.

OMEGA-3 FATTY ACIDS

Some studies have reported that omega-3 fatty acids can contribute to inflammation control and stabilize the tear film by inhibiting pro-inflammatory mediators. They are primarily used for DED and MGD patients.[78] Evidence suggests that compounds containing fish oil and flaxseed oil can effectively improve dry eye symptoms due to high levels of omega-3 fatty acids.[79,80]

FLAXSEED OIL

The effect of flaxseed oil in reducing inflammation in patients with rheumatoid arthritis has been presented in the literature. Furthermore, the oral intake of capsules, containing 1–2 g of flaxseed oil per day, can effectively improve the symptoms of dry eye in patients with Sjögren's syndrome.[81] Moreover, the use of artificial tears containing flaxseed oil has been successful in DED treatment.[79]

AUTOLOGOUS SERUM-BASED EYE DROPS

Autologous serum-based eye drops, with 20% to 100% concentrations, are primarily used against severe DED, neurotrophic keratopathy, and persistent epithelial defects. Albumin and serum growth factors are known to improve the ocular surface condition and reduce apoptosis of corneal and conjunctival epithelial cells.[82] These agents are suitable for ocular surface complications following corneal transplantation. However, these eye drops are associated with complications, such as peripheral corneal infiltration, eyelid eczema, microbial keratoconjunctivitis, scleral vasculitis, and even corneal melting. The high cost and low accessibility of these agents result in their application for more severe cases which show no response to the available therapeutic options.[83,84]

LIFITEGRAST

This relatively new anti-inflammatory agent is a lymphocyte function-associated antigen-1 (LFA-1) antagonist. Lifitegrast 0.5% ophthalmic solution is safe and effective for the treatment of DED and causes a significant improvement in corneal fluorescein staining scores and dry eye.[85] The most common adverse effect is ocular irritation.[86]

The main procedural interventions to address ocular surface problems in the pre-operative period are summarized in Table 27.6.

OCULAR SURFACE COMPLICATIONS FOLLOWING CORNEAL TRANSPLANTATION

We previously discussed the necessity for optimizing the ocular surface condition before PK or anterior lamellar keratoplasty (ALK) in patients with KC and reviewed the therapeutic options. Generally, PK entails the removal of the entire cornea, complete severing of the corneal nerve,

Table 27.6 Procedural Therapies[51,87] for Ocular Surface Complications in Candidates for Corneal Transplantation due to Keratoconus (KC)

Ocular Surface Conditions	Procedural Interventions
MGD and blepharitis	• Meibomian gland thermal pulsation and expression • Intense pulsed light • Eyelid cleansing • Warm compress and eyelid massage
Dry eye disease (DED)	• Punctal occlusion • Intense pulsed light • Lifestyle changes (avoidance of drying conditions) • Eyelid cleansing

intraocular manipulation, and extensive suturing, leading to severe changes in the ocular surface. Ocular surface disorders may even occur after a successful procedure. Dry eye and superficial punctate keratopathy are two common side effects of corneal denervation following PK and ALK.[47] It was previously reported that DED parameters, such as TBUT results, corneal fluorescein stain, Schirmer's I test, corneal esthesiometry, and meibomian gland parameters, may deteriorate following keratoplasty.[44]

During the first few post-transplantation weeks, an ideal treatment approach primarily involves appropriate corneal re-epithelialization, inflammation management, and infection prevention. During this period, clinicians should be highly attentive to conditions that can disrupt the ocular surface homeostasis, including eyelid function disorders (e.g., lagophthalmos), blepharitis, dry eye, MGD, and suture-related complications, such as suture exposure, suture loosening, suture-related immune infiltration, and suture-related infection.[21,46,49]

Long-term post-transplantation ocular surface complications are commonly attributed to prolonged eye drop use, systemic drug toxicity, corneal sensory denervation, corneal surface irregularity, and suture-related complications. After extended use, eye drops containing preservatives may cause epithelial cell damage and inflammation, leading to punctate epithelial erosion and PED. In addition, local ocular surface immunodeficiency predisposes patients to infectious corneal ulcers. Damaged corneal sensory innervations lead to a neurotrophic cornea, which is characterized by PED, corneal surface irregularities, and mild corneal stromal haziness.[21,46,49] The common ocular surface complications following PK and ALK are presented in Table 27.7.[88]

As discussed earlier in this chapter, the ocular surface is affected by structural and inflammatory changes in keratoconus. In addition, allergic conjunctival disorders, especially AKC and VKC, are more prevalent in KC patients, compromising the ocular surface homeostasis. Furthermore, using contact lenses or procedures such as CXL lead to more ocular surface complications in these patients. Ocular surface health is essential in the outcome of surgical procedures, such as corneal transplantation. It is crucial to consider the therapeutic options for optimizing the ocular surface before and after surgery to achieve the most outstanding corneal transplant surgery outcomes.

Table 27.7 Treatment Options and Common Ocular Surface Complications of Penetrating Keratoplasty (PK) and Anterior Lamellar Keratoplasty (ALK) in Patients with Keratoconus

Persistent epithelial defect and corneal melt	The donor's epithelium is frequently destroyed or removed during surgery, which can cause failure to recover, as well as corneal ulcers.	• Bandage contact lens • Preservative-free artificial tears • Autologous serum eye drops • Prophylactic topical antibiotics • Anti-herpetic treatment • Surgical interventions, including tarsorrhaphy and amniotic membrane transplantation
Microbial keratitis	Microbial keratitis is usually suture-related and associated with transplant failure due to endothelial rejection in PK.	• Frequent use of fortified antibiotic eye drops • Intra-stomal antimicrobial injections • Lowering or discontinuing topical corticosteroid use • Considering the use of systemic antimicrobials, such as fluoroquinolones
Postsurgical inflammation (e.g., scleritis)	Surgery can result in excessive post-operative inflammation, including scleritis, which affects roughly 2% of people with keratoconus.[88]	• Preservative-free corticosteroid eye drops • Topical immunomodulatory therapy (cyclosporine A and tacrolimus) • Systemic corticosteroids • Systemic immunomodulatory treatment (T cell inhibitors and alkylating agents)
Neurotrophic cornea	The corneal nerves are severed in each procedure, occasionally resulting in delayed epithelialization, epithelial instability, and persistent corneal epithelial disruption. Within three years, 40% of sensation is regained.	• Bandage contact lens • Preservative-free artificial tears • Autologous serum eye drops • Prophylactic topical antibiotics • Anti-herpetic treatment • Surgical interventions, including tarsorrhaphy and amniotic membrane transplantation

REFERENCES

1. Santodomingo-Rubido J, Carracedo G, Suzaki A, Villa-Collar C, Vincent SJ, Wolffsohn JS. Keratoconus: An updated review. *Contact Lens and Anterior Eye.* 2022;45(3):101559.

2. Keane M, Coster D, Ziaei M, Williams K. Deep anterior lamellar keratoplasty versus penetrating keratoplasty for treating keratoconus. *Cochrane Database of Systematic Reviews.* 2014(7).

3. D'Souza S, Nair AP, Sahu GR, Vaidya T, Shetty R, Khamar P, et al. Keratoconus patients exhibit a distinct ocular surface immune cell and inflammatory profile. *Scientific Reports.* 2021;11(1):1–16.

4. de Almeida Borges D, Alborghetti MR, Franco Paes Leme A, Ramos Domingues R, Duarte B, Veiga M, et al. Tear proteomic profile in three distinct ocular surface diseases: keratoconus, pterygium, and dry eye related to graft-versus-host disease. *Clinical Proteomics.* 2020;17(1):1–16.

5. Tong L, Lan W, Petznick A. Definition of the ocular surface. *Ocular Surface.* 2012. https://doi.org/10.1201/b13153-3

6. Beuerman RW, Mircheff A, Pflugfelder SC, Stern ME. *The lacrimal functional unit. Dry eye and ocular surface disorders.* New York: Marcel Dekker. 2004:11–39.

7. Stern ME, Gao J, Siemasko KF, Beuerman RW, Pflugfelder SC. The role of the lacrimal functional unit in the pathophysiology of dry eye. *Experimental Eye Research.* 2004;78(3):409–16.

8. Javadi M-A, Feizi S. Dry eye syndrome. *Journal of Ophthalmic & Vision Research.* 2011;6(3):192.

9. Lemp MA, Bron AJ, Baudouin C, Del Castillo JMB, Geffen D, Tauber J, et al. Tear osmolarity in the diagnosis and management of dry eye disease. *American Journal of Ophthalmology.* 2011;151(5):792–8.e1.

10. Yagci A, Gurdal C. The role and treatment of inflammation in dry eye disease. *International Ophthalmology.* 2014;34(6):1291–301.

11. Grubbs Jr JR, Tolleson-Rinehart S, Huynh K, Davis RM. A review of quality of life measures in dry eye questionnaires. *Cornea.* 2014;33(2):215.

12. Zeev MS-B, Miller DD, Latkany R. Diagnosis of dry eye disease and emerging technologies. *Clinical Ophthalmology (Auckland, NZ).* 2014;8:581.

13. McMonnies CW. Inflammation and keratoconus. *Optometry and Vision Science.* 2015;92(2):e35–e41.

14. Cingu AK, Cinar Y, Turkcu FM, Sahin A, Ari S, Yuksel H, et al. Effects of vernal and allergic conjunctivitis on severity of keratoconus. *International Journal of Ophthalmology.* 2013;6(3):370.

15. Balasubramanian SA, Pye DC, Willcox MD. Effects of eye rubbing on the levels of protease, protease activity and cytokines in tears: relevance in keratoconus. Clinical and Experimental Optometry. 2013;96(2):214–8.

16. Ferrari G, Rama P. The keratoconus enigma: A review with emphasis on pathogenesis. *The Ocular Surface.* 2020;18(3):363–73.

17. Wheater MK, Kernacki KA, Hazlett LD. Corneal cell proteins and ocular surface pathology. *Biotechnic & Histochemistry.* 1999;74(3):146–59.

18. Sorkhabi R, Ghorbanihaghjo A, Taheri N, Ahoor MH. Tear film inflammatory mediators in patients with keratoconus. *International Ophthalmology*. 2015;35(4):467–72.

19. Taurone S, Ralli M, Plateroti A, Scorcia V, Greco A, Nebbioso M, et al. Keratoconus: the possible involvement of inflammatory cytokines in its pathogenesis. An experimental study and review of the literature. *European Review for Medical and Pharmacological Sciences*. 2021;25(13):4478–89.

20. Stevenson W, Chauhan SK, Dana R. Dry eye disease: an immune-mediated ocular surface disorder. *Archives of Ophthalmology*. 2012;130(1):90–100.

21. Singh R, Gupta N, Vanathi M, Tandon R. Corneal transplantation in the modern era. *The Indian Journal of Medical Research*. 2019;150(1):7.

22. Zhang X-H, Li X. Effect of rigid gas permeable contact lens on keratoconus progression: a review. *International Journal of Ophthalmology*. 2020;13(7):1124.

23. Moreddu R, Vigolo D, Yetisen AK. Contact lens technology: from fundamentals to applications. *Advanced Healthcare Materials*. 2019;8(15):1900368.

24. Alipour F, Khaheshi S, Soleimanzadeh M, Heidarzadeh S, Heydarzadeh S. Contact lens-related complications: a review. *Journal of Ophthalmic & Vision Research*. 2017;12(2):193.

25. Dhawan S, Rao K, Natrajan S. Complications of corneal collagen cross-linking. *Journal of Ophthalmology*. 2011;2011:869015.

26. Uysal BS, Akcay E, Kilicarslan A, Mutlu M, Hondur G, Kosekahya P, et al. Tear function and ocular surface changes following corneal collagen cross-linking treatment in keratoconus patients: 18-month results. *International Ophthalmology*. 2020;40(1):169–77.

27. Acar Eser N, Dikmetas O, Kocabeyoglu S, Tan C, Irkec M. Evaluation of keratoconus disease with tear cytokine and chemokine levels before and after corneal cross-linking treatment. *Ocular Immunology and Inflammation*. 2023;1–7.

28. Moore JE, Atkinson SD, Azar DT, Worthington J, Downes CS, Courtney DG, et al. Protection of corneal epithelial stem cells prevents ultraviolet A damage during corneal collagen cross-linking treatment for keratoconus. *British Journal of Ophthalmology*. 2014;98(2):270–4.

29. Dua HS, Saini JS, Azuara-Blanco A, Gupta P. Limbal stem cell deficiency: concept, aetiology, clinical presentation, diagnosis and management. *Indian Journal of Ophthalmology*. 2000;48(2):83.

30. Ehlers WH, Donshik PC. Allergic ocular disorders: a spectrum of diseases. *The CLAO Journal: Official Publication of the Contact Lens Association of Ophthalmologists, Inc*. 1992;18(2):117–24.

31. Sacchetti M, Abicca I, Bruscolini A, Cavaliere C, Nebbioso M, Lambiase A. Allergic conjunctivitis: current concepts on pathogenesis and management. *Journal of Biological Regulators and Homeostatic Agents*. 2018;32(1 Suppl. 1):49–60.

32. Mehta JS, Chen W-L, Cheng AC, Dualan IJ, Kekunnaya R, Khaliddin N, et al. Diagnosis, management, and treatment of vernal keratoconjunctivitis in asia: recommendations from the management of vernal keratoconjunctivitis in Asia expert working group. *Frontiers in Medicine*. 2022;9.

33. Guglielmetti S, Dart JK, Calder V. Atopic keratoconjunctivitis and atopic dermatitis. *Current Opinion in Allergy and Clinical Immunology*. 2010;10(5):478–85.

34. Ibrahim OMA, Matsumoto Y, Dogru M, Adan ES, Wakamatsu TH, Shimazaki J, et al. In Vivo confocal microscopy evaluation of meibomian gland dysfunction in atopic-keratoconjunctivitis patients. *Ophthalmology*. 2012;119(10):1961–8.

35. Akasaki Y, Inomata T, Sung J, Nakamura M, Kitazawa K, Shih KC, et al. Prevalence of comorbidity between dry eye and allergic conjunctivitis: a systematic review and meta-analysis. *Journal of Clinical Medicine*. 2022;11(13):3643.

36. Shoji J. Ocular allergy test and biomarkers on the ocular surface: clinical test for evaluating the ocular surface condition in allergic conjunctival diseases. *Allergology International*. 2020;69(4):496–504.

37. Solomon A. Corneal complications of vernal keratoconjunctivitis. *Current Opinion in Allergy and Clinical Immunology*. 2015;15(5):489–94.

38. Feizi S, Javadi MA, Alemzadeh-Ansari M, Arabi A, Shahraki T, Kheirkhah A. Management of corneal complications in vernal keratoconjunctivitis: a review. *The Ocular Surface*. 2021;19:282–9.

39. Gadhvi KA, Romano V, Cueto LF-V, Aiello F, Day AC, Allan BD. Deep anterior lamellar keratoplasty for keratoconus: Multisurgeon results. *American Journal of Ophthalmology*. 2019;201:54–62.

40. Brierly SC, Izquierdo Jr L, Mannis MJ. Penetrating keratoplasty for keratoconus. *Cornea*. 2000;19(3):329–32.

41. Ang M, Mehta JS. Deep anterior lamellar keratoplasty as an alternative to penetrating keratoplasty. *Ophthalmology*. 2011;118(11):2306–7.

42. Melles GR, Lander F, Rietveld FJ, Remeijer L, Beekhuis WH, Binder PS. A new surgical technique for deep stromal, anterior lamellar keratoplasty. *British Journal of Ophthalmology*. 1999;83(3):327–33.

43. Thompson RW, Price MO, Bowers PJ, Price FW. Long-term graft survival after penetrating keratoplasty. *Ophthalmology*. 2003;110(7):1396–402.

44. Fu Y, Liu J, Tseng SC. Ocular surface deficits contributing to persistent epithelial defect after penetrating keratoplasty. *Cornea*. 2012;31(7):723–9.

45. Müller LJ, Marfurt CF, Kruse F, Tervo TM. Corneal nerves: structure, contents and function. *Experimental Eye Research*. 2003;76(5):521–42.

46. Price FW, Whitson WE, Collins KS, Marks RG. Five-year corneal graft survival: a large, single-center patient cohort. *Archives of Ophthalmology*. 1993;111(6):799–805.

47. Hara S, Kojima T, Dogru M, Uchino Y, Goto E, Matsumoto Y, et al. The impact of tear functions on visual outcome following keratoplasty in eyes with keratoconus. *Graefe's Archive for Clinical and Experimental Ophthalmology*. 2013;251(7):1763–70.

48. Chuang J, Shih KC, Chan TC, Wan KH, Jhanji V, Tong L. Preoperative optimization of ocular surface disease before cataract surgery. *Journal of Cataract & Refractive Surgery*. 2017;43(12):1596–607.

49. Sugar A, Gal RL, Kollman C, Raghinaru D, Dontchev M, Croasdale CR, et al. Factors associated with corneal graft survival in the cornea donor study. *JAMA Ophthalmology*. 2015;133(3):246–54.

50. Kim KY, Chung B, Kim EK, Seo KY, Jun I, Kim T-i. Changes in ocular surface and Meibomian gland after penetrating keratoplasty. *BMC Ophthalmology*. 2021;21(1):1–8.

51. Amescua G, Akpek EK, Farid M, Garcia-Ferrer FJ, Lin A, Rhee MK, et al. Blepharitis preferred practice pattern®. *Ophthalmology*. 2019;126(1):P56–P93.

52. Sakassegawa-Naves FE, Ricci HMM, Moscovici BK, Miyamoto DA, Chiacchio BB, Holzchuh R, et al. Tacrolimus ointment for refractory posterior blepharitis. *Current Eye Research*. 2017;42(11):1440–4.

53. Nichols KK, Foulks GN, Bron AJ, Glasgow BJ, Dogru M, Tsubota K, et al. The international workshop on meibomian gland dysfunction: executive summary. *Investigative Ophthalmology & Visual Science*. 2011;52(4):1922–9.

54. Thomas J, Guel DA, Thomas TS, Cavanagh HD. The role of atopy in corneal graft survival in keratoconus. *Cornea*. 2011;30(10):1088.

55. Craig JP, Nichols KK, Akpek EK, Caffery B, Dua HS, Joo C-K, et al. TFOS DEWS II definition and classification report. *The Ocular Surface*. 2017;15(3):276–83.

56. Bron AJ, de Paiva CS, Chauhan SK, Bonini S, Gabison EE, Jain S, et al. Tfos dews ii pathophysiology report. *The Ocular Surface*. 2017;15(3):438–510.

57. Epidemiology D. Subcommittee. The epidemiology of dry eye disease: Report of the epidemiology subcommittee of the international dry eye workshop (2007). *Ocular Surface*. 2007;5(2):93–107.

58. Zhou L, Beuerman RW. Tear analysis in ocular surface diseases. *Progress in Retinal And Eye Research*. 2012;31(6):527–50.

59. Labetoulle M, Benitez-del-Castillo JM, Barabino S, Herrero Vanrell R, Daull P, Garrigue J-S, et al. Artificial tears: biological role of their ingredients in the management of dry eye disease. *International Journal of Molecular Sciences*. 2022;23(5):2434.

60. Pucker AD, Ng SM, Nichols JJ. Over the counter (OTC) artificial tear drops for dry eye syndrome. *Cochrane Database of Systematic Reviews*. 2016;2(2):CD009729. doi: 10.1002/14651858. CD009729.pub2. PMID: 26905373; PMCID: PMC5045033.

61. Bielory L, Meltzer EO, Nichols KK, Melton R, Thomas RK, Bartlett JD, editors. *An algorithm for the management of allergic conjunctivitis. Allergy and asthma proceedings*; 2013: OceanSide Publications, Inc.

62. Baudouin C, Labbé A, Liang H, Pauly A, Brignole-Baudouin F. Preservatives in eyedrops: the good, the bad and the ugly. *Progress in Retinal And Eye Research*. 2010;29(4):312–34.

63. Leonardi A. Management of vernal keratoconjunctivitis. *Ophthalmology and Therapy*. 2013;2(2):73–88.

64. Muraro A, Dubois A, DunnGalvin A, Hourihane JOB, De Jong N, Meyer R, et al. EAACI Food Allergy and Anaphylaxis Guidelines. Food allergy health-related quality of life measures. *Allergy*. 2014;69(7):845–53.

65. Yanni J, Sharif N, Gamache D, Miller S, Weimer L, Spellman J. A current appreciation of sites for pharmacological intervention in allergic conjunctivitis: effects of new topical ocular drugs. *Acta Ophthalmologica Scandinavica*. 1999;77:33–7.

66. Welch D, Ousler G, Nally L, Abelson M, Wilcox K. *Ocular drying associated with oral antihistamines (loratadine) in the normal population-an evaluation of exaggerated dose effect*. Lacrimal Gland, Tear Film, and Dry Eye Syndromes 3: Springer; 2002. p. 1051–5.

67. Fauquert JL. Diagnosing and managing allergic conjunctivitis in childhood: the allergist's perspective. *Pediatric Allergy and Immunology*. 2019;30(4):405–14.

68. Cook E, Stahl J, Barney N, Graziano F. Mechanisms of antihistamines and mast cell stabilizers in ocular allergic inflammation. *Current Drug Targets-Inflammation & Allergy*. 2002;1(2):167–80.

69. Rigas B, Huang W, Honkanen R. NSAID-induced corneal melt: clinical importance, pathogenesis, and risk mitigation. *Survey of Ophthalmology*. 2020;65(1):1–11.

70. Cutolo CA, Barabino S, Bonzano C, Traverso CE. The use of topical corticosteroids for treatment of dry eye syndrome. *Ocular Immunology and Inflammation*. 2019;27(2):266–75.

71. Sheppard JD, Comstock TL, Cavet ME. Impact of the topical ophthalmic corticosteroid loteprednol etabonate on intraocular pressure. *Advances in Therapy*. 2016;33:532–52.

72. De Paiva CS, Pflugfelder SC, Ng SM, Akpek EK. Topical cyclosporine A therapy for dry eye syndrome. *Cochrane Database of Systematic Reviews*. 2019;9(9):CD010051. doi: 10.1002/14651858. CD010051.pub2. PMID: 31517988; PMCID: PMC6743670.

73. Erdinest N, Ben-Eli H, Solomon A. Topical tacrolimus for allergic eye diseases. *Current Opinion in Allergy and Clinical Immunology*. 2019;19(5):535–43.

74. Fukushima A, Ohashi Y, Ebihara N, Uchio E, Okamoto S, Kumagai N, et al. Therapeutic effects of 0.1% tacrolimus eye drops for refractory allergic ocular diseases with proliferative lesion or corneal involvement. *British Journal of Ophthalmology*. 2014;98(8):1023–7.

75. Zhai J, Gu J, Yuan J, Chen J. Tacrolimus in the treatment of ocular diseases. *BioDrugs*. 2011;25:89–103.

76. Thode AR, Latkany RA. Current and emerging therapeutic strategies for the treatment of meibomian gland dysfunction (MGD). *Drugs*. 2015;75(11):1177–85.

77. Yoo S-E, Lee D-C, Chang M-H. The effect of low-dose doxycycline therapy in chronic meibomian gland dysfunction. *Korean Journal of Ophthalmology*. 2005;19(4):258–63.

78. Bhargava R, Kumar P, Kumar M, Mehra N, Mishra A. A randomized controlled trial of omega-3 fatty acids in dry eye syndrome. *International Journal of Ophthalmology*. 2013;6(6):811.

79. Downie LE, Hom MM, Berdy GJ, El-Harazi S, Verachtert A, Tan J, et al. An artificial tear containing flaxseed oil for treating dry eye disease: A randomized controlled trial. *The Ocular Surface*. 2020;18(1):148–57.

80. Kawakita T, Kawabata F, Tsuji T, Kawashima M, Shimmura S, Tsubota K. Effects of dietary supplementation with fish oil on dry eye syndrome subjects: randomized controlled trial. *Biomedical Research*. 2013;34(5):215–20.

81. Pinheiro Jr MN, Santos PMd, Santos RCRd, Barros JdN, Passos LF, Cardoso Neto J. Oral flaxseed oil (Linum usitatissimum) in the treatment for dry-eye Sjögren's syndrome patients. *Arquivos Brasileiros de Oftalmologia*. 2007;70:649–55.

82. Shtein RM, Shen JF, Kuo AN, Hammersmith KM, Li JY, Weikert MP. Autologous serum-based eye drops for treatment of ocular surface disease: a report by the American academy of ophthalmology. *Ophthalmology*. 2020;127(1):128–33.

83. Kojima T, Higuchi A, Goto E, Matsumoto Y, Dogru M, Tsubota K. Autologous serum eye drops for the treatment of dry eye diseases. *Cornea*. 2008;27:S25-S30.

84. Ali TK, Gibbons A, Cartes C, Zarei-Ghanavati S, Gomaa M, Gonzalez I, et al. Use of autologous serum tears for the treatment of ocular surface disease from patients with systemic autoimmune diseases. *American Journal of Ophthalmology*. 2018;189:65–70.

85. Haber SL, Benson V, Buckway CJ, Gonzales JM, Romanet D, Scholes B. Lifitegrast: a novel drug for patients with dry eye disease. *Therapeutic Advances in Ophthalmology*. 2019;11:2515841419870366.

86. Zhong M, Gadek TR, Bui M, Shen W, Burnier J, Barr KJ, et al. Discovery and development of potent LFA-1/ICAM-1 antagonist SAR 1118 as an ophthalmic solution for treating dry eye. *ACS Medicinal Chemistry Letters*. 2012;3(3):203–6.

87. Jones L, Downie LE, Korb D, Benitez-del-Castillo JM, Dana R, Deng SX, et al. TFOS DEWS II management and therapy report. *The Ocular Surface*. 2017;15(3):575–628.

88. Tan DT, Dart JK, Holland EJ, Kinoshita S. Corneal transplantation. *The Lancet*. 2012;379(9827):1749–61.

28 Post-Keratoplasty Infectious Keratitis

Mehrnaz Atighehchian

INTRODUCTION

The main procedure for visual rehabilitation of the patient with keratoconus for who sufferers with contact lens intolerance is corneal transplantation.[1] Keratoplasty has been changed from full-thickness toward o the lamellar technique and the main indicator of deep anterior lamellar keratoplasty (DALK) is keratoconus. Compared with penetrating keratoplasty (PKP), DALK has improved graft outcomes and decreased some complications, including endothelial rejection, endophthalmitis, etc.[2]

Infectious keratitis is an important complication after corneal transplantation that affects the viability and clarity of corneal grafts.[3] Clinical presentation of infectious keratitis may present in different patterns and locations as central, paracentral, or peripheral cornea at the graft–host interface.[3,4] Keratoconus eyes with corneal grafts are susceptible to infection because of long-term topical corticosteroid use, suture-related problems, donor tissue contamination, chronic corneal epithelial defects, dry eye, graft hypoesthesia, and the use of soft contact lenses. Unlike PKP, a corneal interface between the donor and the recipient cornea in DALK is a potential space for the growth of microorganisms. In addition, this space causes poor drug penetration so the treatment of infiltration is difficult.[5]

The time presentation of post-keratoplasty infectious keratitis is variable and can present in the early or late post-operative period from the first day to several months after uncomplicated surgery.[5,6] Diagnosis and treatment of post-keratoplasty infectious keratitis are challenging.[4] Microbiological diagnosis is based on corneal scrapings and microorganisms are commonly cultured on a special medium to diagnose the causes of pathogens for early diagnosis and better management.[3,5,6]

MICROORGANISMS

Bacteria

Generally, Gram-positive bacteria are the most widespread microorganisms in post-keratoplasty infectious keratitis due to the normal ocular surface flora.[3] Coagulase-negative *Staphylococcus* spp. and *Staphylococcus aureus* are the most common Gram-positive graft infection microorganisms. Other less common Gram-positive cocci include *Streptococcus pneumoniae*, *Streptococcus viridans*, and other alpha-hemolytic streptococci.[7,8] In high-income countries, *S. aureus* is more common, whereas, in middle- to low-income countries, a greater prevalence of *S. pneumoniae* and coagulase-negative Staphylococcus have been reported from post-keratoplasty infectious keratitis (Figure 28.1 left).[3,8,9]

The most commonly diagnosed Gram-negative bacterium in both high- and middle- to low-income countries is *Pseudomonas aeruginosa*. In addition, high-income countries report cases caused by *Serratia marcescens* and *Klebsiella pneumoniae* (Figure 28.2).[3]

Presentation

Microbial keratitis (MK) can occur in the early or late postoperative period after keratoplasty. Early MK is usually due to ocular surface diseases in the recipient, contamination of the donor cornea, and intraoperative contamination, whereas later MK is due to environmental pathogens.[5,6] Bacterial keratitis is often associated with acute suppurative reactions.[9,10] The corneal infiltration is usually accompanied by stromal infiltration and anterior chamber reaction and can occur in different locations such as the central, paracentral, or graft–host interface. Infections related to sutures typically cause peripheral keratitis, while central and paracentral ulcers are more common when the predisposing factor is an epithelial defect.[3,7-8]

Fungi

Fungal keratitis is uncommon but is the second most common cause of infectious keratitis following keratoplasty. Corneal transplantation increases the risk of fungal keratitis, while the use of topical corticosteroid eye drops increases the risk of fungal growth.[11-13] Additionally, the donor–host fungal transmission is higher when the donor cornea and sclera rim test positive for fungus.[14] Post-keratoplasty fungal keratitis is more challenging to treat and has a lower success rate

DOI: 10.1201/9781003371601-28

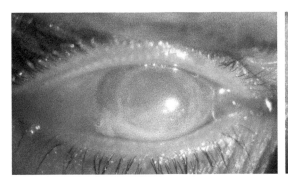
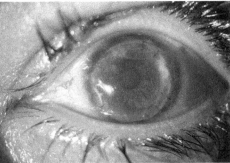

Figure 28.1 (left) A 45-year-old man with a history of deep lamellar keratoplasty (DALK) ten years ago. The smear result from the corneal specimen was Gram-positive cocci and the culture was *Staphylococcus aureus*. (right) A 32-year-old man with a history of deep lamellar keratoplasty (DALK) two months ago.

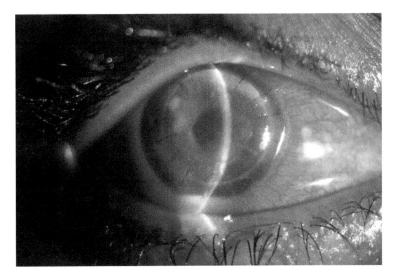

Figure 28.2 A 22-year-old man with a history of DALK three weeks ago. The smear result from the corneal specimen was negative for bacilli.

compared to bacterial graft infections, as it can lead to corneal melting in the early postoperative period.[15] *Candida* species are the majority of cases of post-keratoplasty fungal keratitis. These may occur due to donor corneal contamination or long-term corneal epithelial defects that are contaminated by the microflora of the conjunctiva, the ocular surface, and adnexa.[4,14,16]

The onset of fungal keratitis usually presents in the late postoperative period.[14] However fungal infection after DALK should be considered among the differential diagnosis in patients who present with early interface infiltration.[15] The corneal interface between the donor graft and recipient bed in DALK is a potential space for the growth of microorganisms, such as fungi, and causes an uncommon interface infectious keratitis (IIK). Although the rate of IIK is low, reported at 0.052%, it is a serious complication due to its location, challenges in sample collection for testing, limited drug penetration, and resistance to treatment.[16]

The presentation of IIK may be unchanged for a long period due to the slow growth of the microorganisms, especially fungi.[5] In addition, small interface infiltrations may be mistaken for non-infectious debris or epithelial ingrowth, leading to delayed diagnosis. This delay in diagnosis causes corneal melt, development of haze, and visual loss, especially with fungal pathogens such as Candida and Aspergillus.[7,12-13]

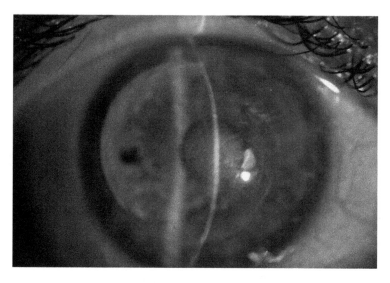

Figure 28.3 Fungal keratitis after DALK.

Clinical Presentation

Post-keratoplasty fungal keratitis has a similar pattern in the form of one or multiple small round white colonies at the edge of the graft–host corneal junction in the deep corneal stroma with or without hypopyon.[3,5] Also, diffuse, scattered, and dense white-to-cream-colored infiltrations can be present at the corneal interface space in the DALK keratitis (Figure 28.3).[5]

Viruses

Viral keratitis is a less common cause of post-keratoplasty infectious keratitis in eyes with keratoconus (KCN). The main risk factor for herpes simplex virus (HSV) keratitis is a preexisting ocular HSV infection. Reactivation of a latent HSV-1 may also lead to persistent corneal epithelial defects or even corneal graft failure after penetrating keratoplasty.

In addition, it has been reported that herpetic keratitis can occur after penetrating keratoplasty in patients with no history of herpetic disease and has been hypothesized that graft-to-host transmission of HSV-1 may cause post-keratoplasty herpetic keratitis.[3,17]

Infectious Crystalline Keratopathy

Post-keratoplasty crystalline keratopathy is a less inflammatory condition in which colonies of microorganisms produce branching crystalline opacities within the corneal stroma. Most eyes with infectious crystalline keratopathy are less inflamed and respond to use of topical corticosteroids. Most cases of infectious crystalline keratopathy are associated with Gram-positive bacteria, especially *Streptococcus viridans*. Other bacteria, fungi, and Gram-negative microorganisms are rare causes of crystalline keratopathy. Additionally, viral pathogens, especially HSV, have been reported to cause crystalline keratopathy[10] (Figures 28.4 and 28.5).

Investigation

Corneal scraping should be obtained and sent for smear and culture for both bacterial and fungal examination. Another diagnostic method is Polymerase Chain Reaction (PCR). PCR involves a repeating cycle of replication to amplify small segments of deoxyribonucleic acid (DNA). A novel application of this technique used microbial, viral, and fungal identification in infectious keratitis. PCR is more sensitive than biological stains and culture, which may be considered the gold standards for diagnosing infectious keratitis.[18]

In-vivo confocal microscopy (IVCM) is a modality to diagnose the post-keratoplasty keratitis. With IVCM, bacteria are visible as highly refractile bodies in the epithelium and superficial to the deep corneal stroma. Branching fungal hyphae are also identified as filaments structures.[7]

The donor-to-host-related infectious keratitis is present at the deep corneal graft interface and sampling these infiltrates is difficult without surgical intervention. So, to obtain a sample for

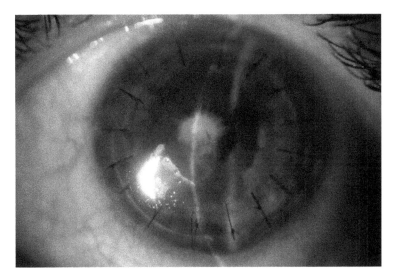

Figure 28.4 Crystalline keratitis. A 41-year-old woman with a history of DALK 2 years ago. The smear result from the corneal specimen was Gram-positive cocci and the culture result after 48 hours was no growth.

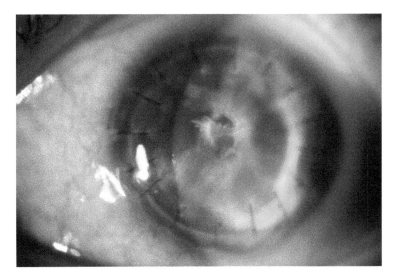

Figure 28.5 Crystalline keratitis after treatment.

microbiological evaluation, in the deep stroma infection in penetrating or lamellar keratoplasty, a corneal biopsy is done and microbiological or histopathological evaluations of the biopsy specimen are performed.

Microbial donor rim cultures are crucial for diagnosing fungal keratitis, while bacterial culture-positive donor rims have a higher reported but poorer correlation with post-operative keratoplasty infectious keratitis.[5,19] At the time of transplantation, the outer edge of the corneal tissue is removed and sent for culture. The transplantation proceeds, and 24–72 hours later, culture result will be reported. This is a crucial period, as any infection may occur during this time. Positive donor rim fungal cultures are rare, but they help identify which patients are at high risk of developing donor-related keratitis. Clinicians provide prophylactic therapy in all cases of culture-positive donor rims. Unfortunately, sometimes the culture results may not return in time to start treatment.[19]

MEDICAL MANAGEMENT

Overall, post-keratoplasty infectious keratitis is treated in an in-patient setting and out-patient treatment happens for the light infection of patients who visited continually.[3] The successful medical treatment for microbial post-keratoplasty infectious keratitis depends on the microorganism's type and the size and depth of infection.[7]

Post-keratoplasty Bacterial Keratitis

The primary treatment is empiric because the culture results can take more than 48 hours. Empirical therapy is based on intensive broad–spectrum topical antibiotics covering both Gram-positive and Gram-negative micro-organisms and should be modified based on clinical response and positive culture and antibiogram results. For central or severe infection, an initial frequent application of topical antibiotic dosage every five to 15 min is recommended followed by hourly applications.[1,20]

Overall, the empirical treatment uses monotherapy with topical fluoroquinolones such as ciprofloxacin 0.3%, ofloxacin 0.3%, moxifloxacin 5 mg/ml, levofloxacin 15 mg/ml, gatifloxacin 3 mg/ml, or besifloxacin 6 mg/ml).[3,20] If the infection appears to be worsening, the clinician can change the topical fluoroquinolones to fortified broad-spectrum antibiotics. On the other hand, an alternative treatment includes a combination of cephalosporin agents or vancomycin to provide a Gram-positive coverage, and aminoglycoside or fluoroquinolone to achieve a Gram-negative coverage.[20]

Although fortified antibiotics are effective at controlling corneal infection, the corneal toxicity with a broad-spectrum fortified antibiotic is an important factor for delaying corneal epithelial healing in lamellar and penetrating keratoplasty, so it is necessary to decrease and taper the duration of topical fortified antibiotics.[1,21]

The use of topical corticosteroids is controversial for managing post-keratoplasty bacterial keratitis. Topical corticosteroids improve visual outcomes by reducing inflammation, corneal scar, neovascularization, and a stromal corneal melt and prevent graft rejection. However, corticosteroids can affect corneal healing and cause delayed corneal epithelial healing and may even worsen infection, so they must be used carefully.[21]

Post-Keratoplasty Fungal Keratitis

Management of fungal keratitis after lamellar or penetrating keratoplasty includes topical and systemic antifungal agents, cycloplegic, and antibiotics for secondary bacterial infection. The selection of antifungal medications may depend on drug availability and clinician presentation. Topical natamycin 5% is associated with better outcomes for *Fusarium* keratitis. Topical voriconazole and amphotericin B 0.15% can also be considered alternative treatment, but voriconazole's limitations involve its high price and its lower effectiveness than topical natamycin. Topical amphotericin can be used as the first choice for yeasts and is an alternative for filamentous fungi.[20] Oral medications such as voriconazole, ketoconazole, itraconazole, and fluconazole can be added to topical antifungal medication.[20-21]

Herpes Simplex Keratitis

Since PKP or DAILK are performed for keratoconus eyes, recurrent herpes simplex virus (HSV) keratitis is not common, but if the patients have a history of previous HSV keratitis, a clinician must consider HSV keratitis. The current treatment recommendations for recurrent HSV post-keratoplasty keratitis are based on the results of the Herpetic Eye Disease Study (HEDS) group clinical trials conducted in the 1990s.[20,22] Oral acyclovir, famciclovir, and topical trifluridine are appropriate medications and are easily accessible in most countries.[20,22]

SURGICAL MANAGEMENT

Localized Scraping

Sub-epithelial and superficial central, paracentral, or donor-recipient infections may be managed by scraping off the overlying infected corneal epithelium to decrease the infectious load and can be effective in enhancing the penetration of topical antimicrobial drugs, especially in fungal keratitis.[1,22]

Intrastromal Antimicrobial Injection

Intrastromal antimicrobial and antifungal injection is recommended when the infection expands to the deep corneal stromal layers in penetrating keratoplasty or interface infection in lamellar keratoplasty (DALK).[20] Also, interface irrigation with antibiotics or antifungal agents is beneficial for IIK in post-DALK keratitis.[22]

Intracameral antimicrobial or antifungal injection may be considered in obvious anterior chamber reaction, significant fungal ball in the anterior chamber, or when the corneal infiltration does not respond to topical and oral medication, especially for fungal infiltrations.[20]

Repeat DALK

It is not recommended to repeat lamellar grafts in cases of post-DALK infectious keratitis with infection in the interface, because the interface provides a potential space for sequestration of the microorganisms and causes recurrent infection in repeated corneal grafts. Hence, if the repeated operation is necessary, full-thickness keratoplasty is the better surgical intervention for these patients. In the superficial infection in which infections are completely removed during surgery and the interface space is not infiltrated; a repeated DALK procedure is performed to decrease the risks of open sky complications.[1,23]

Repeated Penetrating Therapeutic Keratoplasty

Therapeutic penetrating keratoplasty (T-PKP) is required in more than one-third of cases with infectious keratitis following DALK to preserve the anatomical integrity.[1] Therapeutic PKP is performed in the infected lamellar graft that does not respond to medical therapy or cases with impending graft perforation. Sometimes, emergency T-PKP may be needed for the Descemet membrane rupture during interface irrigation for IIK in post-DALK keratitis.

A large diameter T-PKP that circumscribes the previous graft–host junction is performed to ensure complete removal of the infective tissue, especially in fungal keratitis.[19,24]

REFERENCES

1. Namrata Sharma MD, Manpreet Kaur MD, Jeewan S. Infectious keratitis following lamellar keratoplasty. *J Surv Ophthalmol.* 2020.11.001

2. Abdelaal AM, Alqassimi AH, Malak M, Hijazi HT, Hadrawi M, Khan MA. Indications of keratoplasty and outcomes of deep anterior lamellar keratoplasty compared to penetrating keratoplasty. *Cureus.* 2021 Mar 11;13(3):e13825.

3. Sharma N, Kaur M, Titiyal JS, Aldave A. Infectious keratitis after lamellar keratoplasty. *Surv Ophthalmol.* 2021 Jul–Aug;66(4):623–643.

4. Fontana L, Moramarco A, Mandarà E, Russello G, Iovieno A. Interface infectious keratitis after anterior and posterior lamellar keratoplasty. Clinical features and treatment strategies. A review. *Br J Ophthalmol.* 2019 Mar;103(3):307–314.

5. Gao Y, Li C, Bu P, Zhang L, Bouchard CS. Infectious interface keratitis (IIK) following lamellar keratoplasty: A literature review. *Ocul Surf.* 2019 Oct;17(4):635–643.

6. Kodavoor SK, Dandapani R, Kaushik AR. Interface infectious keratitis following deep anterior lamellar keratoplasty. *Indian J Ophthalmol.* 2016 Aug;64(8):597–600.

7. Rasik B. Vajpayee, MS, FRCSEd, Namrata Sharma, MD. Infectious keratitis following keratoplasty. *Surv Ophthalmol.* 2007;52:1–12.

8. Sharma N, Jain M, Sehra SV, Maharana P, Agarwal T, Satpathy G, Vajpayee RB. Outcomes of therapeutic penetrating keratoplasty from a tertiary eye care centre in northern India. *Cornea.* 2014 Feb;33(2):114–118.

9. Al-Hazzaa SA, Tabbara KF. Bacterial keratitis after penetrating keratoplasty. *Ophthalmology.* 1988 Nov;95(11):1504–1508.

10. Khater TT, Jones DB, Wilhelmus KR. Infectious crystalline keratopathy caused by gram-negative bacteria. *Am J Ophthalmol.* 1997 Jul;124(1):19–23.

11. Sati A, Wagh S, Mishra SK, Kumar SV, Kumar P. Post-corneal transplant Candida keratitis - Incidence and outcome. *Indian J Ophthalmol*. 2022 Feb;70(2):536–541.

12. Fontana L, Caristia A, Cornacchia A, Russello G, Moramarco A. Excisional penetrating keratoplasty for fungal interface keratitis after endothelial keratoplasty: Surgical timing and visual outcome. *Int Ophthalmol*. 2021 Jan;41(1):363–373.

13. Otaif W, Al Somali AI, Almulhim A. Corneal perforation as a complication of fungal interface infectious keratitis after deep anterior lamellar keratoplasty. *Middle East Afr J Ophthalmol*. 2021 Dec 31;28(3):184–188.

14. Bahadir AE, Bozkurt TK, Kutan SA, Yanyali CA, Acar S. Candida interface keratitis following deep anterior lamellar keratoplasty. *Int Ophthalmol*. 2012 Aug;32(4):383–386.

15. Sadigh AL, Shenasi A, Mortazavi SZ, Morsali SM. Aspergillus keratitis after deep anterior lamellar keratoplasty. *J Ophthalmic Vis Res*. 2014 Jul-Sep;9(3):392–394.

16. Kodavoor SK, Rathi N, Dandapani R. Complications in deep anterior lamellar keratoplasty: A retrospective interventional analysis in a large series. *Indian J Ophthalmol*. 2022 Oct;70(10):3501–3507.

16. Kodavoor SK, Rathi N, Dandapani R. Complications in deep anterior lamellar keratoplasty: A retrospective interventional analysis in a large series. *Indian J Ophthalmol*. 2022 Oct;70(10):3501–3507.

17. Gatzioufas Z, Hasenfus A, Gyongyossy B, Stavridis E, Sauter M, Smola S, Seitz B. Repeat corneal graft failure due to graft-to-host herpetic infection. *J Ophthalmic Inflamm Infect*. 2013 Jan 28;3(1):24.

18. Liu HY, Hopping GC, Vaidyanathan U, Ronquillo YC, Hoopes PC, Moshirfar M. Polymerase chain reaction and Its application in the diagnosis of infectious keratitis. *Med Hypothesis Discov Innov Ophthalmol*. 2019 Fall;8(3):152-155.

19. Vislisel JM, Goins KM, Wagoner MD, Schmidt GA, Aldrich BT, Skeie JM, Reed CR, Zimmerman MB, Greiner MA. Incidence and outcomes of positive donor corneoscleral rim fungal cultures after keratoplasty. *Ophthalmology*. 2017 Jan;124(1):36–42.

20. Cabrera-Aguas M, Khoo P, Watson SL. Infectious keratitis: A review. *Clin Exp Ophthalmol*. 2022 Jul;50(5):543–562.

21. Austin A, Lietman T, Rose-Nussbaumer J. Update on the management of infectious keratitis. *Ophthalmology*. 2017 Nov;124(11):1678–1689.

22. Cabrera-Aguas M, Robaei D, McCluskey P, Watson S. Clinical translation of recommendations from randomized trials for management of herpes simplex virus keratitis. *Clin Exp Ophthalmol*. 2018 Dec;46(9):1008–1016.

23. Egrilmez S, Palamar M, Sipahi OR, Yagci A. Extended spectrum beta-lactamase producing Klebsiella pneumoniae-related keratitis. *J Chemother*. 2013 Apr;25(2):123–125.

24. Kanavi MR, Foroutan AR, Kamel MR, Afsar N, Javadi MA. Candida interface keratitis after deep anterior lamellar keratoplasty: clinical, microbiologic, histopathologic, and confocal microscopic reports. *Cornea*. 2007 Sep;26(8):913–916.

29 New International Achievements in Modern Modalities of Keratoconus Treatment

Khosrow Jadidi and Seyed Aliasghar Mosavi

INTRODUCTION

Keratoconus is a progressive bilateral non-inflammatory ectatic corneal disease, the cause of which is not known. It affects visual function because of corneal thinning and protrusion.[1] Ethnicity plays a role in the extreme differences in the prevalence of keratoconus. Assessing Caucasian and Asian individuals living in similar geographic zones showed an unequal distribution of keratoconus. The incidence of this disease is four times higher among Asian people than Caucasians.[2] In the last two decades, advancements were made in the treatment of keratoconus. From being limited merely to using penetrating keratoplasty and hard gas-permeable contact lens for cases of advanced keratoconus, to various alternatives to treat/postpone the need for a corneal transplant, and also to delay disease progression with high levels of safety and efficacy. Several studies mentioned the effectiveness of the segmented rings as an additive refractive surgical method for low to moderate myopia, to improve visual acuity and decrease the average keratometry (K) value and refractive error in patients with keratoconus.[3–7] However, intrastromal corneal ring (ICR) is developed into a main instrument for the management of corneal ectatic disorders such as keratoconus but can rarely be used for severe keratoconus,[7] and is not a solution for all keratoconus cases. According to direct observation by the authors, all existing ICRs may cause corneal melting[8,9] and, therefore, development of new devices and methods can provide further help in treating keratoconus on a wider scale. With these problems in mind, new corneal surgical approaches have been developed, such as surgical techniques available for corneal grafting in keratoconus.[10]

We present a summary of the main findings obtained by our group regarding using these new technologies in the ocular tissue reinforcements along with other modern modalities in the treatment of keratoconus.

SURGICAL CORRECTION OF KERATOCONUS

Background: The surgical correction of keratoconus has attracted considerable attention and has led to the development of various surgical procedures. While this article primarily focuses on presenting new technologies in the reinforcement of ocular tissues as a treatment for keratoconus, the main objective of keratoconus treatment has recently evolved. The emphasis has shifted from solely improving visual acuity with keratoplasty to incorporating several novel procedures aimed at preventing disease progression. Additionally, these procedures seek to support or restore contact lens tolerance, ensuring comfortable wear for patients

FEMTOSECOND-ASSISTED INTRASTROMAL CORNEAL GRAFT (FAISCG)

Background: Keratoconus as a multifactorial disease has no known etiology. Nonetheless, biomechanical instability has been among the main causes.[11] Considering disease severity, there are several modalities for the treatment of keratoconus. Adding volume to the peripheral cornea through the implantation of ring segments can decrease central corneal steepening in keratoconus.[12,13] Nonetheless, there are some complications.[14] Also, the highly irregular cornea shape in cases with advanced keratoconus is a challenge. Thus, corneal grafts can be considered for treatment of the disease at a more advanced stage.[15]

Surgical Technique

Epithelium of donor eyes from the whole globe were removed with a blade number 15. Subsequently, a desirable corneal lenticule with precise diameter, depth, and shape was created using a Ziemer LDV femtosecond laser. To create the donor grafts, corneoscleral donor tissue was removed from storage solution and mounted on an artificial anterior chamber. The proper depth of the cornea was defined by subtracting the normal corneal depth measure from the thinnest part of the recipient cornea. The shape of the lenticule was determined on the basis of keratoconus types; in central keratoconus, a circular shape was chosen; in inferior keratoconus, a crescent shape was chosen; and in asymmetric bow-tie keratoconus, mesopic pupil size and round shape were selected. When the intrastromal pocket is created by a small incision while opening the pocket easily via a dissecting spatula, implantation of the intrastromal corneal graft into the

DOI: 10.1201/9781003371601-29

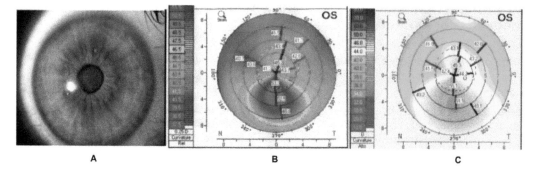

A   B   C

Figure 29.1 Slit-lamp photograph taken seven days after graft implantation (A), pre-operative (B), and 12-month post-operative topographies (C) after graft implantation showing a kind of "regularization" of the corneal surface post-operatively in the study case.

corneal pocket was done quickly and was easily achievable. A Sinskey hook can be used for the implantation as well as for graft adjustment in the pocket

Clinical Data

There were no intra-operative or post-operative complications. Seven days after surgery, the grafts were clear and all eyes seemed quiet and white. Also, 12 months after surgery, there was an improvement in uncorrected visual acuity. An increase in corneal thickness was detected using optical slit scanning topography in addition to no graft folds or interface complications after surgery (Figure 29.1). The corneal surface geometry showed an improvement into a generally regular shape. However, no significant biomechanical improvement and topography change was detected

This approach can be done easily and is safe and effective, especially for the treatment of irregularly shaped corneas, as in keratoconus. Nonetheless, corneal lenticule insertion alone in treating keratoconus, despite having no graft folds or interface complications during a five-year follow-up, was not effective, which may point to a lack of limbal support and visible change in the biomechanics of the cornea.

FEMTOSECOND-ASSISTED INNOVATIVE INTRACORNEAL RING-SUPPORTED GRAFT: RinGraft surgery

Background: Therapeutic options for corneal ectasia are evolving, with an emphasisis on the intrastromal corneal ring (ICR) for delaying or eliminating the need for penetrating keratoplasty. Moreover, ICR can be used only for mild to moderate keratoconus, and is not a solution for all keratoconus cases, and therefore, development of new devices and methods can provide further help for treating keratoconus on a wider scale. In parallel to that, we designed a coupling method to achieve more posterior cornea stress comfort for the ectatic disorder. The suture-coupled ICR and graft generated a 360° ring complex (Figure 29.2A), which, in the present study, was placed into the mid-stromal part of the cornea.

Surgical Procedure

The surgical procedure, with slight changes, have the following steps which has been described in detail previously.[16] In brief, a corneal lenticule was created as a graft from a donor eye with the exact diameter and thickness as required by VICTUS Femtosecond Laser (Bausch + Lomb). Then, our innovative ring, RinGraft,[9] with a base angle of 20–25 degrees, to prevent corneal melting at the cornea ring interface (Figure 29.2A), was sutured to the natural corneal graft lenticule. Afterward, a corneal pocket was created in the recipient's eye using a femtosecond laser. Subsequently, the RinGraft was inserted into the mid-stromal part of the cornea in the corneal pocket. Next, the pocket was irrigated with BSS. Then, the cornea was covered with the silicone-hydrogel bandage contact lens (Alcon Laboratories, Fort Worth, TX, USA), which was removed three days post-operatively. Treatment following surgery included betamethasone drops and ciprofloxacin antibiotic 0.3% drops (Sina Darou Laboratories, Tehran, Iran) four times each day, and preservative-free artificial tears (Artelac Rebalance; Bausch & Lomb, Inc, Bridgewater, NJ, USA) six times per day. One week after the operation, the Ciprofloxacin drops were stopped, whereas the betamethasone dose was tapered off over four to six months.

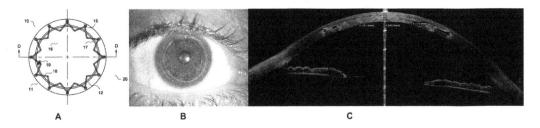

Figure 29.2 Top view of a donor corneal graft sutured peripherally to the inner opening of the RinGraft (A), slit-lamp photograph five days after corneal RinGraft insertion (B), AS-OCT images from the CASIA SS-1000 of study, six months after RinGraft insertion (C).

Clinical Data

Six months after implantation of the RinGraft, the ring, centered at the corneal reflex, and the eye were white and quiet, and the graft was clear. The implant appeared similar to a normal cornea and no graft folds or interface-related problems were found (Figure 29.2B). Moreover, corneal keratometry of the eye after the procedure demonstrated a significant decrease in the mean topographic K values ($P = 0.025$).

Likewise, using optical slit-scanning topography, enhanced corneal thickness was found (Figure 29.2C). Also, after providing the intervention, some sort of "regularization" of the corneal surface was observed. Intraocular pressure (IOP) changes were significantly more after than before the operation, according to the Corvis measurement. Also, 6 months after RinGraft implantation, Corvis-ST measurement revealed diminished CST parameters except for the highest radius of curvature. Additionally, corneal stiffness increased significantly postoperatively ($P = 0.004$). Anterior and posterior corneal aberrometry data collected over a 5-mm diameter revealed a significant decrease in frequency of higher-order aberrations, spherical aberration, primary coma, and trefoil 6 months after surgery ($P = 0.019$). The patients were very satisfied and didn't mention any problem (either during the day or night), most probably related to a decrease in abrasion. The confocal scan of the cornea demonstrated hyperreflective debris more prominent at the level of the posterior interface between the donor lenticule and the recipient stroma. Since our patients were pleased with the quality of their vision, no more augmentation was performed.

COMBINED PROCEDURE OF INTRASTROMAL CORNEAL RINGRAFT INSERTION AND TRANSEPITHELIAL PHOTOREFRACTIVE KERATECTOMY

Background: Refractive surgery in an ectatic cornea is associated with a cost of further worsening biomechanical instability. Therefore, strategies using a combination of the Intrastromal Corneal RinGraft insertion and transepithelial photorefractive keratectomy, the RinGraft/tPRK method, have been designed.

Clinical Data

Favorable findings were found regarding safety and efficacy in the correction of refractive errors along with significant improvements in UDVA, CDVA and effective significant reductions in K_{max} compared with RinGraft alone (unpublished results).

FEMTOSECOND-ASSISTED INTRASTROMAL CORNEAL LINKCOR (FAISCL) SURGERY

Background: Visual impairment caused by corneal stromal disease influences millions all over the world. In advanced stages, transplantation is needed to prevent blindness, although graft rejection, complications after surgery because of wound healing and sutures, corneal neovascularization and/or infection, a need for long-term patient follow-up and immunosuppression, and high astigmatism following the removal of sutures are part of the associated limitations.[17] Therefore, less invasive and newer approaches have been introduced.[18,19] In a pilot feasibility investigation in Iran, a cell-free, sterilized bioengineered corneal substitute made from medical-grade collagen in two advanced keratoconus cases was implanted to reshape the native corneal stroma without removal of existing tissue or sutures.

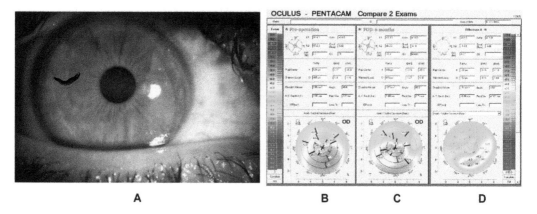

Figure 29.3 Slit-lamp photograph seven days after Bioenginered LinkCor insertion (A), pre-operative (B), one month post-operative (C), and three month post-operative (D) topographies after Bioengeenered LinkCor insertion.

Surgical Technique

The surgical procedure has been described in detail previously.[10] The implant was cut into a crescent shape and inserted into a pocket created in the cornea.

Clinical Data

The intra-stromal graft was safe. However, no significant biomechanical improvement and no significant topographic change was observed (Figure 29.3).

IMPLANTATION OF CELL-FREE ENGINEERED CORNEAL TISSUE, BIOENGINEERED PORCINE CONSTRUCT, DOUBLE CROSS-LINKED (BPCDX)

Background: To overcome the limitations of recombinant human collagen, type I medical-grade porcine dermal collagen was used.

Surgical Procedure

A femtosecond laser was used to create a mid-stromal pocket (9 mm). The pocket dissection was performed by the spatula for the SMILE procedure. The McPherson forceps were used to insert the Gebauer™ Corneal Lenticule into the pocket, and the lenticule was then centered using the spatula.[20]

Clinical Outcomes

There were no adverse events or intra- or post-operative complications within a 24-month follow-up period. Stable and significant corneal thickening and flattening of keratometry, maintenance of corneal transparency, and improved best-corrected visual acuity (BCVA), using 7.6 logMAR lines to a mean of 20/58 in Iran and using 15.1 logMAR lines to a mean of 20/26 in India, were obtained. Slit-lamp photographs showed improved transparency, and the cases were assessed using *in-vivo* confocal microscopy and showed intact sub-basal nerves as well as sufficient endothelial cell density.

BOWMAN'S LAYER TRANSPLANTATION

Background: Keratoconus is associated with Bowman's membrane fragmentation. Bowman's membrane plays a key role in providing biomechanical support to preserve corneal shape, so it is suggested that replacement of this tissue can stop further deterioration and preserve vision.

Clinical Outcomes

Studies have shown that Bowman's layer transplantation provides flattening of approximately 8 D on average within the first post-operative month and stabilizations of five to seven years post-operative.[21] BSCVA seems to remain stable after an initial improvement from pre-operative to 12-months post-operatively, while BCLVA remains unchanged up to five to seven years post-operatively. HOAs, such as spherical aberration, decreased for both anterior and posterior corneal surfaces, whereas corneal backscattering increased. Endothelial cell density also remained unchanged up to five to seven years post-operatively and no allograft rejection episodes have been reported to date. Moreover, Kaplan–Meier analysis showed an estimated success rate of 84% at five years post-operative.

INTRASTROMAL IMPLANTATION OF AUTOLOGOUS ADIPOSE-DERIVED ADULT STEM CELLS (ADASCS) ALONE
Methodology

Standard liposuction under local anesthesia was performed and ~250 mL of adipose tissue was obtained from each patient. Processing of adipose tissue was performed and 3×10^6 cells per patient were prepared in phosphate-buffered saline (PBS), and the cells were transplanted directly into the stroma pocket using a 25-G cannula. No corneal sutures were used.[22]

Clinical Outcomes

No complications were observed during the 3-year follow-up. New collagen production was observed as patchy hyperreflective areas at the level of the stromal pocket. All cases presented an improvement in UDVA and in their CDVA. Results of anterior mean-K evaluation presented a modest improvement of mean values of 1 D to 12-months post-operative and another 1 D at 36 months post-operative compared with the pre-operative mean-K values.

RECOMBINANT CROSS-LINKED COLLAGEN FOR CORNEAL ENHANCEMENT
Implant Characteristics and Surgical Technique

After anterior lamellar keratoplasty (ALK) under general or local anesthesia, the recombinant human cross-linked collagen III, fabricated into substitutes with the dimensions of a human cornea, was transplanted into the anterior stroma. Patients received these biomimetic substitutes anchored with three to four overlying 10–0 Nylon sutures and covered with a bandage lens. Bandage lenses and sutures were removed five weeks after surgery.[23]

Results

At 24 months follow-up, they showed stable biointegration and corneal re-epithelialization, but localized implant thinning in thickness and fibrosis was observed in several patients. Vision improved in six out of ten patients. Four years after the grafting, patient CDVA was 20/54 on average.At four years, the biosynthetic corneas showed steeper surface curvatures and were more irregular than donor corneas, showing increased astigmatism.

LENTICULAR IMPLANTATION COMBINED WITH COLLAGEN CROSS-LINKING
Methodology

Only lenticules with spherical myopic refractive errors were chosen for cryopreservation. The tissue was soaked in 0.25% riboflavin and kept aside and a 3-mm corneal trephine was used to punch the center of the lenticule to obtain a donut-shaped tissue. After that, topical anesthesia was applied. A pocket was created. with a VISUMAX femtosecond laser, with 7.0–8.0 mm diameter at 100 μm depth, then the donut-shaped lenticule was inserted gently into the pocket through the 4 mm superior incision, and, finally, the eye was exposed to ultraviolet radiation (UV-A) using the Avedro Cross-linking (CXL) system.

Clinical Outcomes

The authors did not observe any adverse reaction during the three-year post-operative follow-up. Clinical improvement was observed in all patients: no loss of eye lines of CDVA, and amelioration was detected in UDVA, CDVA, and manifest spherical equivalent. There was flattening of K_{max} in the 3- and 5-mm zones. Also, the mean pachymetry in the central and mid-peripheral zones increased. All patients showed improvements in high-order aberrations, especially in coma.

CORNEAL ALLOGENIC INTRASTROMAL RING SEGMENTS (CAIRS)
Surgical Procedure

The femtosecond laser platform is used to create a circular mid-stromal dissection with an inner diameter of 6.5 mm and an outer diameter of 8 mm. Two entry incisions are made into the channel opposite to one another on the topographic steep axis. Both incisions are then opened using a symmetric glide. An 8-0 Nylon suture threaded through the positioning hole of an Intacs is passed through one end of a CAIRS and tied down. The Intacs is passed through the channel on one side and used to pull the CAIRS after it into the channel. The Intacs is brought out through the opposite incision, using a reverse Sinskey hook. Once the CAIRS is positioned within the channel, the Nylon loop is cut and removed, detaching the Intacs from the CAIRS. The same procedure is repeated on the other side with the second CAIRS.

Outcomes

Significant improvements in UDVA, CDVA, SE, topographic astigmatism, maximum keratometry, steepest keratometry, anterior and posterior BFS, and mean power were reported. No cases of melt or corneal necrosis were encountered. AS-OCT also showed well-placed segments at mid-stromal depth without signs of incompatibility, such as necrosis, edema, or inflammation of the segment or the surrounding host stroma.

INTRACORNEAL CONCAVE LENTICULE IMPLANTATION SFII
Methodology

The donor cornea was placed into an artificial anterior chamber, and a lamellar incision was made with a femtosecond laser. An anterior incision was made with a diameter of 7.5 mm and was located at a depth of 320 μm, then a myopia correction of −4.00 D was executed (69.59 μm thickness) with an excimer laser. The lenticule was then separated from the stromal bed and used as a graft. Then, SMILE treatment with a myopic correction of −0.75 D (28 μm thickness) was effected in the recipient cornea with 160 μm cap thickness, 7.8 mm cap diameter, and 7.8 mm lamellar cornea diameter. Finally, the graft was implanted into the stromal pocket.[24]

Conclusion

At three months post-operative in the SFII group, all patients showed improved UDVA and CDVA, then they remained stable to 24 months. Minimum and maximum central keratometry improved, but less than with PKP results. An increased in the corneal thickness was better in the SFII group than in the PKP group at three months after the surgery. Confocal microscopy study revealed the presence of dendritic cells in the subepithelial region, and dendritic and inflammatory cells could be observed among the graft and the host cornea up to one month with the group SFII and up to three months with the PKP group.

CORNEAL STROMAL CELL THERAPY

Background: Corneal stromal cell therapy for treatment of keratoconus was proposed in some studies. For this purpose, different cell sources, including bone marrow mesenchymal stem cells, corneal stromal stem cells, umbilical cord mesenchymal stem cells, adipose-derived adult mesenchymal stem cells, embryonic stem cells, induced pluripotent stem cells (iPSCs), were used in *in-vitro* or animal studies.[25]

Results

In our previous study, Wharton's jelly-derived mesenchymal stem cells (MSCs) were seeded into the human corneal lenticule and implanted in the rabbit's corneal stroma. Three months follow-up showed that this recellularized implant was stable and did not induce severe complications in the rabbit's cornea. Real time quantitative-PCR showed that keratocyte-specific gene expression, including keratocan, lumican, CD34, and ALDH3A1, was increased in the cell-injected group rather than the decellularized one. These results indicated that MSC can be differentiated into keratocytes in the cornea.[26]

In-vitro differentiation of MSCs into keratocytes can be an interesting method for keratocyte providing. In a recent study, we used conditional medium from keratocytes for differentiation of adipose-derived adult mesenchymal stem cells into corneal keratocytes. Keratocytes were isolated and cultured in an optimized medium and its conditional medium was prepared. This medium was added to the MSC culture to induce differentiation. Immunohistochemical analysis showed that treated stem cells expressed lumican and keratocan and so differentiated into keratocytes (Figure 29.4). After further evaluations in animal and clinical studies, these cells could be proposed for treatment of keratoconus.

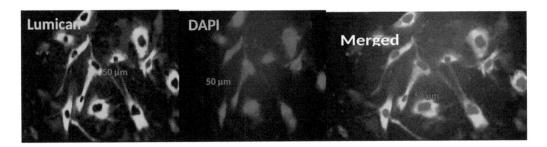

Figure 29.4 Immunocytochemistry of MSC differentiated to keratocytes by conditional medium. The cells were stained with anti-lumican antibody. The green signals indicate the presence of lumican.

NON-SURGICAL CORRECTION OF KERATOCONUS
Gene Therapy

Background: The pathogenesis of keratoconus remains a mystery. Keratoconus is a complex disorder involving an interaction of environmental and genetic factors. Detecting a gene responsible for keratoconus is important and it can help surgeons because keratoconus is a contraindication for corneal refractive surgery, although the identification of a gene would help to elucidate the disease pathogenesis

Conclusion

International assessments should indicate crucial affected pathways, although more effort is needed to understand the disease development. Genetic susceptibility is very important in the occurrence of keratoconus, but, in spite of many studies, no contributing gene has been identified.

Summary

Several modalities were made in the treatment of keratoconus in the past two decades and it is very likely that, in the future, corneal ectasia can be stopped at an early stage and perhaps the need for keratoplasty avoided altogether. However, due to the rising trend of the incidence of keratoconus, especially among Asian people, and the mystery of the pathogenesis of keratoconus in highly irregular corneas, there are still challenges and currently there is no definitive treatment modality. The studies described in this chapter include most of the treatments for this disease, in addition to the introduction of some of the research conducted in our center that will be needed in the future. So, further randomized, prospective, and long-term follow-up studies should provide pivotal evidence regarding the efficacy and safety of the various procedures and their role in managing the progression of keratoconus or the possibility of delaying or even replacing keratoplasty in keratoconus patients.

REFERENCES

1. Rabinowitz YS. Keratoconus. *Surv Ophthalmol.* 1998;42:297–319. [PubMed] [Google Scholar]

2. Pearson AR, Soneji B, Sarvananthan N, Sandford-Smith JH. Does ethnic origin influence the incidence or severity of keratoconus? *Eye.* 2000;14:625–628.

3. Burris TE. Intrastomal corneal ring technology: results and indications. *Curr Opinion Ophthalmol.* 1998;9(4):9–14.

4. Jadidi K, Mosavi SA, Nejat F, Naderi M, Janani L, Serahati S. Intrastromal corneal ring segment implantation (keraring 355) in patients with central keratoconus: 6-month follow-up. *J Ophthalmol.* 2015;2015(1):916385.

5. Naderi M, Karimi F, Jadidi K, Mosavi SA, Ghobadi M, Tireh H, Khorrami-Nejad M. Long-term results of MyoRing implantation in patients with keratoconus. *Clin Exp Optom.* 2021;104(4):499–504.

6. Jadidi K, Mosavi SA, Nejat F, Alishiri A, Aghamolaei H, et al. Aberrometric outcomes of intrastromal corneal ring segment (KeraRing 355) implantation using pocket-maker microkeratome in patients with keratoconus. *J Clin Exp Ophthalmol*. 2017;8:640. doi:10.4172/2155-9570.1000640

7. Jadidi K, Nejat F, Mosavi SA, Naderi M, Katiraee A, Janani L, Aghamollaei H. Full-ring intrastromal corneal implantation for correcting high myopia in patients with severe keratoconus. *Medical Hypothesis, Discovery and Innovation in Ophthalmology*. 2016;5(3):89.

8. Jadidi K, Mosavi SA, Nejat F, Alishiri A. Complications of intrastromal corneal ring implantation (keraring 355) using a femtosecond laser for channel creation. *Inter J Kerato Ect Cor Dis*. 2011;3(2):53.

9. Nejat F, Naderi M, Janani L, Aghamollaei H, Mosavi SA, Jadidi K. Clinical outcomes after continuous intracorneal ring implantation in post-lasik ectasia: long-term follow-up. *J Ophth Opto Sci*. 2017;1(3).

10. Jadidi K, Mosavi SA. Keratoconus treatment using femtosecond-assisted intrastromal corneal graft (FAISCG) surgery: a case series. *Inter Med Case Rep J*, 2018;11:9.

11. Daxer A, Fratzl P. Collagen fibril orientation in the human corneal stroma and its implication in keratoconus. *Invest Ophthalmol Vis Sci*. 1997;38:121–129.

12. Ertan A, Colin J. Intracorneal rings for keratoconus and keratectasia. *J Cataract Refract Surg*. 2007;33:1303–1314.

13. Miranda D, Sartori M, Francesconi C, Allemann N, Ferrara P, Campos M. Ferrara intrastromal corneal ring segments for severe keratoconus. *J Refract Surg*. 2003;19:645–653.

14. Jadidi K, Mosavi SA, Nejat F, Alishiri A. Complications of intrastromal corneal ring implantation (Keraring 355) using a femtosecond laser for channel creation. *Int J Kerat Ectatic Corneal Dis*. 2014;3(2):53.

15. Funnell CL, Ball J, Noble BA. Comparative cohort study of the outcomes of deep lamellar keratoplasty and penetrating keratoplasty for keratoconus. *Eye (Lond)*. 2006;20:527–532.

16. Jadidi K, Mosavi SA, Nejat F, Aghamolaei H, Pirhadi S. Innovative intracorneal ring supported graft surgery for treatment of keratoconus and cornea regeneration: surgical technique and case report. *Indian J Ophthalmol*. 2022;70:3412–3415.

17. Parker JS, van Dijk K, Melles GR. Treatment options for advanced keratoconus: a review. *Surv Ophthalmol*. 2015;60:459–480.

18. Mastropasqua L, Nubile M, Salgari N, Mastropasqua R. Femtosecond laser-assisted stromal lenticule addition keratoplasty for the treatment of advanced keratoconus: a preliminary study. *J Refract Surg*. 2018;34:36–44.

19. van Dijk K, et al. Bowman layer transplantation to reduce and stabilize progressive, advanced keratoconus. *Ophthalmol*. 2015;122:909–917.

20. Koulikovska M, et al. Enhanced regeneration of corneal tissue via a bioengineered collagen construct implanted by a nondisruptive surgical technique. *Tissue Eng. Part A*. 2015;21:1116–1130.

21. van Dijk K, Parker JS, Baydoun L, et al. Bowman layer transplantation: 5-year results. *Graefes Arch Clin Exp Ophthalmol*. 2018;256:1151–1158.

22. El Zarif M, Alió JL, Alió Del Barrio JL, Jawad KA, Palazón-Bru A, Jawad ZA, De Miguel MP, Makdissy N. Corneal stromal regeneration therapy for advanced keratoconus: long-term outcomes at 3 years. *Cornea*. 2021;40(6):741–754.

23. Koh, LB, Islam MM, Mitra D, Noel CW, Merrett K, Odorcic S, Fagerholm P, et al. Epoxy cross-linked collagen and collagen-laminin peptide hydrogels as corneal substitutes. *J Funct Bio*. 2013;4(3):162–177.

24. Wei, Q, Ding H, Nie K, Jin H, Zhong T, Yu H, Yang Z, Hu S, He L, Zhong X. Long-term clinical outcomes of small-incision femtosecond laser-assisted intracorneal concave lenticule implantation in patients with keratoconus. *J Ophthalmol*. 2022;2022.

25. Ghiasi, M, Jadidi K, Hashemi M, Zare H, Salimi A, Aghamollaei H. Application of mesenchymal stem cells in corneal regeneration. *Tissue Cell*. 2021;73:101600.

26. Aghamollaei H, Hashemian H, Safabakhsh H, Halabian R, Baghersad M, Jadidi, K, Safety of grafting acellular human corneal lenticule seeded with Wharton's Jelly-Derived Mesenchymal Stem Cells in an experimental animal model. *Exp Eye Res*. 2021;205:108451.

30 New Horizons for Regenerative Medicine and Gene Therapy for Keratoconus

Sara Taghizadeh and Seyed Farzad Mohammadi

INTRODUCTION

Keratoconus is a progressive eye disease in which the cornea, the clear front surface of the eye, thins and bulges out in the shape of a cone. This can result in blurred vision, distortion, and light sensitivity.[1]

Although the precise causes of keratoconus are unknown, a number of factors are believed to cause its development, either alone or in combination. Genetic factors, hormonal imbalances, environmental factors such as excessive sun exposure or living in an area with high levels of air pollution, and having other conditions such as Down syndrome, weak collagen, or other connective tissue disorders such as Ehlers–Danlos syndrome, are all possible causes of keratoconus. Although understanding the cause of the disease is complicated, learning it can aid disease management and treatment.[2]

There are several types of therapy that can be used for keratoconus treatments, including surgical and non-surgical therapies. Keratoconus is treated using both traditional and novel surgical techniques. Non-surgical methods include both traditional and comparatively new methods. Glasses and contact lenses are traditional methods, and novel methods include bioengineered corneal implants, regenerative methods or tissue engineering, and cell-based and gene therapies.[3–8]

The severity of the disease, the patient's age and overall health, and the particular symptoms and complications associated with the disease are all factors that determine the choice of therapy. Traditional and novel surgical therapies are discussed in other chapters and in this chapter we are going to learn more about emerging treatment methods for keratoconus.

NON-SURGICAL THERAPIES FOR KERATOCONUS

These are non-surgical treatments that can be used to manage symptoms of the disease or improve vision. Glasses and contact lenses are the most prevalent non-surgical treatments for keratoconus. Keratoconus symptoms can be effectively managed with glasses and contact lenses, particularly in the early stages of the disease. However, as the condition grows more severe, these treatments can cease to be effective, and surgical treatments might be required to manage the disease and restore vision.[6]

BIOENGINEERED CORNEAL IMPLANTS FOR KERATOCONUS

Advanced keratoconus patients could benefit from bioengineered corneal implants, which substitute the damaged cornea with artificial or bioengineered tissue. Compared with conventional corneal transplantation, which has a high risk of rejection and other complications, these implants are intended to provide a more durable and long-lasting option.[7] There are several types of bioengineered corneal implants that are being investigated for the treatment of keratoconus, namely synthetic corneas, decellularized corneal scaffolds, and bioengineered corneal tissue.

1. **Synthetic corneas**. Synthetic corneas, also known as keratoprostheses, are artificial structures that are implanted to replace damaged corneas when traditional corneal transplantation is either not possible or has failed. The process of using synthetic corneas for keratoconus treatment involves surgically implanting the device into the eye, either in front of or behind the damaged cornea. The artificial cornea then replaces the damaged tissue, restoring vision and decreasing the chance of further damage.

   Synthetic corneas are produced from a variety of materials, including polymers, collagen, and silicone.

   The use of synthetic corneas for keratoconus treatment is still in its early stages, with limited clinical data on their efficacy. However, some studies have shown promising results, especially when biocompatible synthetic corneas, made of materials such as silk fibroin, were used.

   For years, synthetic corneas have been studied as a possible treatment option for a variety of corneal diseases, including keratoconus.[9]

2. **Decellularized corneal scaffolds** can be used to treat keratoconus by supplying a natural template for corneal tissue regeneration. The procedure is as follows. To start, corneal tissue is

DOI: 10.1201/9781003371601-30

acquired from a donor and processed to remove all cellular components, leaving a "decellularized" scaffold behind. Second, patient-derived corneal cells, such as epithelial or stromal cells, are inserted onto the scaffold. The seeded scaffold is then incubated in a bioreactor to enable the corneal tissue to grow and develop. Finally, once the tissue has matured and grown to an appropriate size, it can be transplanted into the patient's eye to replace damaged or diseased corneal tissue.[10–12]

There are no clinical trials or reports of successful therapy in humans at this time, and research on the use of decellularized corneal scaffolds for the treatment of keratoconus is still in the preclinical stage. Several studies, however, have shown that decellularized corneal scaffolds can promote corneal regeneration and healing in animal models. These findings indicate that decellularized corneal scaffolds may be used as an alternative to traditional corneal transplant techniques, but additional research is required to determine their safety and efficacy in human patients.

3. **Bioengineered corneal tissue** can be used to treat keratoconus by creating a scaffold that mimics the corneal structure and seeding it with corneal cells or stem cells using various techniques. To replace the damaged corneal tissue, the bioengineered corneal tissue can be transplanted into the patient's eye.

   Because this method is mainly constructed from tissues and cells, we can regard this group as being separate from tissue and cell engineering and regenerative methods. A collagen-based scaffold, that is shaped to fit the patient's eye, is one method for creating bioengineered corneal tissue. Corneal or stem cells are then seeded onto the scaffold and permitted to develop and differentiate into the desired cell types. Once produced, the bioengineered tissue can be transplanted into the patient's eye.[12,13]

   Another approach is to use 3-D bioprinting technology to create a bioengineered cornea that closely matches the shape and structure of the patient's cornea. Before transplantation, the 3-D-printed scaffold is seeded with corneal or stem cells and allowed to mature.[14–16] Studies concentrate on different methods of producing bioengineered corneal tissue, such as the use of decellularized corneal scaffolds, induced pluripotent stem cells, and injectable collagen-genipin gel. These techniques have the ability to be used in the treatment of keratoconus.

REGENERATIVE METHODS OR TISSUE ENGINEERING AND CELL-BASED THERAPIES

Tissue engineering is a field in which cells, biomaterials, and growth factors are used to make functional tissues or organs. Tissue engineering in keratoconus treatment aims to produce functional corneal tissue that can replace the damaged cornea in patients with advanced keratoconus.[12]

Tissue engineering methods for keratoconus treatment include cell therapy, collagen-based scaffolds, and 3-D bioprinting. Despite the fact that tissue engineering for keratoconus treatment is still in the early stages of development, it offers several advantages over traditional corneal transplantation, including the ability to create personalized tissue that is customized to the patient's specific needs, a reduced risk of rejection, and improved long-term results.

Cell-Based Therapies for Keratoconus

Keratoconus cell-based therapies use stem cells or other types of cells to regenerate and repair damaged corneal tissue. The goal of these procedures is to restore the normal structure and function of the cornea to improve vision in keratoconus patients.

Limbal stem cell transplantation, cultivated epithelial stem cell transplantation, amniotic membrane transplantation, and corneal endothelial cell transplantation are some of the cell-based therapies being investigated for the treatment of keratoconus.[17–19]

While cell-based therapies for keratoconus are still in the early stages of development, they show promise for potential treatments for the condition. These therapies have the potential to regenerate and repair damaged corneal tissue over time, potentially improving vision and reducing the need for other interventions, such as corneal transplantation.

Stem Cell Therapy for Keratoconus Treatment

Stem cell therapy has been investigated as a potential treatment for keratoconus. The general concept behind keratoconus stem cell therapy is to use stem cells to regenerate and repair damaged corneal tissue. The following are the basic steps involved in using stem cell therapy to treat keratoconus:

1. Stem cell harvesting: Stem cells are usually harvested from the patient's own body, most commonly from bone marrow or adipose tissue. Stem cells can be obtained from a donor in some situations.

2. Culturing and expanding stem cells: To increase their numbers, harvested stem cells are cultured and expanded in the laboratory.

3. Implantation: The expanded stem cells are then surgically inserted into the patient's eye. The stem cells should differentiate into corneal cells to promote corneal regeneration in damaged or diseased corneas.

Stem cell treatment for keratoconus is available in several forms, including the use of mesenchymal stem cells or induced pluripotent stem cells. Several trials have been conducted to investigate the potential of stem cell therapy for the treatment of keratoconus.[17,20–27]

1. **Limbal Stem Cell Transplantation for Keratoconus Treatment**

   Limbal stem cell transplantation (LSCT) is a surgical technique used to treat corneal damage or disease caused by damage to the limbal stem cells, which are responsible for regenerating and maintaining the cornea. Keratoconus causes the cornea to become thin or misshapen, and LSCT can be used to restore the cornea's regular structure and function.

   The process requires transplanting of a small piece of healthy limbal tissue from the patient or a donor onto the damaged region of the cornea. The transplanted cells then migrate and expand throughout the cornea, restoring the cornea's typical structure and function.

   LSCT has been shown to be successful in the treatment of corneal damage caused by a wide range of conditions, including keratoconus. In fact, LSCT is frequently used as a first-line therapy for severe keratoconus cases that are not responding to other treatments, such as contact lenses or corneal collagen cross-linking.

   The findings support the efficacy of LSCT as a treatment option for keratoconus and other corneal diseases.

   However, it is important to remember that LSCT is a complex procedure, and not all patients may be suitable candidates. Before having any surgical procedure, it is also critical to carefully consider the potential risks and benefits.

2. **Cultivated Epithelial Stem Cell Transplantation for Keratoconus Treatment**

   Cultivated epithelial stem cell transplantation (CEST) is a form of stem cell therapy in which epithelial stem cells are grown and transplanted onto the cornea to repair damage and improve vision in keratoconus patients.

   A small sample of the patient's own epithelial stem cells is taken and cultured in a laboratory to create a sheet of healthy corneal epithelium. After that, the sheet is transplanted into the patient's cornea to replace the damaged epithelial layer.

   CEST has been shown to be a successful treatment for keratoconus patients with severe corneal damage and vision loss.

   While there have been some successful cases of CEST transplantation for keratoconus treatment, additional research is required to determine the optimal conditions and techniques for CEST transplantation, as well as the procedure's long-term safety and efficacy. Also, before undergoing treatment, it is critical to thoroughly consider the possible benefits and risks of any surgical procedure.

Amniotic Membrane Transplantation for Keratoconus Treatment

Amniotic membrane transplantation (AMT) is a surgical procedure in which amniotic membrane tissue is transplanted into the cornea to promote healing and decrease inflammation. In the context of keratoconus treatment, AMT can be used to address corneal scarring, thinning, and other disease-related complications.

A thin layer of amniotic membrane tissue is harvested from a placenta and processed for transplantation during the operation. The membrane is subsequently placed onto the cornea, where it can help in epithelial cell development, inflammation reduction, and general corneal healing. The amniotic membrane can additionally act as a scaffold for the growth of new corneal tissue in some instances.[28–30]

Corneal Endothelial Cell Transplantation for Keratoconus Treatment

Corneal endothelial cell transplantation is a surgical procedure that includes the transplantation of healthy endothelial cells into a damaged cornea in order to restore its function and transparency. This procedure is most commonly used to treat Fuchs' endothelial dystrophy, but it may also be used in some instances of keratoconus.

A thin layer of the damaged cornea is removed and replaced with donor tissue having healthy endothelial cells. Typically, donor tissue is acquired from a deceased donor and processed to ensure that it is safe for transplantation.

Descemet's stripping endothelial keratoplasty (DSEK) and Descemet's membrane endothelial keratoplasty (DMEK) are two methods for transplanting corneal endothelial cells. The type and amount of tissue transplanted differs between these techniques.[31–34]

Bowman's Layer Transplantation

This is a surgical procedure for treating keratoconus. The Bowman's layer is a translucent layer that exists between the epithelium and the stroma. Bowman's layer transplantation involves the transplantation of a small section of the Bowman's layer from a healthy donor cornea into the patient's cornea in the area where it has been weakened or thinned due to keratoconus. The procedure's aim is to strengthen and shape the cornea, allowing for clearer vision. The Bowman's layer transplanted can also promote the growth of new, healthy tissue in the cornea. Bowman's layer transplantation is a new method that is still being researched to determine its long-term efficacy. Early findings, however, have been encouraging, with many patients reporting improved vision and corneal stability. It is usually reserved for advanced keratoconus patients who have not responded to other treatments, such as contact lenses or corneal cross-linking.[35,36]

Collagen-Based Scaffolds for Keratoconus Treatment

Collagen-based scaffolds have been studied as a possible keratoconus treatment. The basic concept behind this method is to use a collagen scaffold to promote the regeneration of damaged or diseased corneal tissue. The following are the general stages involved in treating keratoconus with collagen-based scaffolds:

1. Scaffold preparation: In the laboratory, a collagen-based scaffold is prepared using methods such as freeze-drying or electrospinning. The scaffold is made to be the correct shape and size for the patient's eye.

2. Implantation: The scaffold is then surgically placed into the patient's eye. The scaffold is anticipated to provide a framework for corneal tissue regeneration while also promoting cell adhesion, proliferation, and differentiation.

3. Integration: Over time, the patient's own cells will migrate into the scaffold and repopulate it with corneal tissue, resulting in corneal regeneration.[37–39]

While these studies indicate that collagen-based scaffolds may be a promising treatment for keratoconus, additional research is required to thoroughly evaluate this approach and determine the best protocol for collagen-based scaffold therapy in this context. Furthermore, approval by regulators for collagen-based scaffolds can be complicated, and, in some cases, there may be concerns about the safety and efficacy of these products.

3-D Bioprinting for Keratoconus Treatment

Three-dimensional (3-D) bioprinting could be used to treat Keratoconus by creating corneal tissue constructs that can replace damaged or diseased corneal tissue. The following are the general stages in using 3-D bioprinting for Keratoconus treatment:

1. Tissue engineering: First, researchers create a "bioink" through the combination of living cells, biomaterials, and growth factors. The bioink acts as the foundation for the 3-D printing process.

2. Imaging: To identify the size and shape of the damaged or diseased cornea, the patient's eye is imaged using technologies such as optical coherence tomography (OCT) and topography.

3. 3-D printing: The bioink is deposited layer by layer using a 3-D printer to make a customized corneal tissue construct that fits the size and shape of the patient's cornea.

4. Implantation: The corneal tissue construct is then implanted surgically into the patient's eye. The implanted construct is anticipated to integrate with surrounding tissue and promote corneal regeneration in damaged or diseased regions.

Three-dimensional (3-D) bioprinting has emerged as a promising method for producing corneal tissue for the treatment of keratoconus. There are no FDA-approved 3-D bioprinting therapies for keratoconus at the moment. However, some promoting pre-clinical studies on the use of 3-D bioprinting for keratoconus treatment have been conducted.

While these pre-clinical studies indicate that 3-D bioprinting may be a promising treatment for keratoconus, more research is required to fully determine the safety and efficacy of this method, and obtaining regulatory approval for 3-D bioprinting can be complicated. Furthermore, there may be concerns about the long-term safety and durability of bioprinted corneal tissue, and more research is required to resolve these concerns.[16,40,41]

GENE THERAPY FOR KERATOCONUS TREATMENT

Gene therapy is an experimental treatment for keratoconus which involves delivering functional genes to the cornea to correct genetic mutations or defects that contribute to the disease's development. The aim of gene therapy is to restore the gene's normal function. The two primary approaches to gene therapy are gene replacement therapy and gene editing.[5,42-46]

1. **Gene Replacement Therapy** entails delivering a functional copy of the defective gene to the corneal cells. A viral vector, which is a modified virus that can deliver the gene to the target cells, is usually employed to deliver the functional gene. After injecting the recombinant viral vector into the cornea, the functional gene is expressed in the corneal cells, correcting the genetic defect and returning normal corneal function.

2. **Gene Editing** involves directly editing the genetic code of the corneal cells using CRISPR-Cas9 or other gene editing technologies, correcting the mutation that causes keratoconus. Compared with gene replacement therapy, gene editing is a more precise and targeted method.

Keratoconus, as the most prevalent corneal ectatic disorder, affects both sexes and all ethnic groups. It can be caused by both genetic and environmental factors. Evidence from genome-wide association studies, candidate gene analyses, family-based linkage analysis, and fine mapping in linkage regions has been used to evaluate genetic discoveries. At a relatively rapid rate, a number of genes have been identified. Our understanding of keratoconus (KC) will be significantly enhanced as a result of comprehending the molecular mechanism underlying its pathogenesis, which will also aid in the development of potential treatments.[47]

Corneal collagen cross-linking is currently the only fairly reliable treatment that slows down the progression of KC. A corneal transplant may be necessary in extreme cases. This reality alone makes gene therapy treatment for KC a promising remedial methodology. These hopes are bolstered by the straightforward surgical approach to the eye's anterior chamber, the transparent corneal tissue and its *ex-vivo* stability, and the biophysical properties of the corneal tissues, such as the corneal immune privilege status. The prospects for successfully treating KC through gene therapy are also bolstered by recent advancements in vectors and the capability to alter the corneal milieu to prolong the target gene's survival and enable its successful translation.

Throughout the course of recent decades, however, genome-wide association studies and studies on single-nucleotide polymorphisms (SNPs) and hereditary loci have distinguished more than 50 genomic loci that play a role in both the dysregulation of the corneal collagen framework development and the support or the cell separation pathways that support corneal integrity. The *VSX1* gene, which is also involved in posterior polymorphous corneal dystrophy, is one of the most prominent genes in KC; the *SOD1* gene, which controls how reactive oxygen species accumulate; the *ZNF469* gene, which is also responsible for the Brittle Cornea Syndrome; the TGF8 pathway, which regulates the composition of the extracellular matrix; the TGFI quality which plays a part in cell-collagen cooperations. It is necessary to also emphasize the roles played by mitochondrial DNA and microRNAs, particularly miRNA 184.[48,49]

Recently, 24 distinct genes or genetic loci were linked to 18 distinct KC symptoms and clinical signs. It turns out that three to fourteen known KC genes are linked to each of these symptoms. In a similar way, 49 diseases and/or syndromes involving at least some of the KC-implicated genes were identified and linked to these 24 genes. Again, it turns out that between one and 23 KC-implicated genes are linked to each of the 49 diseases and syndromes.[46]

In the past ten years, gene therapy has become one of the most researched subjects. Modern medicine has evolved into a revolutionary therapeutic tool. The process of altering the disease-causing defective gene in host cells is known as gene therapy. It conveys helpful hereditary data by means of adjusted viral or non-viral vectors. Because the eye is a suitable organ for the development of gene therapy, ocular gene therapy has made particular progress in treating inherited retinal diseases. The blood–ocular barrier and the eye's easy accessibility make it an ideal target for gene therapy. Gene therapies for other ocular diseases, such as glaucoma, Usher syndrome, neovascular age-related macular degeneration, and retinitis pigmentosa (RP), are the subject of several ongoing clinical trials. Ocular inflammation and humoral response, infection by viral vectors, and insertional mutagenesis are, however, obstacles. These restrictions are based on a number of factors; whether viral or non-viral vectors are utilized, which viral vectors are utilized, the modes of administration – subretinal, intravitreal, or suprachoroidal – as well as the dose of the vectors and the target tissue are all important considerations. Due to intraocular inflammation, these complications may result in therapeutic failure and vision loss.[50]

In response to the above potentially unfavorable effects, unfortunately, gene therapy is viewed negatively as a viable treatment option for KC due to the numerous genomic loci involved, the large number of comorbidities, and the intricate interrelationships between the various biophysical and biochemical processes involved in KC. There have been a few studies exploring the potential of gene therapy for the treatment of keratoconus. While some of these findings are encouraging, more study is required to assess the safety and efficacy of gene therapy approaches for the treatment of keratoconus in human clinical trials. Furthermore, the development of safe and efficient vectors and gene delivery methods that can precisely target the cornea will be critical to the success of gene therapies for keratoconus.

REFERENCES

1. Santodomingo-Rubido J, Carracedo G, Suzaki A, Villa-Collar C, Vincent SJ, Wolffsohn JS. Keratoconus: An updated review. *Cont Lens Anterior Eye*. 2022;45(3):101559.

2. Daniell M, Sahebjada S. *Etiology and Risk Factors of Keratoconus. Keratoconus: Diagnosis and Treatment*. Springer; 2022. p. 11–22.

3. Emilio P, Chiara C, Bonacci E, Zuliani A, Adriano F, Giorgio M. New treatments for keratoconus. *International Ophthalmology*. 2020;40(7):1619–23.

4. Andreanos KD, Hashemi K, Petrelli M, Droutsas K, Georgalas I, Kymionis GD. Keratoconus treatment algorithm. *Ophthalmology and Therapy*. 2017;6:245–62.

5. Mohammadpour M, Heidari Z, Hashemi H. Updates on managements for keratoconus. *Journal of Current Ophthalmology*. 2018;30(2):110–24.

6. Şengör T, Kurna SA. Update on contact lens treatment of keratoconus. *Turkish Journal of Ophthalmology*. 2020;50(4):234.

7. Rafat M, Jabbarvand M, Sharma N, Xeroudaki M, Tabe S, Omrani R, et al. Bioengineered corneal tissue for minimally invasive vision restoration in advanced keratoconus in two clinical cohorts. *Nature Biotechnology*. 2023;41(1):70–81.

8. Mehta JS, Kocaba V, Soh YQ. The future of keratoplasty: cell-based therapy, regenerative medicine, bioengineering keratoplasty, gene therapy. *Current Opinion in Ophthalmology*. 2019;30(4):286–91.

9. Sevgi DD, Fukuoka H, Afshari NA. 20 Years of Advances in Keratoprosthesis. *Current Ophthalmology Reports*. 2016;4:226–43.

10. Alió del Barrio JL, Alió JL. Cellular therapy of the corneal stroma: a new type of corneal surgery for keratoconus and corneal dystrophies. *Eye and Vision*. 2018;5(1):28.

11. Alió JL, Zarif M, del Barrio JLA. *Cellular Therapy of the Corneal Stroma: A New Type of Corneal Surgery for Keratoconus and Corneal Dystrophies—A Translational Research Experience*. Elsevier; 2023. p. 525–52.

12. El Zarif M, Alió JL, Alió del Barrio JL, De Miguel MP, Abdul Jawad K, Makdissy N. Corneal stromal regeneration: A review of human clinical studies in keratoconus treatment. *Frontiers in Medicine*. 2021;8:650724.

13. Long K, Liu Y, Li W, Wang L, Liu S, Wang Y, et al. Improving the mechanical properties of collagen-based membranes using silk fibroin for corneal tissue engineering. *Journal of Biomedical Materials Research Part A*. 2015;103(3):1159–68.

14. Song Y, Hua S, Sayyar S, Chen Z, Chung J, Liu X, et al. Corneal bioprinting using a high concentration pure collagen I transparent bioink. *Bioprinting*. 2022;28:e00235.

15. Ludwig PE, Huff TJ, Zuniga JM. The potential role of bioengineering and three-dimensional printing in curing global corneal blindness. *Journal of Tissue Engineering*. 2018;9:2041731418769863.

16. Zhang B, Xue Q, Li J, Ma L, Yao Y, Ye H, et al. 3D bioprinting for artificial cornea: Challenges and perspectives. *Medical Engineering & Physics*. 2019;71:68–78.

17. Del Barrio JLA, El Zarif M, de Miguel MP, Azaar A, Makdissy N, Harb W, et al. Cellular therapy with human autologous adipose-derived adult stem cells for advanced keratoconus. *Cornea*. 2017;36(8):952–60.

18. Kitazawa K, Sotozono C, Kinoshita S. Current advancements in corneal cell–based therapy. *The Asia-Pacific Journal of Ophthalmology*. 2022;11(4):335–45.

19. Atalay E, Özalp O, Yıldırım N. Advances in the diagnosis and treatment of keratoconus. *Therapeutic Advances in Ophthalmology*. 2021;13:25158414211012796.

20. Pellegrini G, Traverso CE, Franzi AT, Zingirian M, Cancedda R, De Luca M. Long-term restoration of damaged corneal surfaces with autologous cultivated corneal epithelium. *The Lancet*. 1997;349(9057):990–3.

21. Koizumi N, Inatomi T, Suzuki T, Sotozono C, Kinoshita S. Cultivated corneal epithelial stem cell transplantation in ocular surface disorders. *Ophthalmology*. 2001;108(9):1569–74.

22. Holland EJ, Mogilishetty G, Skeens HM, Hair DB, Neff KD, Biber JM, et al. Systemic immunosuppression in ocular surface stem cell transplantation: results of a 10-year experience. *Cornea*. 2012;31(6):655–61.

23. Mikhailova A, Ilmarinen T, Ratnayake A, Petrovski G, Uusitalo H, Skottman H, et al. Human pluripotent stem cell-derived limbal epithelial stem cells on bioengineered matrices for corneal reconstruction. *Experimental Eye Research*. 2016;146:26–34.

24. Nurković JS, Vojinović R, Dolićanin Z. Corneal stem cells as a source of regenerative cell-based therapy. *Stem Cells International*. 2020;2020.

25. El Zarif M, Jawad KA, Del Barrio JLA, Jawad ZA, Palazón-Bru A, de Miguel MP, et al. Corneal stroma cell density evolution in keratoconus corneas following the implantation of adipose mesenchymal stem cells and corneal laminas: an in vivo confocal microscopy study. *Investigative Ophthalmology & Visual Science*. 2020;61(4):22.

26. Nosrati H, Alizadeh Z, Nosrati A, Ashrafi-Dehkordi K, Banitalebi-Dehkordi M, Sanami S, et al. Stem cell-based therapeutic strategies for corneal epithelium regeneration. *Tissue and Cell*. 2021;68:101470.

27. Samoila O, Samoila L. Stem cells in the path of light, from corneal to retinal reconstruction. *Biomedicines*. 2021;9(8):873.

28. Wylegala E, Tarnawska D. Amniotic membrane transplantation with cauterization for keratoconus complicated by persistent hydrops in mentally retarded patients. *Ophthalmology*. 2006;113(4):561–4.

29. Prajna VN, Devi L, Seeniraj SK, Keenan JD. Conjunctival autograft versus amniotic membrane transplantation following double pterygium excision: a randomized trial. *Cornea*. 2017;36(3):e7–e8.

30. Sasaki T, Ide T, Toda I, Kato N. Amnwiotic membrane transplantation as a treatment for sterile infiltration and corneal melting after corneal crosslinking for keratoconus. *Case Reports in Ophthalmology*. 2018;9(1):185–9.

31. Vira S, Abugo U, Shih CY, Udell IJ, Sperling B, Hannush SB, et al. Descemet stripping endothelial keratoplasty for the treatment of combined fuchs corneal endothelial dystrophy and keratoconus. *Cornea*. 2014;33(1):1–5.

32. Park CY, Lee JK, Gore PK, Lim C-Y, Chuck RS. Keratoplasty in the United States: a 10-year review from 2005 through 2014. *Ophthalmology*. 2015;122(12):2432–42.

33. Cooper E, Parker JS, Parker JS, Melles GR. Descemet membrane endothelial keratoplasty in an eye with Fuchs endothelial dystrophy and keratoconus. *Ophthalmology@ Point of Care*. 2017;1(1):oapoc. 0000002.

34. Kit V, Kriman J, Vasquez-Perez A, Muthusamy K, Thaung C, Tuft S. Descemet membrane detachment after penetrating keratoplasty for keratoconus. *Cornea*. 2020;39(10):1315–20.

35. Dragnea DC, Birbal RS, Ham L, Dapena I, Oellerich S, van Dijk K, et al. Bowman layer transplantation in the treatment of keratoconus. *Eye and Vision*. 2018;5(1):1–6.

36. Parker JS, Dockery PW, Melles GR. Bowman layer transplantation—a review. *The Asia-Pacific Journal of Ophthalmology*. 2020;9(6):565–70.

37. Sheehy E, Cunniffe G, O'Brien F. *Collagen-based Biomaterials for Tissue Regeneration and Repair. Peptides and Proteins as Biomaterials for Tissue Regeneration and Repair*. Elsevier; 2018. p. 127–50.

38. El Zarif M, Del Barrio JA, Arnalich-Montiel F, De Miguel MP, Makdissy N, Alió JL. Corneal stroma regeneration: new approach for the treatment of cornea disease. *The Asia-Pacific Journal of Ophthalmology*. 2020;9(6):571–9.

39. Cheema U, Mudera V. Collagen-based systems to mimic the extracellular environment. *Multifunctional Hydrogels for Biomedical Applications*. 2022:23–36.

40. Lagali N. Corneal stromal regeneration: current status and future therapeutic potential. *Current Eye Research*. 2020;45(3):278–90.

41. Orash Mahmoud Salehi A, Heidari-Keshel S, Poursamar SA, Zarrabi A, Sefat F, Mamidi N, et al. Bioprinted membranes for corneal tissue engineering: a review. *Pharmaceutics*. 2022;14(12):2797.

42. Williams KA, Coster DJ. Gene therapy for diseases of the cornea–a review. *Clinical & Experimental Ophthalmology*. 2010;38(2):93–103.

43. Farjadnia M, Naderan M, Mohammadpour M. Gene therapy in keratoconus. *Oman Journal of Ophthalmology*. 2015;8(1):3.

44. Li B. Updates on managements for keratoconus. *International Eye Science*. 2020:464–7.

45. Pedrotti E, Chierego C, Bonacci E, De Gregorio A, De Rossi A, Zuliani A, et al. New treatments for keratoconus. *International Ophthalmology*. 2020;40:1619–23.

46. Anogeianakis G. Genetics of keratoconus; how realistic is gene therapy? *Acta Ophthalmologica*. 2022;100(S275):Special Issue:Abstracts from the 2022 European Association for Vision and Eye Research Festival, 13-15 October 2022, Valencia.

47. Gordon-Shaag A, Millodot M, Shneor E, Liu Y. The genetic and environmental factors for keratoconus. *BioMed Research International*. 2015;2015:19 pages.

48. Stunf Pukl S. Are miRNAs Dynamic biomarkers in keratoconus? A review of the literature. *Genes*. 2022;13(4):588.

49. Syrmakesi ELKSP, Rafailia ETMOD, Spyridon BMSAK, Zachariadis KZ, Balidis PTNKM, Gatzioufas Z, et al. Genetic aspects of keratoconus: a literature review exploring potential genetic contributions and possible genetic relationships with comorbidities. 2018;7:263–292

50. Wasnik VB, Thool AR. Ocular Gene Therapy: A Literature Review With Focus on Current Clinical Trials. *Cureus*. 2022;14(9).

Index

Page numbers in *italic* indicate figure and **bold** indicate table respectively

For Product Safety Concerns and Information please contact our EU
representative GPSR@taylorandfrancis.com
Taylor & Francis Verlag GmbH, Kaufingerstraße 24, 80331 München, Germany

www.ingramcontent.com/pod-product-compliance
Ingram Content Group UK Ltd.
Pitfield, Milton Keynes, MK11 3LW, UK
UKHW050930180425
457613UK00014B/349